Upper Extremity and Vascular Access

Modern Trends in Vascular Surgery

Upper Extremity and Vascular Access

Modern Trends in Vascular Surgery

Tadaki M. Tomita, MD

Assistant Professor of Surgery (Vascular Surgery)
Professor of Radiology and Cardiology
Chief, Division of Vascular Surgery
Department of Surgery
Northwestern University Feinberg School of Medicine
Chicago, Illinois

Mark K. Eskandari, MD

The James S.T. Yao, MD, PhD, Professor of Vascular Surgery
Professor of Surgery, Radiology, and Medical Education
Chief and Program Director, Division of Vascular Surgery
Department of Surgery
Northwestern University Feinberg School of Medicine
Chicago, Illinois

PMPHUSA
RALEIGH, NORTH CAROLINA
2018

PMPH-USA, LTD.
5711 Six Forks Road, Suite 210
Raleigh, North Carolina 27609
Tel: 919-502-4220
Fax: 919-502-7673
E-mail: info@pmph-usa.com

PMPHUSA
Publishing to Advance
the Practice of Medicine

18 19 20 21/KING/9 8 7 6 5 4 3 2 1

ISBN-13 978-1-60795-292-3
ISBN-10 1-60795-292-0
eISBN-13 978-1-60795-959-5

Printed in the United States of America by King Printing Company.
Editor: Linda Mehta; Copyeditor/Typesetter: diacriTech; Cover designer: Mary McKeon

Library of Congress Cataloging-in-Publication Data
Names: Tomita, Tadaki M., editor. | Eskandari, Mark K., editor.
Title: Upper extremity and vascular access / [edited by] Tadaki M. Tomita, Mark K. Eskandari.
Other titles: Modern trends in vascular surgery.
Description: Raleigh, North Carolina : PMPH USA, Ltd., 2018. | Series: Modern trends in vascular surgery | Includes bibliographical references and index.
Identifiers: LCCN 2018031650 | ISBN 9781607952923 | ISBN 1607952920 | ISBN 9781607959595 (eISBN)
Subjects: | MESH: Upper Extremity—surgery | Vascular Surgical Procedures—methods | Vascular Access Devices
Classification: LCC RD559 | NLM WE 805 | DDC 617.471—dc23 LC record available at https://lccn.loc.gov/2018031650

Sales and Distribution

Canada
Login Canada
300 Saulteaux Cr.
Winnipeg, MB R3J 3T2
Phone: 1.800.665.1148
Fax: 1.800.665.0103
www.lb.ca

Foreign Rights
John Scott & Company
International Publisher's Agency
P.O. Box 878
Kimberton, PA 19442, USA
Tel: 610-827-1640
Fax: 610-827-1671
rights@johnscottco.us

United Kingdom, Europe, Middle East, Africa, Singapore, Thailand, Philippines, Indonesia, Vietnam, Pacific Rim, Korea, Australia, New Zealand, Papua New Guinea, Fiji, Tonga, Solomon Islands, Cook Islands, Malaysia
Eurospan Limited
3, Henrietta Street, Covent Garden,
London WC2E 8LU, UK
Tel: Within the UK: 0800 526830
Outside the UK: +44 (0)20 7845 0868
http://www.eurospanbookstore.com

India, Bangladesh, Pakistan, Sri Lanka, Nepal
Jaypee Brothers Medical Publishers Pvt. Ltd.
4838, 24 Ansari Road, Darya Ganj
New Delhi- 110002, India
Phone: +91 11 23272143
Fax: +91 11 23276490
www.jaypeebrothers.com

People's Republic of China
People's Medical Publishing House
International Trade Department
No. 19, Pan Jia Yuan Nan Li
Chaoyang District
Beijing 100021, P.R. China
Tel: 8610-67653342
Fax: 8610-67691034
www.pmph.com/en

Contents

Preface *xi*

Contributors *xiii*

SECTION I. Northwestern Vascular Surgery Annual Symposium

1. 40th Anniversary of the Northwestern Vascular Symposium—A Reflection 1

James S.T. Yao, MD, PhD

2. 30 Years of Excellence 11

Mark K. Eskandari, MD

SECTION II. Hemodialysis Access Creation

3. Preoperative Planning for Hemodialysis Access 15

Godfrey Parkerson, MD and Karl A. Illig, MD

4. Basilic Vein Transposition for Hemodialysis: A Review 29

Marc H. Glickman, MD

5. Impact of Anastomotic Angles on Vascular Access 35

Nirvana Sadaghianloo, MD and Alan Dardik, MD, PhD

6. Rethinking Arteriovenous Anastomoses: Interrupted Suturing and Nonpenetrating Clips 45

Karl A. Illig, MD

7. Forearm versus Upper Arm Arteriovenous Graft for Dialysis Access: Which is Preferred? 55

Alik Farber, MD and Steven Pike, MD

8. Advances in the Biology of Prosthetic Graft for Dialysis Access 65

Mark G. Davies, MD, PhD, MBA

9. Bioengineered Vascular Access Grafts 77

Ehsan Benrashid, MD; David N. Ranney, MD; and Jeffrey H. Lawson MD, PhD

10. Dialysis Access Coding: New and Upcoming Changes 89

Matthew J. Sideman, MD and Francesco A. Aiello, MD

SECTION III. Management Of Hemodialysis Access

11. Dialysis Vascular Access and Transvenous Cardiac Devices 97

Haimanot Wasse, MD, MPH and Dirk Hentschel, MD

12. Drug-Coated Balloons in Dialysis Access 107

Syed M. Hussain, MD and Nikolous Karagiorgos, MD

13. HeRO Grafts in Patients with Central Vein Occlusions: When and How to Incorporate Them in Your Practice 117

Virginia L. Wong, MD

14. Management of Infected AV Grafts 129

Samir K. Shah, MD and C. Keith Ozaki, MD

15. Arteriovenous Access-Associated Ischemia ("Steal")—A Hemodynamic Analysis and Evaluation of Treatment Options 135

Karl A. Illig, MD

16. Utility of the Venous Window Needle Guide Device in Hemodialysis Access 151

Spencer W. Galt, MD

17. What to Do with Patent Arteriovenous Fistulas after Successful Renal Transplantation? 159

Staci Canterino, MS, PA-C and David Fox, MD

SECTION IV. Upper Extremity Catheters

18. Incidence and Treatment of Central Venous Catheter-Associated Upper Extremity DVT 173

Timothy K. Liem, MD, MBA and Jeffrey D. Crawford, MD

19. Catheter-Directed Thrombolysis for Acute Finger Ischemia 181

Matthew A. Corriere MD, MS

20. Brachial Access for Peripheral Arterial Interventions 201

Matthew Mell, MD, MS

21. Management of Complications after Invasive Upper Extremity Testing and Treatment 207

Katherine E. Hekman, MD, PhD and Andrew W. Hoel, MD

SECTION V. Upper Extremity Compression Syndromes

22. Neurogenic and Vascular Quadrilateral Space Syndromes: A New Classification and Management 219

Arjun Jayaraj, MD and Peter Gloviczki, MD

23. Surgical Approaches to Thoracic Outlet Syndrome: Supraclavicular Versus Transaxillary 229

Robert W. Thompson, MD

24. Patency after Limited Venoplasty and Anticoagulation following First Rib Resection for Venous Thoracic Outlet Syndrome 237

Gabriela Velazquez-Ramirez, MD and Julie A. Freischlag, MD

25. Cervical Ribs and Arterial Thoracic Outlet Syndrome 249

Kaj H. Johansen, MD, PhD

SECTION VI. Upper Extremity Trauma

26. Upper Extremity Trauma and the Advanced Surgical Skills Exposures for Trauma (ASSET) Course 259

Col. (ret.) Mark W. Bowyer, MD, FACS, DMCC

27. Management of Upper Extremity Arterial Civilian Trauma 267

Nicole Toscano, MD and Michael Stoner, MD

28. Outcome Comparison Between Open and Endovascular Repair of Axillosubclavian Arterial Injuries 275

Bruce L. Tjaden, Jr., MD and Naveed U. Saqib, MD

Index 287

Preface

Over the past four decades, the Northwestern Vascular Symposium, held each December in Chicago, has provided a platform for experts at the forefront of vascular surgery to pass on their knowledge and expertise to a diverse audience. During this symposium, a broad range of topics from all aspects of vascular surgery are presented and discussed. To accompany these presentations, a textbook is published each year. This collection of symposium textbooks offers a tremendous resource of interesting topics in vascular surgery. Our current aim is to condense this material down into discrete books to provide the information presented at the symposium to a larger audience. The current collection of books highlights chapters from the Northwestern Vascular Symposium over a three-year period from 2015 through 2017.

This book, divided into five sections, covers a range of unique topics that pertain to hemodialysis access and the upper extremities. The first section of the book discusses the creation of hemodialysis access ranging from preoperative evaluation, to technical aspects of fistula creation including new graft design, and concluding with a chapter on coding and billing. The following section details a variety of hemodialysis access complications and chapters that discuss difficult decision-making with these complex patients. The remaining three sections involve other topics related to upper extremity disease. The first of these discusses issues related to upper extremity catheters in the venous and arterial systems. The following section covers upper extremity compression syndromes including thoracic outlet syndrome. The book closes with a section on the management of upper extremity trauma and covers both open surgical approaches and endovascular options.

Finally, I would like to thank all of the authors who contributed to these very interesting works and those who have contributed to the Northwestern Vascular Symposium. Please enjoy this book; I hope it adds value to your practice.

—Tadaki M. Tomita, MD

Contributors

Francesco A. Aiello, MD
University of Massachusetts Memorial Medical Center
Worcester, Massachusetts

Ehsan Benrashid, MD
Duke University
Durham, North Carolina

Col. (ret.) Mark W. Bowyer, MD
Uniformed Services University
Bethesda, Maryland

Staci Canterino, MS, PA-C
Fox Vascular Access Care
New York, New York

Jeffrey D. Crawford, MD
Oregon Health & Science University
Portland, Oregon

Matthew A. Corriere MD, MS
University of Michigan Health System
Ann Arbor, Michigan

Alan Dardik, MD, PhD
Yale School of Medicine
New Haven, Connecticut

Mark G. Davies, MD, PhD, MBA
University of Texas Health Sciences Center
San Antonio, Texas

Mark K. Eskandari, MD
Northwestern Vascular Symposium
Feinberg School of Medicine
Chicago, Illinois

Alik Farber, MD
Boston University
Boston, Massachusetts

David Fox, MD
Fox Vascular Access Care
New York, New York

Julie A Freischlag, MD
Wake Forest University School of Medicine
Winston-Salem, North Carolina

Spencer W. Galt, MD
Summit Physician Specialists
Murray, Utah

Marc H Glickman, MD
Eastern Virginia Medical School
Norfolk, Virginia

Peter Gloviczki, MD
Mayo Clinic
Rochester, Minnesota

Katherine E. Hekman, MD, PhD
Northwestern University
Feinberg School of Medicine
Chicago, Illinois

Dirk Hentschel, MD
Brigham and Women's Hospital
Boston, Massachusetts

Andrew W. Hoel, MD
Northwestern University
Feinberg School of Medicine
Chicago, Illinois

Syed M. Hussain MD
University of Illinois College of Medicine
at Urbana
Champaign, Illinois

Karl A. Illig, MD
University of Florida
Morsani College of Medicine
Tampa, Florida

Arjun Jayaraj, MD
St. Dominic Hospital,
Jackson, Mississippi

Kaj Johansen, MD, PhD
Vascular and Surgical Care
Northwest
Seattle, Washington

Nikolous Karagiorgos MD
University of Illinois College of Medicine
at Urbana
Champaign, Illinois

Jeffrey H. Lawson, MD, PhD
Duke University
Durham, North Carolina

Timothy K. Liem, MD, MBA
Oregon Health & Science University
Portland, Oregon

Matthew Mell, MD, MS
Stanford University School
of Medicine
Stanford, California

C. Keith Ozaki, MD
Brigham and Women's Hospital
Harvard Medical School
Boston, Massachusetts

Godfrey Parkerson, MD
University of Florida
Morsani College of Medicine
Tampa, Florida

Steven Pike, MD
Boston University
Boston, Massachusetts

David N. Ranney, MD
Duke University
Durham, North Carolina

Nirvana Sadaghianloo, MD
University of Nice Sophia Antipolis
Nice, France

Naveed U Saqib, MD
The University of Texas Health Science
Center at Houston
McGovern Medical School
Houston, Texas

Samir K Shah, MD
Brigham and Women's Hospital
Boston, Massachusetts

Matthew J. Sideman, MD
University of Texas Health System
San Antonio, Texas

Michael C. Stoner, MD
University of Rochester
Rochester, New York

Robert W. Thompson, MD
Washington University School of Medicine
St. Louis, Missouri

Bruce L Tjaden Jr., MD
The University of Texas Health Science Center at Houston
McGovern Medical School
Houston, Texas

Nicole C. Toscano, MD
University of Rochester
Rochester, New York

Gabriela Velazquez-Ramirez, MD
Wake Forest School of Medicine
Winston-Salem, North Carolina

Haimanot Wasse, MD, MPH
Rush Medical College
Chicago, Illinois

Virginia L Wong, MD
University Hospitals Case Medical Center
Cleveland, Ohio

James S.T. Yao, MD, PhD
Northwestern University
Feinberg School of Medicine
Chicago, Illinois

1

40th Anniversary of the Northwestern Vascular Symposium—A Reflection

James S.T. Yao, MD, PhD

According to Webster's dictionary,[1] in ancient Greece, a symposium was an entertainment characterized by drinking, music and intellectual discussion. As it evolved, it became a conference focused on a subject with current significance. The Northwestern Vascular Symposium developed following the pursuit by leaders of the Society for Vascular Surgery (SVS) of better training for vascular surgeons and certification in vascular surgery. E. J. Wylie in his ISCVS-NA presidential address first pointed out the need for better training of vascular surgeons.[2] James DeWeese, who headed the Inter-Society Commission for Heart Disease Resources (ICHD) sponsored by the American Heart Association, also found inadequate vascular care in many hospitals in the United States.[3] In order to improve training and certification in vascular surgery, SVS engaged in negotiation with the American Board of Surgery (ABS) and the Resident Review Committee (RRC) for better training of vascular surgery in surgical residency. At the time, both RRC and ABS showed little interest. SVS and the International Society for Cardiovascular Surgery (ISCVS) set up a committee named Program Evaluation and Endorsement Committee (PEEC) to establish an approval process for one-year vascular fellowship programs. After 17 programs were approved, RRC and ABS decided to get involved and negotiations started, with many past presidents of SVS being involved in the negotiations. It took at least 13 years (1970–1983) of bitter negotiations before the first Certificate of Special Qualification in General Vascular Surgery was awarded to E. J. Wylie.[3]

With vascular surgery emerging as a surgical specialty, educational activities also increased. The first symposium in vascular surgery was sponsored in 1973 by Dr. Henry Haimovici of Montefiore Medical Center in New York. This symposium later became the well-known VEITH Symposium under the leadership of Dr. Frank Veith. Haimovici was a pioneer vascular surgeon. He served as president of the International Society of Angiology and later of ISCVS. A great writer, he wrote several classics including a complete textbook on vascular surgery.[4]

The idea of having a symposium at Northwestern was solely the idea of John Bergan. He strongly believed that vascular surgery was much different from general surgery.[5] He thought the best way to advance the field was to have a scientific exchange among national and international scholar-surgeons. Although I was new on the faculty, Bergan treated me equally in planning the meeting program. We each made a program and then we combined them after an in-depth discussion to finalize the program. The equal partnership exercised by Bergan led to the birth of the Bergan-Yao partnership in vascular surgery that lasted for 16 years (Figure 1-1). December was chosen for the date of the symposium because it is a good time to reflect on what has been done during the year and to chart for the future. With the support of a generous grant from the Scholl Foundation, the first Northwestern Vascular Symposium was held on December 2, 1976, at the Drake Hotel[5] with the topic of *Venous Problems.* It was a 2½ day meeting with a faculty of 33 national and international leaders, pathologists, physiologists and vascular surgeons to provide a multidisciplinary approach to the disease. The symposium represented the first meeting attended by international experts to address a much neglected subject.

We are honored to have had the opportunity to dedicate several symposia to outstanding vascular surgeons. The first symposium was dedicated to Geza de Takats, a Hungarian surgeon who moved to Chicago in 1925 and was invited by Dr. Allan Kanavel, Chairman of Surgery at Northwestern, to join the faculty. De Takats established the first vascular clinic at Northwestern and is considered to be the father of vascular surgery in Chicago. He served as president of SVS in 1953. The meeting was a great success with Chicago Mayor Richard J. Daley in attendance for the opening ceremony and the first day of the meeting. December 2, 1976, was proclaimed the Dr. Geza de Takats Day in Chicago (Figure 1-2). In 1995, we were honored to have Mayor Richard M. Daley, son of the first Mayor Daley, to join us in the symposium to honor yet another pioneer surgeon, Michael E. DeBakey (Figure 1-3). Table 1-1 lists the surgeons to whom symposia have been dedicated.

The format of the Symposium has changed over the span of 40 years. In the beginning, the topic of the symposium was often focused on a specific disorder. As new

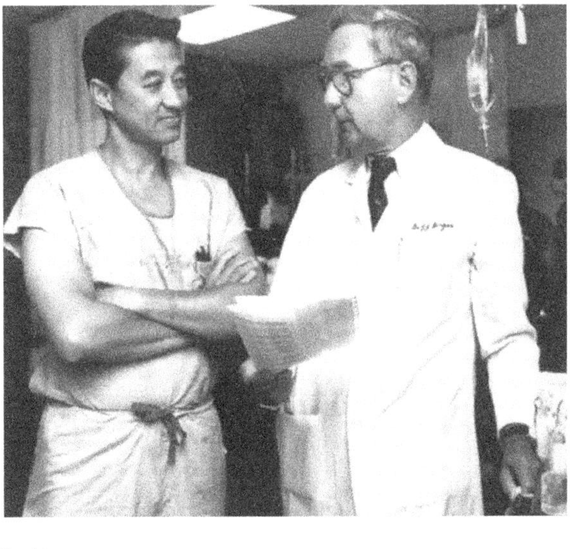

Figure 1-1. The Bergan-Yao team.

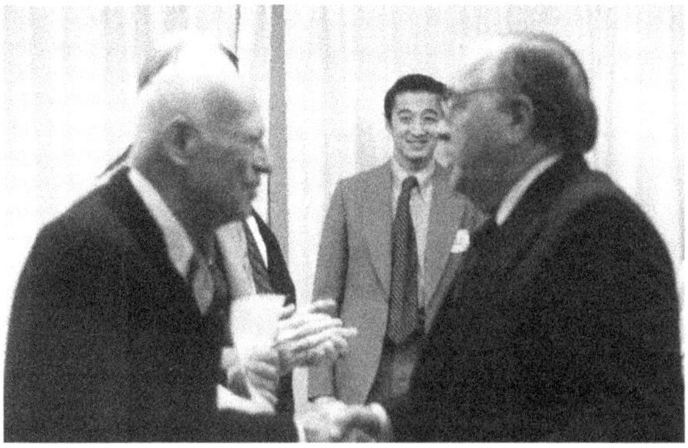

Figure 1-2. Geza de Takats, James Yao, Mayor Richard J. Daley.

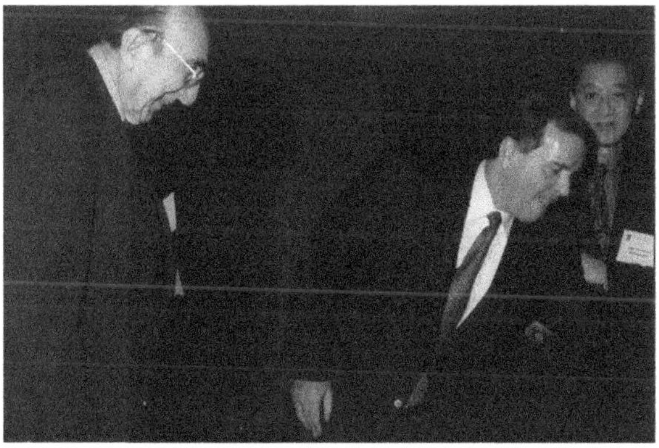

Figure 1-3. Michael DeBakey, Mayor Richard M. Daley, James Yao.

TABLE 1-1. FAMED VASCULAR SURGEONS HONORED BY NORTHWESTERN VASCULAR SYMPOSIUM

Year*	Name	Symposium
1982	Edwin J. Wylie	Cerebral Insufficiency
1993	Stanley Crawford	Aneurysm: New Findings and Treatment
1994	D. Emerick Szilagyi	Advances in Treatment of Ischemic Extremities
1995	Michael E. DeBakey	Arterial Surgery: Management of Challenging Problems
1997	Jesse Thompson	Techniques in Vascular and Endovascular Surgery
2002	James DeWeese	Trends in Vascular Surgery
2008	Robert Rutherford	Techniques and Outcomes in Endovascular Surgery

*Copyright year of the symposium book. The copyright date is often the year after the date of the symposium for which the book was published.

technology evolved, we changed the format to a review covering all aspects of vascular practice. This change was requested by participants of the symposium. In addition, we added morning breakfast meetings on Friday and Saturday with case presentations by our vascular fellows to reflect our interest in clinical surgery.

The Northwestern Vascular Symposium is well known for its ability to produce a book at the time of the symposium, to serve as a permanent record of the presentations at the meeting. The first book, *Venous Problems*, was published 2 years after the meeting, as old printing techniques were still in use. In 1978, Grune and Stratton, using the newly introduced computer typesetting technique, greatly reduce the printing time and the book, *Gangrene and Severe Ischemia of the Lower Extremity*, was distributed at the time of the meeting. In the ensuing years, from 1978 to 2014, we have successfully produced a book containing all presentations at the time of each meeting a total of 38 books published under the editorial leadership of the current Chief of the Division of Vascular Surgery. We are thankful for the many leaders in vascular surgery who have given up their time to join the faculty of the symposia and to prepare manuscripts for the accompanying books.

In 2010, we develop a new series of monographs based on previously published symposia. The series is called *Modern Trends in Vascular Surgery*, with five topics: *Carotid Artery Disease, Endovascular Technology, Venous Disorders, Aorta and Its Body Branches* and *Lower Extremity Ischemia.* We selected chapters published within the past 5 years that were of special interest in each of the categories. These were supplemented with a few new chapters to maintain continuity and ensure complete coverage of each topic. Table 1-2 shows the dates and titles of the books related to the Northwestern Vascular Symposium published over the last 40 years.

TABLE 1-2. BOOKS PRODUCED IN CONJUNCTION WITH THE NORTHWESTERN VASCULAR SYMPOSIUM

Copyright Date*	Title
Editors: John J. Bergan, James S. T. Yao	
1978	*Venous Problems*
1978	*Gangrene and Severe Ischemia of the Lower Extremities*
1979	*Surgery of the Aorta and Its Body Branches*
1980	*Operative Techniques in Vascular Surgery*
1982	*Aneurysms: Diagnosis and Treatment*
1983	*Cerebrovascular Insufficiency*
1984	*Evaluation and Treatment of Upper Extremity Disorders*
1985	*Surgery of the Veins*
1986	*Reoperative Arterial Surgery*
1987	*Vascular Surgical Emergencies*
1988	*Arterial Surgery: New Diagnosis and Operative Techniques*
1989	*Aortic Surgery*
1990	*Techniques in Arterial Surgery*
1991	*Venous Disorders*
Editors: James S. T. Yao, William H. Pearce	
1992	*Technologies in Vascular Surgery*
1993	*Longterm Results in Vascular Surgery*
1994	*Aneurysms: New Findings and Treatment*

(Continued)

TABLE 1-2. *(Continued)*

Copyright Date*	Title
1995	*The Ischemic Extremity: Advances in Treatment*
1996	*Arterial Surgery: Management of Challenging Problems*
1997	*Progress in Vascular Surgery*
1998	*Techniques in Vascular and Endovascular Surgery*
1999	*Practical Vascular Surgery*
2000	*Modern Vascular Surgery*
2001	*Current Techniques in Vascular Surgery*
2002	*Advances in Vascular Surgery*
Editors: William H. Pearce, Jon S. Matsumura, James S. T. Yao	
2003	*Trends in Vascular Surgery*
2004	*Trends in Vascular Surgery*
2005	*Trends in Vascular Surgery*
2006	*Trends in Vascular Surgery*
2007	*Trends in Vascular Surgery*
2008	*Vascular Surgery in the Endovascular Era*
Editors: Jon S. Matsumura, Mark D. Morasch, William H. Pearce, James S. T. Yao	
2009	*Techniques and Outcome in Endovascular Surgery*
Editors: Mark K. Eskandari, Mark D. Morasch, William H. Pearce, James S. T. Yao	
2010	*Vascular Surgery: Therapeutic Strategies*
2011	*New Findings in Vascular Surgery*
2011	*Contemporary Vascular Surgery*
Editors: Mark K. Eskandari, William H. Pearce, James S. T. Yao	
2013	*Current Vascular Surgery: 2012*
2014	*Current Vascular Surgery: 2013*
2015	*Current Vascular Surgery: 2014*
Modern Trends in Vascular Surgery (recompilation books published 2010–2011)	
Endovascular Technology	
Editors: Mark K. Eskandari, Mark D. Morasch, William H. Pearce, James S. T. Yao	
The Ischemic Extremity	
Editors: Heron E. Rodriguez, William H. Pearce, James S. T. Yao	
Surgery of the Aorta and Its Body Branches	
Editors: Mark D. Morasch, William H. Pearce, James S. T. Yao	
Venous Disorders	
Editors: Melina R. Kibbe, William H. Pearce, James S. T. Yao	
Carotid Artery Disease	
Editors: Mark K. Eskandari, William H. Pearce, James S. T. Yao	

*Note: The copyright date is often the year after the date of the symposium for which the book was published.

A TRIBUTE TO JACK HOOVER AND DONALD LASS OF W. L. GORE & ASSOCIATES

The Northwestern Vascular Symposium and its compendium book could not have been possible without the support from an education grant from W. L. Gore & Associates. The grant is unrestricted funding and is designated to be used for postgraduate education for vascular surgeons. The 2½ day symposium program is formulated by members of the Division of Vascular Surgery. W. L. Gore & Associates is not involved nor consulted. We thank Mr. Robert Gore and Ms. Terry Kelly, Chief Executive Officer, for their foresight in the academic-industry alliance to promote advances in the field. More importantly, they assigned two outstanding business executives, Mr. Jack Hoover and Mr. Donald Lass, to work with us. As we cherish these four decades of academic-industry alliance, I, on behalf of past and present members of the Division of Vascular Surgery, pay tribute to Jack and Don.

John T. (Jack) Hoover (Figure 1-4) was born April 22, 1929, an only child. He graduated from Penn State University in 1951 with a BS in chemistry. Jack then served in the US Army from 1951 to 1953. He first worked as a shift supervisor for Squibb in New Brunswick. In 1955, he started working for American Cyanamid and won salesman of the year twice then became regional manager. In 1970, he was working for ICI America and met Bill and Bob Gore. He then was recruited by W. L. Gore in 1975 to develop the medical division. Under the leadership of Jack Hoover, W. L. Gore outperformed all other graft companies. Jack retired in 1992 but remained on the Board until the end of 2010.

Donald Lass (Figure 1-5) was born December 12, 1946, and raised in Chicago. He attended Northern Illinois University in DeKalb from 1964 to 1968 and graduated with a BS in marketing. He then worked for Montgomery Ward and Company as a copy writer.

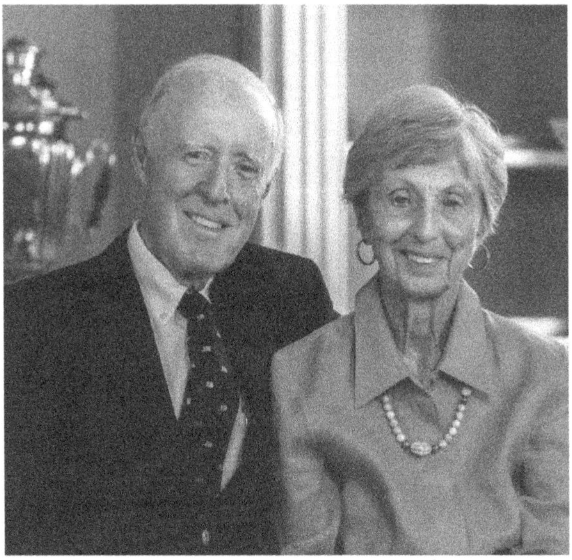

Figure 1-4. John T. and Beverly Hoover.

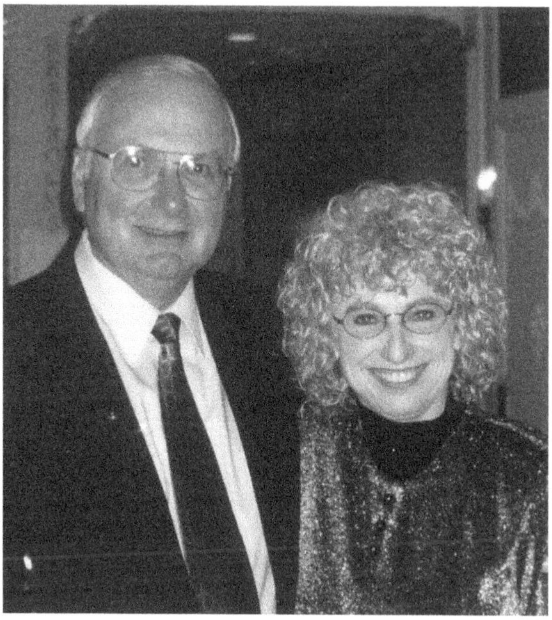

Figure 1-5. Donald and Diana Lass.

In 1968, he served in the US Army Reserve and, from 1968 to 1975, he sold pharmaceuticals for Lederle. In 1975, he was recruited by Jack Hoover to join W. L. Gore and became the first of many sales associates covering 17 states from the Appalachians to the Rockies and from Canada to Texas. Don spent 37 years at Gore and retired in 2011.

Both Jack Hoover and Don Lass are consummate sales representatives. They presented the facts of their product to you and never engaged in hard sell pressure techniques. They supported the idea of an education grant and believed in a close alliance between academic centers and industry as the main force to improve products for patients. Under their leadership, W. L. Gore has supported education programs in many academic centers. At no time did Hoover and Lass demand that we popularize their product.

In addition to the education grant to Northwestern, both Hoover and Lass recognized the need to develop young leaders in vascular surgery. When the concept of a traveling fellowship modeled after the well-known James IV Traveling Fellowship was brought up, they both gave their unconditional support.[6] The SVS E. J. Wylie Traveling Fellowship is supported by donations from W. L. Gore and Associates. The fellowship program has been a great success and young surgeons have benefited from the program. Three Wylie fellows have been elected to the office of president of SVS (Craig Kent, Peter Gloviczki and Julie Freischlag, the first female President of SVS).

EPILOGUE

I am fortunate to have been involved from the beginning of the Northwestern Vascular Symposium and I attended all but one of the meetings. The meeting that I missed I was in China for an invited visit and Don Lass became the only attendee with a perfect

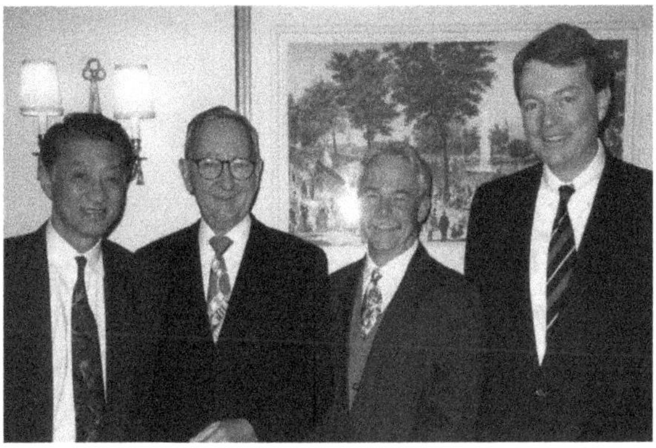

Figure 1-6. James Yao, John Bergan, William Flinn, Walter McCarthy.

score. Unfortunately, hip surgery in 2014 denied him the honor and now, in fact, there is no perfect attendance record.

The past 40 years have taught me that progress in surgical care is an ongoing process and it is largely driven by technology. Care of vascular disease is no longer just an operative craft and technology will play an important role in its future. Academic-industry cooperation is essential for future advances and, as demonstrated here, it is possible.

The success of the symposium is a team effort. I thank Bill Flinn and Walt McCarthy for their unrelenting support (Figure 1-6). After Bergan left the division, William Pearce returned and expanded basic science research. In 1990, when endovascular repair of abdominal aortic aneurysm was introduced, we asked Jon Matsumura to develop the technology. Mark Morasch, Mark Eskandari, Melina Kibbe and Heron Rodriguez were recruited to the Division and, at present, Mark Eskandari is the Chief of the Division. Under his leadership, three young faculty members have joined the Division: Karen Ho, Andy Hoel and Tadaki Tomita. All of these bright young vascular surgeons are leaving their marks on the symposium.

Finally, in the midst of the celebration of our 40 year anniversary, it is with much regret that I report to you that, of 38 speakers at the first symposium, we have identified only 14 faculty members who are still alive. We thank all of them for their valiant effort at the first symposium and assure them that the Northwestern Vascular Symposium will go on.

ACKNOWLEDGEMENT

We thank Janet Goldstein for preparation and editing of this manuscript and Sara Minton for administering the symposium. Both Janet and Sara are indispensable to the symposium.

REFERENCES

1. *Webster's New World Dictionary of American Language—Third College Edition.* New York: Macmillan General Reference, 1994.
2. Wylie EJ. Vascular surgery: A quest for excellence. *Arch Surg* 1970;101:645–648.

3. DeWeese JA. Accreditation of vascular training programs and certification of vascular surgeons. *J Vasc Surg* 1996;23:1043–1053.
4. Veith FJ, Ascher E. A tribute to Henry Haimovici September 7, 1907 – July 10, 2001. *J Vasc Surg* 2001;34:1135–1136.
5. Yao JST. 30th Anniversary of Northwestern Vascular Symposium. In Pearce WH, Matsumura JS, Yao JST, eds. *Trends in Vascular Surgery.* Evanston IL: Greenwood Academic; 2006. pp xvii–xxii.
6. Yao JST, Stoney RJ. The E. J. Wylie traveling fellowship. *J Vasc Surg* 1996;23:1088–1091.

2

30 Years of Excellence

As we enter 2018, I would like to take this opportunity to acknowledge the tremendous contributions over the last three decades of William H. Pearce, MD, the Violet R. and Charles A. Baldwin Professor of Vascular Surgery, to the Department of Surgery and Division of Vascular Surgery at Northwestern University Feinberg School of Medicine (Figure 2-1). A native of Colorado, Dr. Pearce graduated from Harvard University and earned a medical degree from the University of Colorado Medical School. He is an alumnus of the Northwestern Vascular Fellowship (1981–1982) and joined the Northwestern faculty in July 1988 after two years at the University of Cincinnati Medical Center and three years at the University of Colorado Health Sciences Center. The decision by James S. T. Yao, MD, PhD, Emeritus Professor of Vascular Surgery at Northwestern, to recruit Dr. Pearce back to Northwestern in order to develop a comprehensive research program far exceeded his original goal (Figure 2-2). In fact, Dr. Pearce's scope of influence at Northwestern enhanced four primary domains within the Division of Vascular Surgery.

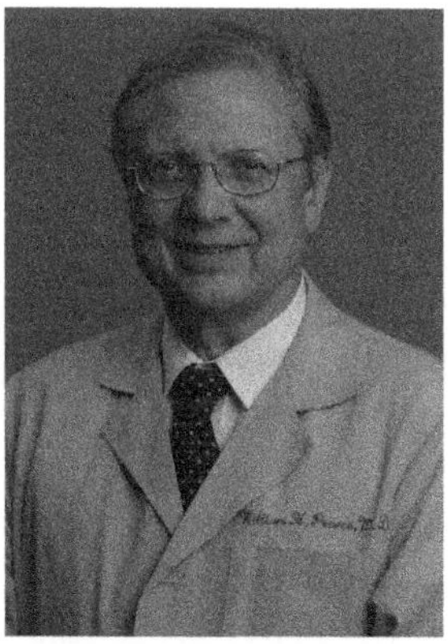

Figure 2-1. William H. Pearce, MD, the Violet R. and Charles A. Baldwin Professor of Vascular Surgery, Northwestern Feinberg School of Medicine.

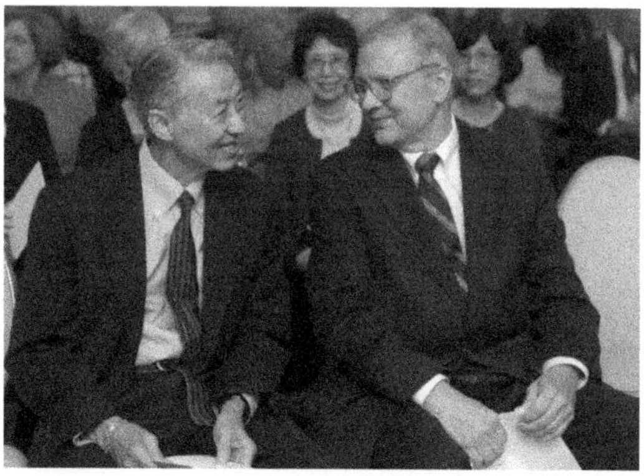

Figure 2-2. James S.T. Yao, MD, PhD, Emeritus Professor of Vascular Surgery, Northwestern University Feinberg School of Medicine, and Dr. William H. Pearce, 2009.

RESEARCH

With nearly 300 publications, more than 120 chapters, and over 40 edited books, Dr. Pearce's impact on the field of vascular surgery has been substantial. He has been the principal investigator (PI) or co-PI on numerous federal and nonfederal grants totaling almost $62,000,000 over the last 30 years at Northwestern. Much of his interest has focused on the pathogenesis of abdominal aortic aneurysms, but his research interests are vast, ranging from stem cell and gene therapy to racial disparities in vascular care. His service to the National Institutes of Health (NIH) has included Chairperson, Special Study Section, Application Review; Reviewer for Small Business Innovation Research; Reviewer for Surgery and Bioengineering Study Section; and NHLBI Institutional Training Mechanism Review Group designee. He has also served on the Swiss National Science Foundation—Division of Biology and Medicine and recently on the Defense Medical Research and Development Program—Vascular Surgery Peer Review Panel. In 2009, Dr. Pearce established the first NIH-funded Vascular Surgery Scientist Training Program (T32) at Northwestern. This successful mentorship program is entering its second competitive renewal under his guidance.

EDUCATION

"Lead by example" is one of Dr. Pearce's mantras and he truly exemplifies a commitment to this philosophy of education. He has been the recipient of five Excellence in Teaching Awards from the Department of Surgery; a Dean's Award for Teaching Excellence at Northwestern; the first Gary A. Mecklenburg Distinguished Physician Award from Northwestern Memorial Hospital; two Faculty Mentor of the Year Awards from the Northwestern Feinberg School of Medicine; the Pioneers in Performance Award from W. L. Gore; the American Heart Association's Council on Cardiovascular Surgery and Anesthesia Surgical Mentoring Award; and the Northwestern Feinberg School of Medicine Teaching Hall of Fame. Throughout his years of service, Dr. Pearce has given over 40 named/visiting professor lectures.

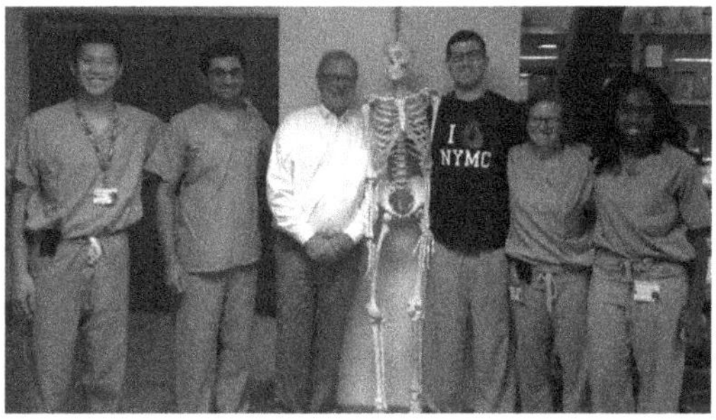

Figure 2-3. Dr. Pearce at the 2016 summer advanced dissection lab with Integrated vascular surgery residents (left to right): Matthew Chia, MD, Neel Mansukhani, MD, Dr. Pearce, Michael Nooromid, MD, Courtney Morgan, MD, and Courtney Furlough, MD.

He is often known for his sense of humor and quick wit. In fact, one of his common questions to residents and medical students relates to venous outflow in the necks of giraffes, which always leads to a few chuckles. It is interesting to review some of his lectures' titles, which demonstrate his creative side: "You Can't Fool Mother Nature," Sterling Edwards Visiting Lecturer, or "Don't Bury Your Head in the Sand," Annual Jonathan B. Towne Lecture. Despite being an lifelong avid tennis enthusiast, Dr. Pearce eschews the benefits of exercise by noting that "trees live a very long time."

Dr. Peace officially served as the Northwestern Vascular Surgery Fellowship Program Director from 1994 to 2005; however, he has been a mentor for faculty, fellows, residents, students, and nurses well beyond those formal years of service. As a result of his continued compassion and support, he has fostered the successful development of countless professionals, and it is with great pride that we can say, "I trained with Dr. Pearce." Even today, he leads an advanced vascular surgery dissection program for the fellows (Figure 2-3).

CLINICAL

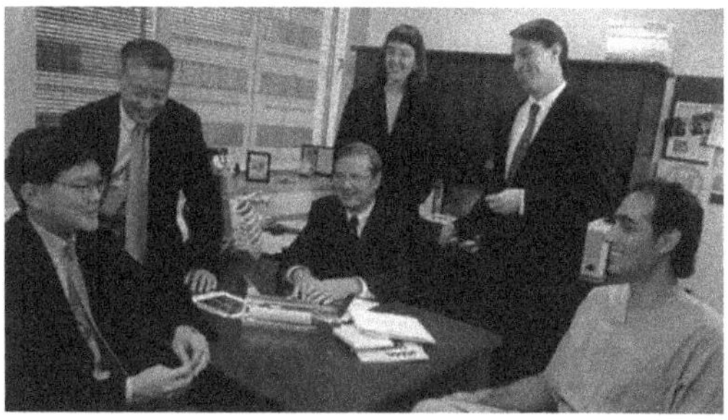

Figure 2-4. Northwestern Vascular Surgery Group in 2010 (left to right): Jon S. Matsumura, MD, James S.T. Yao, MD, PhD, William H. Pearce, MD, Melina R. Kibbe, MD, Mark D. Morasch, MD, and Mark K. Eskandari, MD.

Dr. Peace served as the Chief of the Division of Vascular Surgery from 1998 to 2010, and during that time he hired me—current Chief and Fellowship Program Director, Northwestern University; Melina R. Kibbe, MD—Chair of Surgery, University of North Carolina; and Heron E. Rodriguez—Professor and Integrated Vascular Residency Program Director, Northwestern University (Figure 2-4). In addition, he previously served as Chief of Vascular Surgery, Veterans Administration Chicago Health Care System—Lakeside Division (1988–1999); Vascular Medicine Fellowship Program Director (1993–1996); Medical Director, Vascular Laboratory (1995–2012); Vice Chairman, Department of Surgery (2000–2001); and Acting Trauma Director (2000–2001). In addition, Dr. Pearce was the President of the American Association for Vascular Surgeons (subsequently the Society for Vascular Surgery) from 2000 to 2001.

While these achievements are remarkable, what truly sets Dr. Pearce apart from other surgical leaders in our field is his unwavering commitment to his patients—not just his meticulous care and surgical expertise, but also his personal interest and involvement with his patients, exemplified by his actually providing his personal phone number to patients and even making house calls. As a result, he personally connects with each and every patient and can recall everyone he has ever treated, which translates into an exceptional level of patient care.

HUMANITARIAN

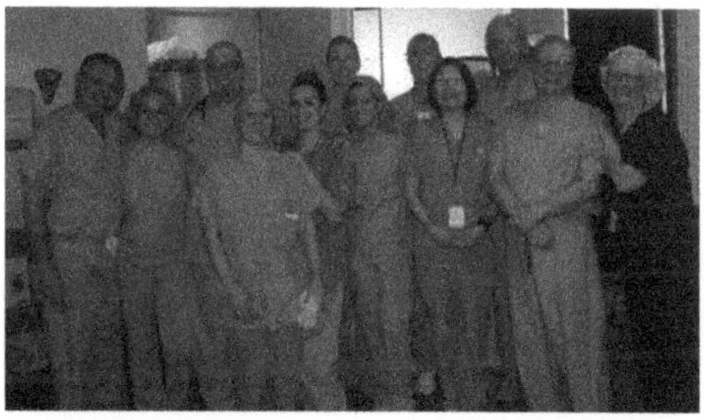

Figure 2-5. Dr. Pearce at the 2014 Faith in Practice Medical Mission in Guatemala pictured with the surgical team including his daughter, Annie Pearce.

The ongoing conflict in Iraq and Afghanistan was associated with a shortage of vascular surgeons in United States military hospitals as well as abroad. Dr. Pearce served as a Red Cross Volunteer at Walter Reed Medical Center, Washington D.C., in 2006 and at Landstuhl Regional Medical Center, Landstuhl, Germany, in 2008 and 2011, taking care of military personnel injured in the war. In 2009, Dr. Pearce received the first Dr. Martin Luther King, Jr. Humanitarian Award from Northwestern Memorial Hospital in appreciation of his local, regional, and national humanitarian efforts. Then in 2013 and 2014, he served as a volunteer surgeon in the Faith In Practice Medical Missions to Guatemala to provide care to underserved individuals (Figure 2-5). Oftentimes, Dr. Pearce is away dedicating time nationally and internationally to underserved populations, broadening his scope to include the building of housing in Kentucky this past summer.

Words alone cannot completely express the deep gratitude that I and all the members of the Division (faculty, fellows, residents, nurses, and staff) have for the privilege of working with Dr. Pearce (Figure 2-6). While he has taught us how to be accomplished professionals, his greatest effect has been exemplifying the essentials of compassionate care. Congratulations, Dr. Pearce, and thank you for 30 years of excellence.

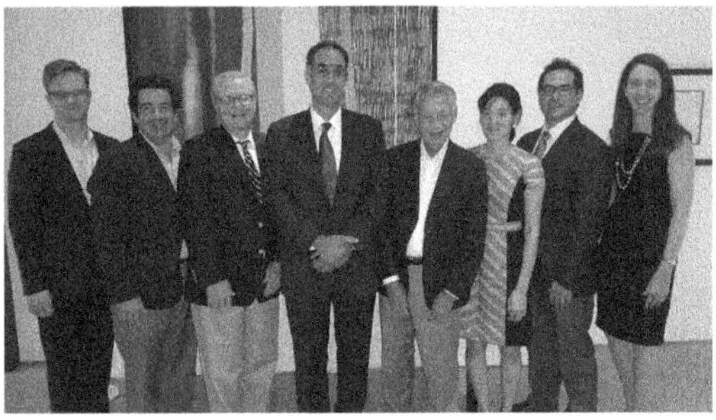

Figure 2-6. Northwestern Vascular Surgery Group in 2016 (left to right): Andrew W. Hoel, MD, Heron E, Rodriguez, MD, William H. Pearce, MD, Mark K. Eskandari, MD, James S.T. Yao, MD, PhD, Karen J. Ho, MD, Tadaki M. Tomita, MD, and Melina R. Kibbe, MD.

With heartfelt appreciation and admiration,

Mark

3

Preoperative Planning for Hemodialysis Access

Godfrey Parkerson, MD and Karl A. Illig, MD

Too many surgeons view construction of arteriovenous access (AV access) as a chore, often delegated to junior partners, faculty, or residents. As such, when approached in such a manner, results can be poor. The modern approach to AV access planning emphasizes careful preoperative evaluation including, critically, ultrasonic vein mapping to plan the access choice that has the greatest chance of working in the short-term, while keeping in mind the long-term potential sequence of events to keep the patient as healthy as possible.

It is best to consider access choices as a series of preferences, although certain conditions MUST be met. A general algorithm is presented in Table 3-1, but the following is a useful guide in determining the choice of access:

Absolute requirements:

- Adequate arterial inflow to provide at least 500cc/min flow, and
- Unobstructed venous outflow to the right atrium

General preferences, in rough order of significance (note that exceptions to each exist):

- Establishing AV access is better than relying on a catheter in the long-term
- An autologous fistula is better than a prosthetic graft
- The nondominant arm is preferable to the dominant arm
- Start distally and work proximally

HISTORY AND RISK FACTORS

Patients being considered for AV access are seen for a thorough history and physical exam. Several components of the patient's medical and surgical situation can have a large impact on pre-operative planning and post-operative expectations. With the multiple comorbidities and hospitalizations common in the patient with end-stage renal disease (ESRD), it is important that surgeons investigate each patient's medical history to optimize success of the operation.[1]

TABLE 3-1. GENERAL ALGORITHM FOR AV ACCESS DECISION-MAKING

Mandatory for either side to be used:

- Adequate arterial inflow (absence of significant stenosis, ideally arterial size greater than 2–3 mm at the wrist (undefined higher) with minimal calcification at site(s) of anastomosis)
- Unobstructed venous outflow (or realistic endovascular or surgical options to achieve it); ideally no pacemaker or AICD in place

Next steps, in rough order of preference (although the order may vary according to patient factors):

- Cephalic vein at wrist and centrally >3 mm? Use better arm if so; if equally good, use nondominant arm. RADIOCEPHALIC AVF
- Cephalic vein at upper arm and centrally >3 mm? Use better arm if so; if equally good, use non-dominant arm. BRACHIOCEPHALIC AVF
- No usable cephalic vein?
  - — Patient acceptable risk, reasonable life expectancy?
    - » Basilic vein >3 mm? Use better arm if so; if equally good, use non-dominant arm.
      - If >4 mm, ONE STAGE TRANSPOSED BRACHIOBASILIC FISTULA
      - If <4 mm, TWO STAGE BRACHIOBASILIC FISTULA
  - — Patient poor risk, unusually poor life expectancy, or tenuous catheter dependence:
    - » Consider AVG (ACUSEAL if immediate access of benefit)
- All steps above: If vein borderline consider AVG

If cephalic and basilic veins are not usable in either arm, or if patient has unusual risk or unusually limited life expectancy:

- AVG – forearm to brachial veins, upper arm (we prefer axillary-based loop)

If arterial inflow is adequate, but veins are obstructed and cannot easily be decompressed and reconstructed:

- HeRO

If arterial inflow and venous outflow adequate only on opposite sides:

- Chest wall/necklace AVG

If venous outflow stenotic ONLY at costoclavicular junction:

- Consider anterior thoracic outlet decompression with plasty/stent, AVF or AVG as above

If central veins stenotic but catheter in place:

- HeRO/ACCUSEAL combination

If SVC is occluded:

- Leg AVF (preferred) or AVG
- Exotic recanalization

End Stage Renal Disease

It's obvious that patients being evaluated for AV access will have Chronic Kidney Disease (CKD), but the degree and duration of their renal disease is an important factor when evaluating a patient for AV access creation. According to KDOQI guidelines, ideally patients should have AVF placed at least 6 months prior to anticipated hemodialysis (HD) therapy, and 3–6 weeks earlier if an AV graft is to be placed. These guidelines are set to allow for use of the permanent AV access at the start of HD therapy, thus avoiding the need for catheter-based access and associated complications. Placement of AV access before progression to HD therapy also allows for fistula maturation in a healthier environment not subjected to the oxidative stress associated with uremia and dialysis. Lower failure-to-mature rates and increased patency rates have been shown in AV access placed before commencing dialysis versus those placed afterward.[2] While the intervals set by the KDOQI guidelines are usually enough time for maturation and wound-healing, they may not be appropriate for all patients. A retrospective cohort study of 150 patients with late-stage CKD and preemptive AVF creation found that only 49% of the patients were actually receiving HD at mean follow-up of 10 months. Of the patients on HD therapy, 65% were using their AVF while 35% were not because of failure to create a working fistula. In the patients not on HD, 55% had their fistula abandoned either due to death, transplant, HD refusal, or AVF failure.[3] Although preemptive AVF creation is advantageous if catheter placement can be avoided, not all patients will benefit as about half of such patients never received HD (at 10 month follow up). The timing of AVF creation is a decision that should be made with awareness of multiple patient-related factors that may affect incidence of HD therapy and success/maturation of the access. Discourse between the surgeon, the nephrologist, and the patient can help refine the decision and timing for AV access creation to optimize success and avoid unnecessary surgery.

Diabetes Mellitus

The prevalence of diabetes is high among the CKD patient population. Patients with diabetes have been shown to have lower AVF patency compared to non-diabetic patients and centers have reported increased use of prosthetic grafts in diabetic patients.[1] The poor patency rates reported are presumably due to increased vessel calcification and decreased vessel compliance predominantly with regard to the arterial supply. Certain preoperative strategies can help to reduce these deleterious effects and achieve satisfactory maturation and patency rates. In their comprehensive review, Smith et al. found that the use of careful preoperative vessel imaging contributed to similar primary AVF outcomes in diabetic versus nondiabetic patients.[1] Although diabetic patients may require more proximal access than nondiabetic patients, studies have yielded primary access survival rates comparable to that of nondiabetic patients.[4] One important risk in diabetic patient is the increased incidence of ischemic complications after AV access creation. Although rare, ischemic monomelic neuropathy is a complication occurring exclusively in diabetic patients. It occurs almost exclusively with AV access created above the brachial artery bifurcation. In addition, steal occurs more commonly in patients with diabetes, particularly those with small and calcified forearm vessels.

History of Steal

In patients with a history of prior hemodialysis access, prior complications are thought to predict subsequent events in the contralateral arm. Patients with a history of ischemic steal syndrome on one side are at increased risk for steal with future fistula and graft creation on the other. Surgeons should be particularly cautious in patients who require access creation on their dominant extremity as untreated ischemic complications can have catastrophic effects on patient quality of life. Experience has revealed several strategies to reduce the probability of steal. These strategies include limiting arteriotomy to 0.4–0.7mm in length and the use of more proximal arteriotomy sites.

Age and Life Expectancy

According to the United States Renal Data System (USRDS), the adjusted incidence rate of the ESRD in the U.S. population from 2000 to 2011 has grown by 7.1% in the population aged 75 years and older. Data from meta-analyses have shown that radiocephalic AVFs have reduced patency and increased primary failure rates in elderly patients,[5] and as such a lower threshold to create a brachiocephalic fistula may be warranted. Research has varied regarding the effect of specific access options on quality of life in the elderly population, but patterns in certain cohorts have been identified. Particularly in patients aged >80y who are female and/or had prior hemodialysis access, brachiocephalic fistulas have been shown to provide improved patency and quality of life over radiocephalic fistulas.[6] Consideration of primary AV grafts may be appropriate in elderly patients with comorbidities that predict no long-term life expectancy. Starting with a graft would avoid the complications associated with catheter-based access while awaiting fistula maturation and would provide the patient with a functional access for the remaining months of their lives.

Obesity

Obese patients (defined as those with BMI > 30) can present a challenge for AV access creation. Superficial veins are often difficult to visualize on physical exam, and these patients frequently require duplex ultrasound for evaluation of venous circulation. With the use of duplex vein mapping, obese patients have the same frequency of suitable venous anatomy as non-obese patients.[1] In a study comparing 1486 patients with BMI >30 and those <30, BMI was not found to be a predictor of AVF revision or failure. On the other hand, patients with BMI >35 had increased risk of failure to mature.[7] Historically, many surgeons have avoided creation of AV fistulas in obese patients preferring graft-based AV access options, the argument being that veins in obese patients often require increased operative time and/or multiple operations to superficialize the venous outflow. This is particularly true for super-obese patients and autogenous access requiring venous transposition such as brachial-basilic and brachial-brachial fistulas. When performing these procedures in obese patients, we generally plan for longer operative times and often opt for general over regional anesthesia. We have found substantial success with autogenous access creation even in obese patients and have actually tended to steer away from prosthetic access if possible due to an observed increased incidence of re-intervention. We do discuss superficialization at initial evaluation with the patient.

Hypotension

Diastolic hypotension (defined as diastolic pressure <60mmHg) has been associated with decreased 12-month survival of AVFs even after exclusion of patients with early fistula failure.[1] The same trend holds true for both AVF and AV grafts in pre-dialysis patients with diastolic hypotension.[1] As such early attempts at more proximal access locations may be warranted in patients with diastolic hypotension to avoid thrombosis and necessary return to the OR for revision or creation of subsequent access. Hypotensive patients may also have decreased baseline Doppler signals at the wrist, which surgeons must be aware of when evaluating Doppler signals for steal syndrome after completion of the AV anastomosis.

ARTERIAL AND VENOUS EXAM

Traditionally, Allen's test has been performed (or at least recommended) as an integral part of the physical exam. Most high-volume access centers and surgeons, however, have failed to find any prognostic benefit with this maneuver, especially in the age of widespread availability of duplex ultrasound. What is probably more important than patency of the Palmer arch is patency of the radio and/or owner arteries. If both of these are patent, but the arch is occluded, in fact, this may be protective of steal after radiocephalic fistula creation. If duplex examination shows that both form vessels are not patent, consideration may be strong to start higher.

Examination is useful for assessing venous patency in patients without much subcutaneous body fat, but can be very misleading in the obese. A visible antecubital cephalic vein predicts upper arm cephalic patency, but, again, ultrasound is critical to ensure that everything is wide open. A palpable radial pulse suggests adequate inflow, but if any question arises, hemodynamic assessment should be undertaken. Finally, attention should obviously be paid to evidence of venous outflow obstruction, including scars suggestive of prior catheter placement, dilated chest wall and shoulder veins, and, obviously, a swollen arm or pacemaker in place.

IMAGING

Duplex Ultrasound

The modern cornerstone of presurgical evaluation is now thorough duplex ultrasound (DUS) examination of the arteries and veins ("vein mapping"). Randomized controlled trials have shown 10–20% increased success of AVF creation with DUS over physical examination in radiocephalic fistula creation.[1] The KDOQI guidelines now recommend preoperative duplex ultrasound for all patients undergoing evaluation for AV access creation. Multiple studies have shown an increase in the rate of autogenous access creation with the use of preoperative DUS, but the effect on maturation and functional patency rates remains uncertain.

Factors obtainable using DUS that have been shown to affect early patency include arterial diameter, venous diameter, and presence of anatomic anomalies. Small arterial diameters <1.5–3.0 mm are associated with increased rates of nonmaturation, but agreement on minimum diameters has not been established.[8] For radiocephalic fistulas (RCF) at the wrist, radial artery diameters >2 mm were shown to have significantly higher success rate than radial artery diameters <2 mm (59% vs. 40%).[1] Criteria for minimum venous diameter range greatly, typically judged to be from 2.0 to 4.0 mm. Success rates for cephalic vein diameters <2 mm are significantly less than those with diameter >2 mm (29% vs. 71%).[1]

Venography

Duplex ultrasound has become the preferred imaging modality for most surgeons prior to AV access creation, but the sensitivity and specificity of DUS still falls short of digital subtraction angiography (DSA). DSA provides direct visualization of the selected veins, especially those that make up the central venous circulation. Reports have shown sensitivities less than 80% for DUS compared to DSA in detection of central venous stenoses.[8] While venous waveforms may help suggest the presence of central stenosis or occlusion, DUS has a limited ability to precisely locate these abnormalities. Adequate assessment of central venous circulation is especially important for patients with history of central venous catheterization (in whom the prevalence of central venous stenosis or obstruction can be as high as 40%).[8] The use of iodinated contrast in patients who are not yet on dialysis is the obvious drawback. For patients with eGFR <30 mL/min/1.73 m^2, the risk of contrast induced AKI is 30–40%, with a 2–8% risk of precipitating the need for dialysis, and in patients with diabetes and eGFR < 60 mL/min/1.73 m^2 the incidence of contrast-induced AKI has been reported as high as 50%.[9] We do not routinely obtain venography, but save this for people with relatively high suspicion of venous outflow abnormalities (visible dilated veins, pacemaker in place, any degree of arm swelling, or a history of subclavian or multiple jugular central venous catheters). If venography is obtained, it's important to use superficial tourniquets, both to dilate the superficial veins peripheral to the tourniquets and also to better visualize the deep veins.

ARTERIAL FACTORS

Arterial diameter and degree of atherosclerosis measured on DUS have significant effects on patency of AV fistulas. While arterial diameter has not been shown to affect patency at more proximal sites, radial artery diameters of less than 2 mm have been correlated with decreased fistula success rates at the wrist. Additionally, the degree of atherosclerosis has been correlated with increased rates of thrombosis and inability to support dialysis at 1 year post-fistula creation.[1] Awareness of anatomic variants such as a high radial take-off may help surgeons avoid potential ischemic complications in patients with poor collateral ulnar circulation, and/or choose the best vessel for inflow. In our vascular lab, every evaluation for hemodialysis access includes bilateral brachial pressures (with optional forearm and finger pressures if any question exists as to perfusion), duplex evaluation of brachial, radial, and ulnar artery sizes, documentation of the presence or absence of atherosclerosis and calcification, and documentation of anatomic abnormalities or anomalies.

VENOUS FACTORS

Diameter has served as the primary venous trait assessed in the planning stages of AV access for decades, even before the widespread availability of duplex ultrasound. As discussed above, the cut-off for a minimum vein diameter for successful creation of other AV access configurations has not been agreed upon. A recent single center retrospective review of patients who had undergone brachiocephalic and brachiobasilic AVF demonstrated that minimum vein diameter of <2.7mm was associated with significantly increased failure rates (> 33%) and decreased long-term patency compared to those a minimum diameter of ≥3.3 mm. Models adjusting for age, diabetes, gender, and preoperative dialysis status found that increased minimum vein diameter alone was associated with decreased risk of failure to mature and increased long term patency in brachiocephalic and brachiobasilic fistulas.[10] In our lab the venous evaluation for hemodialysis access includes direct duplex imaging of the axillosubclavian veins for patency, venous diameter of cephalic vein measured from its origin to its termination noting evidence of phlebosclerosis and anatomic abnormalities, and venous diameter of the basilic vein measured from its origin to its insertion into the deep system noting evidence of phlebosclerosis and anatomic abnormalities (the length of the true basilic vein is noted, but we use the entire basilic and brachial/axillary venous complex dissected high into the axilla for routine brachiobasilic transposed AV fistulas, so this is not critical). Patients with previous failed access may also have assessment of the brachial veins for possible brachial–brachial AVF. Although the ideal cut-off for minimum vein diameter has yet to be established, utilization of imaging still allows surgeons stratify the venous outflow options for each individual patient and plan the access configuration that has the greatest chance of success.

ANESTHESIA

Before making the incision, every patient undergoing AV access creation must be evaluated for appropriate anesthesia. The choice of anesthesia has traditionally been a joint decision between surgeon and anesthesiologist based on the given patient's tolerance of general anesthesia and endotracheal intubation. Regional anesthesia (brachial plexus block) produces significant vasodilatation, which may improve maturation and short term patency rates. Malinzak and Gan have documented that regional anesthesia improved vasodilation in cephalic and basilic veins as well as increased AVF blood flow in the immediate post-operative period compared to general and local anesthesia.[11] This advantage of regional anesthesia has led us to steer away from local anesthesia and utilize regional anesthesia (brachial plexus block) whenever patients can tolerate it. In our experience, the most common factors limiting the utilization of regional anesthesia have been patient anxiety and inability to lie still or lie flat, and our practice of dissecting well into the axilla to eliminate a tethered "swing point" in patients requiring transposed brachiobasilic fistula creation. Although no prospective randomized trials have been completed, the collection of evidence suggests that regional anesthesia may be preferred in any patient willing to have their surgery performed while awake.

PUTTING IT ALL TOGETHER: CHOICE OF ACCESS

The optimal location or configuration of initial autogenous fistula creation remains a hotly debated and intensely researched subject in the field of hemodialysis access, and one that is surprisingly difficult to construct an algorithm for. The KDOQI guidelines attempt to standardize the selection of initial autogenous AV access, ranking forearm/wrist radiocephalic fistulas as the first preferred configuration for AV access followed by elbow brachiocephalic and finally transposed brachiobasilic fistulas. While the evidence presented in the KDOQI guidelines provides adequate support for these recommendations, it fails to take into account several of the factors that we have discussed so far. In addition, "value judgments" such as utilization of a good cephalic vein vs. arm dominance, forearm grafts vs. transposed fistulas, the value of staging certain fistulas, and so on are not addressed.

Radiocephalic Fistula

The radiocephalic fistula (RCF) has traditionally been the first option for permanent AV access. The KDOQI guidelines recommend a wrist radiocephalic fistula (Cimino) as the preferred option for primary AV access creation, and many surgeons feel confident attempting RCF in patients who meet the minimum vein diameter of ≥2 mm (although many would use 3.0 mm as a better predictor of success). The main benefits of RCF's lie in the simplicity of the operation (low risk) and excellent patency rates after maturation. A major problem encountered with RCFs is, however, their poor initial maturation rates. Diabetic and elderly patients are two groups in which RCF creation should be approached with caution. Patients with diabetes have been shown to have lower maturation rates of RCF's (30%) compared to brachiocephalic and brachiobasilic fistulas (73%, 100%) with cumulative patency rates as much as 45% lower as compared to upper arm fistulas.[12] A recent meta-analysis of RCFs fistulas in elderly patients has likewise documented decreased 12 and 24 months patency rates as compared to upper arm AV access.[5] Additionally, a factor that surgeons sometimes fail to consider is patient preference and cosmetic concerns. Some patients, particularly the young, may be highly concerned about appearance and the ability to conceal their access sites. For these patients, more proximal configurations should be considered to allow the fistula or graft to be hidden under the sleeve.

Brachiocephalic Fistula

According to the KDOQI, the preferred site for primary autogenous access if a RCF is not possible is the brachiocephalic fistula (BCF) at the elbow. This fistula offers the advantages of a single short incision for creation as well as good maturation (66–75%) and patency rates. The main drawback in creation of BCF over RCF is the increased incidence of ischemic symptoms and median nerve injury. Although BCFs have increased risk with regard to RCFs, the risk remains low. In comparison to other brachial artery based access configurations, the creation of a BCF requires less time and dissection and offers equal if not superior patency. While there is no consensus agreement on anatomic criteria for BCFs, we use 3 mm as the minimum vein diameter to consider creation of a BCF.

Transposed Brachiobasilic Fistulas

The last choice of AV access configuration addressed by the KDOQI guidelines is the transposed brachiobasilic fistula (TBBF). If creation of an RCF or BCF is not likely to succeed, this is the next option. The main disadvantage of TBBF creation lies in the obligation to widely expose the basilic (and usually brachial/axillary) vein to allow for transposition. As general anesthesia is more commonly required, the patient's medical comorbidities and physical exam findings can have significant effects on the success and ease of TBBF creation. Obese patients may require more time for exposure, transposition, and superficialization around/through large amounts of adipose tissue. The incision required for TBBF is larger, and wound complications are thus greater. The larger dissection also results in increased time required to complete the operation (although the operation is easily performed in less than 90 min). To address some of these concerns, some have advocated that the procedure be done in two stages, saving transposition (i.e., most of the morbidity) for only those who achieve initial patency. This approach may be useful for obese patients or patients with marginal anatomy to hopefully allow for vein dilation and lengthening to ease maturation and transposition, but preliminary results have not shown overwhelming benefit. Two recent meta-analyses have shown no differences in terms of overall maturation rate or post-operative complications in one- versus two-stage TBBF.[13,14] Although TBBF is traditionally not attempted unless options for RCF or BCF have been precluded, the performance of TBBF in terms of patency is excellent, and perhaps the best-performing fistula of all. Koksoy et al. randomized patients with prior failed distal access to receive either BCF or TBBF. All patients had minimum vein diameter of >3 mm. Their study showed no statistically significant difference in primary or secondary patency at 42 months between BCF and TBBF.[15] The largest series reporting outcomes of TBBFs shows maturation rates of almost 90%.[16] Patient-specific risk factors mentioned previously should be considered and may be the deciding factor in patients with marginal cephalic vein and suitable basilic vein. While more distal access options may offer shorter and less demanding operations, the TBBF remains an excellent access option that should be considered when anatomy is suitable.

Transposed Brachial-Brachial Fistula

In patients with absolutely no suitable superficial vein, many will proceed to nonautogenous upper extremity access using prosthetic graft. Although not traditionally thought of as a first line autogenous access option, a brachial artery to brachial vein fistula (transposed in one stage or two) can serve as an excellent autogenous access option. Data have suggested that brachial-brachial fistulas have equal patency to TBBF and improved primary patency and functional patency compared to prosthetic upper arm AV access.[17,18] The decision for staged versus unstaged brachial-brachial access creation depends on patient-specific factors (overlying tissue depth, vein length) and surgeon preference, but the brachial vein is more often highly branched and inherent to the artery, and we thus prefer a staged approach in virtually all circumstances.

Prosthetic Upper Extremity AV Access

When autogenous AV access in the upper extremity has been exhausted or is unavailable, the only upper extremity option for most patients is a non-autologous upper extremity AV graft (AVG). Although it is axiomatic that long-term function is less when compared with autologous access, there are some clear advantages to prosthetic access. Standard PTFE-based AVG's can be cannulated within 3-6 weeks of creation, and with varying degrees of success several previous graphs and the new trilayer prosthetic (ACUSEAL; Gore, Inc; Flagstaff Arizona) can be cannulated within 24 hours. Because "maturation" is nearly certain, an AVG serves as a good first option for patients with limited life expectancy, fast-approaching dialysis needs, or unusually urgent need for catheter removal. Rosas and Fieldman conducted a cost-utility analysis evaluating autogenous vs prosthetic access and found a difference of only 0.13 QALY's. They also found that cost-effectiveness of the fistula first strategy was significant only when fistula maturation rate was >36%.[19] The configuration of upper extremity AVGs is largely based on patient preference and physician experience. Patients who are not concerned about the appearance of their access site may receive forearm straight or loop grafts. Those who prefer a more discrete AV access usually receive curved or loop brachial artery based grafts. Finally, grafts derived from bovine, ovine, porcine, and cultured human cell sources are all available or will soon be; although no clear evidence of benefit exists, the possibilities are encouraging that we will have better options in the near future.

CHALLENGES AND SOLUTIONS

Central Vein Stenosis

Early access failure is often due to venous outflow stenosis. While the vein itself can be stenotic, this is usually identifiable by preoperative imaging and easily corrected. By contrast, stenosis or occlusion of the more central veins has been reported to be present in up to 40% of patients with history of central venous catheterization,[8] and in our experience seems to be surprisingly prevalent even in those without. Patients with symptomatic CVS in the setting of a functioning AV access typically present with prolonged post-cannulation bleeding, arm swelling, failed maturation, or even access thrombosis. When access sites opposite to the side of stenosis are not available, surgeons are forced address the central vein stenosis directly in order to create upper extremity AV access. The KDOQI recommends percutaneous transluminal venoplasty with or without stenting as the first line treatment for central venous stenosis, but results of this therapy have been disappointing as a whole. Treatment of asymptomatic CVS should be avoided as studies have shown that it results in faster progression of CVS.[20] For stenosis occurring at the costoclavicular junction (CCJ) the cause is often due extrinsic bony compression which is less amenable to PTA and stenting alone. These cases should be considered dialysis-associated venous thoracic outlet syndrome. The treatment of venous thoracic outlet syndrome generally requires bony decompression in the form of first rib resection.[21] In patients with symptomatic CCJ stenosis recognized after AV access creation, several small studies have found satisfactory rates of access salvage after first rib resection.[22,23] In patients with confirmed symptomatic CCJ stenosis and history of failed AV Access, we have found success performing first rib resection with simultaneous new AV access creation to relieve symptoms of CVS. Despite the available treatments for CVS, some patients still fail to achieve functional upper extremity AV access by standard autogenous or prosthetic configurations. For these patients, surgeons should be prepared to offer more complex AV access options.

HeRO Grafts

The Hemodialysis Reliable Outflow (HeRO) graft (Cryolife Inc., Kennesaw, GA) has become an increasingly popular option for catheter-dependent patients with central venous occlusion or stenosis preventing upper extremity AV access. The driving force behind the graft's approval and use has been the 69% lower incidence of infection shown in HeRO grafts compared to tunneled dialysis catheters.[24] The patency and infection rate of the HeRO graft compared to alternate lower extremity AVG has been similar, but with more interventions (2.21/year) required to maintain HeRO patency.[25] Preoperatively, surgeons should measure each patient's ability and willingness to undergo interventions to maintain patency after implantation. Patients with poor follow up and those with a history of steal may be better candidates for alternate AV access options in the trunk or lower extremities.

Lower Extremity AV Access

Conventionally patients seeking permanent dialysis access without upper extremity options have received lower extremity AV access. The typical lower extremity autogenous access involves transposition of the femoral vein to the lateral thigh with anastomosis to the distal SFA. Prosthetic lower extremity access arrangements vary greatly. Surgeons have typically avoided lower extremity AV access in obese patients as they tend to require several interventions often for infection post-operatively. The greatest drawback of lower extremity prosthetic AV access is the increased infection rate compared to upper extremity. Antiniou et al. performed an extensive review of the literature regarding lower extremity prosthetic and autogenous AV access and divided patients into three groups based on configuration: autogenous, prosthetic upper thigh, and prosthetic mid-thigh. As expected, infection rates were significantly greater at 18.39% for prosthetic thigh access. The data also revealed a greatly increased primary patency of autogenous fistula (83%) over upper (48%) and mid-thigh (43%) prosthetic. Rates of secondary patency were significantly greater for autogenous as well. While autogenous access provided greater patency, the rate of steal syndrome resulting in limb ischemia with autogenous access was three times greater at 20.7% compared to prosthetic access. Ischemic complications were particularly high in elderly diabetic patients with a long history of ESRD.[26] For this subset of patients, avoidance of lower extremity access creation is likely the best strategy. While lower extremity access may provide durable access options for some patients, physicians must be able to weigh the benefits with impact of potential complications on each patient's current state of health.

Chest Wall or Truncal AV Access

As medical technology has expanded and guidelines set in place, the longevity of patients with ESRD has increased. This has challenged surgeons to provide vascular access for patients in whom upper extremity access has been exhausted. One example for patients with patent central venous circulation is the prosthetic axilloaxillary loop access. In a prospective cohort study, Kendall et al placed prosthetic axilloaxillary loop grafts in both non-obese and obese patients seen as high risk for thigh AV access. They achieved 59% secondary patency at 1 year overall with no infections in the non-obese cohort.[27] The axilloaxillary loop graft serves as a viable alternative for patients with open central venous circulation in whom lower extremity AV access for whatever reason (amputation, history of lower extremity steal, severe PAD, etc.) cannot be attempted. Several other prosthetic complex access configurations have been studied in small numbers, but strong data supporting when and how to employ them has been lacking. Ultimately, the decision to embark on more complex AV access options is a joint decision between the physician and patient with the appropriate strategy determined by the patient's history, imaging, and physical exam.

AN ALGORITHM FOR PLANNING ACCESS

Multiple algorithms have been published to address optimization of the success of AV-access patient populations. Although the validity of these algorithms have not all been verified by reproduction in separate studies, each algorithm incorporates important facets that should be considered when planning AV access. In their scoring system to predict autogenous AV access maturation Lok et al. used age > 65yo, white race, presence of peripheral vascular disease, and presence of coronary artery disease to assign points 445 patients who had their first fistula creation for HD access. They found a correlation between scores and rates of successful maturation in their patient series.[28] It is important to note that the scoring system fails to identify a significant number of the previously discussed risk factors which may confound their results. Table 3-1 presents the general algorithm used in our practice encompassing the major factors discussed above.

SUMMARY

The exact choice of access is not currently definable: too many variables exist. In general, autologous access is preferred over prosthetic, which in turn is preferred over catheter use, but exceptions exist. Additionally, distal access is preferred over proximal access, and superficial veins over deep, but veins and arteries don't always cooperate. What is probably certain is that preoperative examination of the arterial inflow, venous conduit, and venous outflow using duplex ultrasound is critically important, and that the decision should be made by an experienced access surgeon in conjunction with the patient. Finally, the "access whisperer" will think several steps ahead. This is not a one-time surgical event, but a relationship between the physician and the patient. There must be a plan B, a plan C, and so on, if one is to keep these patients alive.

REFERENCES

1. Smith GE, Gohil R, Chetter IC. Factors affecting the patency of arteriovenous fistulas for dialysis access. *J Vasc Surg*. 2012;55:849–55.
2. Kalantarinia K, Campbell A, Mourad S, et al. Timing of hemodialysis vascular access placement determines access outcomes. *Am J Kidney Dis*. 2010;55:B67.
3. Kimball TA, Barz K, Dimond KR, et al. Efficiency of the kidney disease outcomes quality initiative guidelines for preemptive vascular access in an academic setting. *J Vasc Surg*. 2011;54(3):760–6.
4. Konner K, Hulbert-Shearon TE, Roys EC, Port FK. Tailoring the initial vascular access for dialysis patients. *Kidney Int*. 2002;62:329–38.
5. Lazarides MK, Georgiadis GS, Antoniou GA, Staramos DN. A meta-analysis of dialysis access outcome in elderly patients. *J Vasc Surg*. 2007:45:420–6.
6. Weale AR, Bevir P, Neary, et al. Radiocephalic and brachiocephalic arteriovenous fistula outcomes in the elderly. *J Vasc Surg*. 2008;47:144–50.
7. Chan MR, Young HN, Becker YT, Yevzlin AS. Obesity as a predictor of vascular access outcomes: Analysis of the USRDS DMMS Wave II study. *Semin Dial*. 2008;21:274–9.
8. Planken RN, Tordoir JHM, Duijm LEM, et al. Current techniques for assessment of upper extremity vasculature prior to hemodialysis vascular access creation. *Eur Radiol*. 2007;17:3001–11.
9. Goldfarb S, McCullough PA, McDermott J, Gay SB. Contrast-induced acute kidney injury: Specialty-specific protocols for interventional radiology, diagnostic computed tomography radiology, and interventional radiology. *Mayo Clin Proc*. 2009;84(2):170–9.
10. Dageforde LA, Harms KA, Feurer ID, Shaffer D. Increased minimum vein diameter on preoperative mapping with duplex ultrasound is associated with arteriovenous fistula maturation and secondary patency. *J Vasc Surg*. 2015;71:170–6.
11. Malinzak EB, Gan TJ. Regional anesthesia for vascular access surgery. *Anesth Analg*. 2009;109(3):976–80.

12. Hakaim AG, Nalbandian M, Scott T. Superior maturation and patency of primary brachiocephalic and transposed basilic vein arteriovenous fistulae in patients with diabetes. *J Vasc Surg*. 1998;27(1):154–7.
13. Cooper J, Power AH, DeRose G, et al. Similar failure and patency rates when comparing one- and two-stage basilic vein transposition. *J Vasc Surg*. 2015;61(3):809–16.
14. Wooster M, Dansey K, Gabbard W, Illig KA. One- versus two-stage brachiobasilic arteriovenous fistulae: A meta-analysis. *Ann Vasc Surg*. 2015; in press.
15. Koksoy C, Demirci RK, Balci D, et al. Brachiobasilic versus brachiocephalic arteriovenous fistula: A prospective randomized study. *J Vasc Surg*. 2009:171–7.
16. Glass C, Porter J, Singh M, et al. A large scale study of the upper arm basilic transposition for hemodialysis. *Ann Vasc Surg*. 2010;24(1):85–91.
17. Casey K, Tonnessen BH, Mannava K, et al. Brachial versus basilic vein dialysis fistulas: A comparison of maturation and patency rates. *J Vasc Surg*. 2008;47:402–6.
18. Greenberg JI, May S, Suliman A, Angle N. The brachial artery-brachial vein fistula: expanding the possibilities for autogenous fistulae. *J Vasc Surg*. 2008;48:1245–50.
19. Rosas SE and Fieldman HI. Synthetic vascular hemodialysis access vs native arteriovenous fistula: A cost-utility analysis. *Ann Surg*. 2012;255(1):181–6.
20. Renaud CJ, Francois M, Nony A, et al. Comparative outcomes of treated symptomatic versus non-treated asymptomatic high grade central stenosis in the outflow of predominantly dialysis fistulas. *Nephrol Dial Transplant*. 2012;27:1631–8.
21. Illig KA. Management of central vein stenoses and occlusions: the critical importance of the costoclavicular junction. *Semin Vasc Surg*. 2011;24(2): 113–8.
22. Glass C, Dugan M, Gillespie D, et al. Costoclavicular venous decompression in patients with threatened arteriovenous hemodialysis access. *Ann Vasc Surg*. 2011;25(5):640–5.
23. Illig KA, Gabbard W, Calero A, et al. Aggressive costoclavicular junction decompression in patients with failing AV access. *Ann Vasc Surg*. 2015;29(4):698 703.
24. Katzman HE, McLafferty RB, Ross JR, et al. Initial experience and outcome of a new hemodialysis access device for catheter-dependent patients. *J Vasc Surg*. 2009;50:600–7.
25. Steerman SN, Wagner J, Higgins JA, et al. Outcomes comparison of HeRO and lower extremity arteriovenous grafts in patients with long-standing renal failure. *J Vasc Surg*. 2013; 57:776–83.
26. Antiniou GA, Lazarides MK, Georgiadis GS, et al. Lower-extremity Arteriovenous Access for Haemodialysis: A systematic Review. *Eur J Vasc Endovasc Surg*. 2009;38:365–72.
27. Kendall TW, Cull DL, Carsten CG, et al. The role of prosthetic axilloaxillary loop access as a tertiary arteriovenous access procedure. *J Vasc Surg*. 2008;48:389–93.
28. Lok CE, Allon M, Moist L, et al. Risk equation determining unsuccessful cannulation events and failure to maturation in arteriovenous fistulas (REDUCE FTM I). *J Am Soc Nephrol*. 2006;17(11):3204–12.

4

Basilic Vein Transposition for Hemodialysis: A Review

Marc H. Glickman, MD

The basilic vein transposition was first described by Dagher[1] in 1976 and since then several modifications and changes have been described. The basilic vein lies deep in the upper arm and several different techniques have been described to superficialize this vein for puncture for dialysis. In 2001 this procedure became more common and became part of the KDOQI guidelines in recommendation for access in patients to maintain" the fistula first" concept. After failure of either a radial cephalic fistula or brachial cephalic fistula, the guidelines recommend placement of a brachial basilica vein transposition for hemoaccess. There are several techniques that have been described to obtain satisfactory results with this method of access creation. These include placing the fistula in two stages rather than one stage. There are also techniques also described in elevation of the vein as opposed to transposition that recent data appears to show improvement in outcomes. These various techniques will be discussed in this review article. New concepts also to improve outcomes with this procedure will also be part of the discussion as well.

ONE-STAGE VERSUS TWO-STAGE TECHNIQUE

There have been multiple reports and articles concerning the advantages and disadvantages of performing the basilic vein operation for dialysis access. This includes the presence of a long upper arm incision, which can be fraught with complications such as wound breakdown and infection, poor maturation and often-lengthy times to cannulation due to creation of edema from the transposition portion of the procedure. There have been numerous articles demonstrating the advantages or disadvantages of this procedure over using prosthetic grafts. However, concurrence in the literature demonstrates a lower incidence of infection and the need for fewer interventions over its superiority to prosthetic grafts for access. A disadvantage noted in the literature is its higher rate of nonmaturation, running up to 38% in the literature.

There may be several reasons for this high nonmaturation rate. The major reason could be technical as a smaller, friable vein may be more difficult to handle and thereby resulting in torque of the vessel. This torque can result in stenosis and early graft failure and could be the result of such a high rate of fistula nonmaturation. Another reason, described by Anaya-Ayala et al.[2] could be related to anatomical variation of the basilic vein. They describe three variations of the anatomy of the basilic vein. Only 66% of all patients have "normal" anatomy, which is described as the basilic vein entering one of two paired brachial veins close to the axilla. 17% of patients have a type 2 anatomy which describes the basilica vein entering one of the paired brachial veins low in the arm. The last type, three, was seen in 17% of patients where the basilic vein enters a single brachial vein low in the arm. This last type of anatomy could have a confounding influence on fistula maturation and complications including venous hypertension. Their findings suggest that 34% of all patients have abnormal anatomy of the basilic vein and this reason alone could account for the reason for a high nonmaturation rate of this fistula.

The basilic vein fistula can be formed in either a one-stage or a two-stage method. The theoretical concept of a two-stage procedure was to allow for the basilic vein to mature and with a larger vein, the hopes would be that this could reduce technical complications and result in improved outcomes. The one-stage method offers benefits of one procedure and can result in a shorter duration for access cannulation. Also patients are more satisfied with one procedure rather than with two procedures. As stated, the advantage of the two-stage, theoretically, is technical with the ease of mobilizing a larger, thicker and arterialized vein. To date, however, there is no clear-cut report demonstrating the superiority of one method over the other. The purpose of this report is to summarize present data on the comparison of one-stage vs. two-stage basilic vein transposition

Agarwal et al.[3] reported a retrospective study of 144 patients at one center. Forty-two percent had a one-stage procedure, and 58% had a two-stage procedure. There was no direct reason why one group underwent one-stage vs. two-stage except for surgeon preference. Results demonstrated that 90% of one-stage procedures matured compared to 75% of two-stage ($P = 0.92$). Mean time to initiation of cannulation was similar in the two groups, 142 days for one-stage and 146 days for two-stage. Secondary patency rates were similar between the two groups ($P = 0.12$) (Table 4-1) Their conclusion from this report demonstrated that basilic vein transposition in two stages confers only a modest reduction in maturation rates and secondary patency and should only be used considered if a prosthetic conduit is being considered due to a small basilic vein.

Kakkos et al.[4] reported on a retrospective study of 173 patients, 76 patients receiving a one-stage and 98 patients receiving a two-stage procedure. Failure to mature was equivalent in groups, 15% for one-stage and 18% for two-stage. Time to fistula access was decreased for the one-stage at 68 days vs. 132 days for the two-stage ($P < 0.001$). However, there was a significantly lower complication rate for the two-stage procedure including reduction in wound hematomas, venous hypertension when compared to the one stage procedure ($P < 0.001$). This study demonstrated that a two-stage procedure produced a functioning access with less morbidity but at a cost of longer time to cannulation.

In a more recent study, Kakkos[5] reported on a randomized, prospective controlled trial comparing primary and staged basilic vein transposition. In this study, 16 patients

TABLE 4-1. STUDIES COMPARING PATENCY OF A ONE-STAGE VERSUS A TWO-STAGE PROCEDURE FOR FORMING A BASILICA VEIN FISTULA

Agarwal	1 year: Secondary patency	2 year	3 year	4 year	
One stage	86%	75%	69%	57%	
Two stage	76%	71%	49%	25%	
Vrakas	1 year: assisted primary patency	2 year: assisted primary patency	1 year secondary patency	2 year: Secondary patency	
One Stage	77%	57%	79%	57%	
Two Stage	95% $P = 0.017$	77% $P = 0.026$	95% $P = 0.026$	77% $P = 0.026$	
Syed	1 year primary patency	2 year primary patency	3 year primary patency	1 year secondary patency	2 year secondary patency
One stage	82%	81%	51%	91%	80%
Two Stage	67%	27%	18%	81%	61%
Reynolds	Primary Functional Patency—1 year	Primary Functional patency—2 years	Secondary functional patency—1 year	Secondary functional patency—2 years	
One stage	61% p = .047	34%	80% p = .015	41%	
Two Stage	88%	88%	94%	94%	

who had basilic veins greater than 2.5 mm were randomized with primary placement of the fistula ($N = 9$) and staged ($N = 7$). This small study was concluded early due to the significant maturation difference between the two groups. The primary procedure had a maturation rate of 33% (3/9) while the staged procedures had a maturation rate of 100% (7/7, $P = .011$, Fisher's exact test). Their conclusion noted higher maturation rates with staged procedures and this reflected in improved secondary patency rates due to a higher number of patients that matured.

Vrakas et al.[6] in 2013 reported on a retrospective study looking at 149 patients. Again these patients were not randomized and underwent their procedure due to surgeon preference. Sixty-five patients underwent a one-stage procedure, and 84 patients underwent a two- stage procedure. Primary failure was similar in both groups. Results are in Table 4-1.

They did not see any difference in complication rates between the two procedures. Their conclusion from this study demonstrated improved functional patency rates with a two-stage procedure over a one-stage both at the one-year and two-year time frames.

Syed et al.[7] reported a retrospective review of 106 patients: 29 patients who underwent a one-stage procedure, and 77 patients who underwent a two-stage procedure. Primary failure was found to be similar in both groups. Primary patency and secondary patency rates are demonstrated in Table 4-1. Their conclusion was that the one-stage procedures provided better patency rates but at the primary and secondary rates for all years.

Reynolds et al.[8] in 2011 presented 90 patients in a retrospective review of basilic vein transpositions. Sixty patients underwent the one-stage procedure, whereas 30 patients underwent the two-stage procedure. The primary procedure was performed by different surgeons than the two-stage procedure. Also, the second part of the two-stage procedure was more of an elevation rather than a transposition. They demonstrated no difference in early failures between the two groups. However, primary patency and secondary patency as well as functional patency were improved with the two-stage procedure (Table 4-1).

Lastly, Glickman et al.[9] presented their data for a comparison of one-stage vs. two-stage procedures for basilic vein transposition. This again was a retrospective study of 316 patients, 270 patients who underwent one-stage and 46 patients who underwent a two-stage procedure. The one-stage group had an 83% maturation rate and the two-stage group had an 89% maturation rate. The one-stage group had a 7.4% complication rate and the two-stage had a 2.27% complication rate (P = 0.075). One year primary patency rate for one-stage was 33% and two-stage was 45% (P = 0.01). Secondary patency rates at one year was 63.9% for one-stage and 73.9% for two-stage (P = 0.26): 0.98 procedures per year were required to maintain patency in one-stage patients, whereas 0.63 procedures per year were required to maintain patency in two-stage patients (P = 0.08). They concluded from this study, that a two-stage procedure provided statistically improved primary patency and trended in improvement in secondary patency, reduced interventions to maintain patency and fewer complications post operatively.

ELEVATION AND NEW FRONTIERS

Dagher1 described the basilic vein techniques with one long incision and the vein being rerouted laterally through a subdermal tunnel. Another method that is used to utilize the basilic vein is an elevation method, where after the anastomosis is performed, the vein is elevated within the incision by closing the subcutaneous fascia beneath the skin and over the vein. Another potential method for elevation is also to perform a lipectomy in the same area of the vein.

Korkut et al.[10] reported a series of 350 cases over a 4-year period that used the elevation technique. Mean time to first puncture was 52 days. They describe a primary patency rate of 92%, 78%, 64%, and 54% at 1, 2, 3, and 4 years, respectively. Secondary patency rates were 93%, 81%, 66% and 56% at 1, 2, 3, 4 years. This technique suggests that reducing the angle of the basilic vein/axillary area can reduce intimal hyperplasia.

Effat et al.[11] performed a randomized prospective study comparing the elevation technique with standard basilic vein transposition. The study was performed from October 2010 to December 2011. One hundred and four patients were randomized within this study. Although there was no statistical difference in patency rates, the patients who underwent elevation technique had improved primary and secondary patency rates at 1 and 2 years over the standard transposition technique. The elevation technique did require a slightly longer time to cannulation than the standard operation.

A new device approved by the FDA, the Venous Window Guide or V wing, may offer another alternative to the transposed portion of the basilic vein procedure or elevation technique. This device is composed of a single piece of titanium allowing for repeated access of the AVF through a single puncture site, similar to a buttonhole technique. This device would be implanted and sewn to the mature basilic vein and placed subcutaneously in the vein's natural bed. Although this device was not used in this fashion in the majority of the original trial, several cases in the trial were used in this fashion.[12] Using this device would allow the vein to lie in its natural bed, reduce any torque and allow earlier use of the basilic vein for cannulation.

The NEAT clinical study in Canada is providing exciting potential for use in basilic vein access creation. The trial utilizes the EVERLINQ catheters and system to create a percutaneous fistula in the forearm region. Small bursts of radiofrequency energy are used to connect the artery to the vein to create a small fistula in the forearm area. This creation may allow for a "percutaneous "first stage and create a large basilic vein for either an elevation, transposition or V wing procedure. Although the data is not complete as of this writing, the potential seems significant to the author.

CONCLUSION

Defined data on whether to perform a one-stage over a two-stage procedure is not apparent, although Kakkos' small but significant prospective data adds some clarity to the debate. Technical advantages of a two-stage procedure are apparent to the surgeon, using a larger thicker vein can create a better conduit to perform and create the functional fistula. Patient satisfaction needs to be considered as well as many ESRD patients get "surgical fatigue" and often do not show up for the second procedure or delay it significantly. The new endovascular approach to fistula creation may result in not only creating improved patient satisfaction but also improve both long-term and short-term results.

REFERENCES

1. Dagher F, Gelber R, Ramose E, Sadler J. The use of the basilic vein and brachial artery as an A-V fistula for long term hemodialysis. *J Surg Res.* 1976;20:373–6.
2. Anaya-Ayala JE, Younes HK, Kaiser CL, et al. Prevalence of variant brachial-basilic vein anatomy and implications for vascular access planning. *J Vasc Surg.* 2011;53:3,720–3.
3. Agarwal A, Mantell M, Cohen R. Outcomes of single-stage compared to two-stage basilic vein transposition fistulae. *Semin Dial.* 2014;27(3):298–302. doi:10.1111/sdi.12170, 2013.
4. Kakkos S, Haddad GK, Weaver RK. Basilic vein transposition: What is the optimal technique? *Eur J Vasc Endovasc Surg.* 2010;39(5):612–9.
5. Kakkos S, Tsolakis I, Papadoulas S, et al. Randomized controlled trial comparing primary and staged basilic vein transposition. *Front Surg.* 2015; 2:14. doi: 10.3389/fsurg.2015.00014.
6. Vrakas G, Defigueiredo F, Turner S. A comparison of the outcomes of the one-stage and two-stage brachiobasilic arteriovenous fistula. *J Vasc Surg.* 2013;58:5: 1300–4.
7. Syed F, Smolock C, Duan C. Comparison of outcomes of one-stage basilic vein transpositions and two-stage basilic vein transposition. *Ann Vasc Surg.* 2012; 26(6):852–7.
8. Reynolds T, Zayed M, Kim K, et al. A comparison between one-and two-stage brachiobasilic arteriovenous fistulas. *J Vasc Surg.* 2011;53(6):1632–9.
9. Chen B, Glickman M. Basilic vein transposition. *VASA* 2010, Las Vegas.
10. Korkut AK, Kosem M. Superficialization of the basilica vein technique in brachiobasilic arteriovenous fistula: Surgical experience with 350 cases during 4 years. *Ann Vasc Surg.* 2010;24(6):762–7.
11. Effat M. Staging of brachiobasilic arteriovenous fistulae, is it worth the effort? VSE9–EVC9, May 29– June 1, 2013, Hurghada Egypt.
12. Hill AA, Vasudeven T, Young NP, et al. Use of an implantable needle guide to access difficult or impossible to cannulate arteriovenous fistulae using the buttonhole technique. *JVA.* 2013;14(2):164–9.

5

Impact of Anastomotic Angles on Vascular Access

Nirvana Sadaghianloo, MD and Alan Dardik, MD, PhD

Although the upper limb autogenous arteriovenous fistulae (AVF) is generally considered to be superior to other types of vascular accesses such as grafts or catheters, AVF have relatively high rates of early and late failure, requiring multiple reinterventions and hospitalizations, as well as adding morbidity and economic burden to both patients and health care systems.[1,2] In a recent meta-analysis by Al-Jaishi et al., the rate of primary failure for autogeneous upper limb fistulae was 23%, and the rate of primary patency was 55% in forearm fistulae and 65% in upper-arm fistulae.[3] In addition, the most recent U.S. Renal Data System Annual Data Report included data that 35.9% of AVF failed to be mature, with a mean of 135 days to first dialysis.[4] Early primary failure and failure to mature are frequently due to juxta-anastomotic stenosis, particularly in forearm fistulae, with literature reports of 54% to 77% that develop juxta-anastomotic stenosis in these configurations.[5,6] As such, the development of juxta-anastomotic stenoses appears to be a critical factor in the ability to use an AVF for hemodialysis, and understanding how juxta-anastomotic stenoses develop may lead to the ability to diminish their incidence and thereby improve AVF usage.

WHY DOES THE ANGLE MATTER? UNDERSTANDING THE HEMODYNAMICS WITH COMPUTATIONAL MODELING

AVF are inherently non-physiological constructs that disrupt the hemodynamic and rheological rules that characterize arteries and veins. By creating a high-flow, low-pressure system, the fistula anastomosis allows dilation and remodeling of both arterial and venous limbs of the AVF, up to the limit of their plasticity.[7] Vessel remodeling is necessary for the vein to accommodate the high flow of the arterial circulation, and any factor that precludes this remodeling will prevent the AVF from clinical usage, the desired outcome. Thus it is not surprising that experienced vascular access surgeons know that the outcomes of AVF access procedures are determined by several geometrical parameters such as the type of anastomosis (e.g. side-to-side, end-to-end, end-to-side), the characteristics of arterial and venous wall, the length of the anastomosis, and the angle between the artery and the vein.[8] The common effect of all these parameters is the alteration of the pattern of the blood flow through the AVF.

Several authors have examined the effects of the anastomotic configuration on the outcomes of AVF. Soon after Brescia et al. published the first report describing the use of the radial-cephalic fistula for hemodialysis,[9] the end-vein to side-artery configuration became the favorite configuration, often replacing the side-to-side anastomosis reported in the original description of the procedure. As such, the anastomotic angle between the dissected and mobilized vein and the artery has become an important subject of research.

In 1999, Sivanesan et al. studied the pattern of progressive and non-progressive stenosis in 24 radial-cephalic fistulae, and showed that progressive stenosis develops at the juxta-anastomotic segment rather than at the anastomosis itself. However, the mean anastomotic angle was approximately 45° and the authors could not make conclusions regarding the significance of the angle on the development of stenosis.[10]

Following this first insight on the role of anastomotic angle, other researchers studied the flow pattern in *in vitro* AVF models using three-dimensional grids and computational modeling. Van Canneyt et al. used a conduit with an arterial diameter of 4 mm connected to a 6 mm diameter venous conduit; blood flow conditions were set to be non-pulsatile, laminar, Newtonian and incompressible. A range of 600 to 1200ml/min flow was imposed for the system. The cross-sectional area (12.6 to 23.6 mm^2) and the angle of the anastomosis (27°, 34°, 45°, 53°, 63°, 76°, 90°) were treated as variables, and their roles on hemodynamics were studied. The authors concluded that a narrow anastomosis with an angle between 27-45° would create fewer low magnitude flow zones, whereas a wide anastomosis and angles >58° could cause reversed flow, potentially associated with a risk of hand ischemia.[11]

In 2012, Ene-Iordache and Remuzzi associated the low flow and oscillating shear stress to the sites of development of stenosis. These authors used computational fluid dynamics to compare two AVF configurations, the end-to-end anastomosis with the end-to-side anastomosis with a specific angle of 49°. On the venous side of the fistula, besides the flow effects on blood distribution, there was formation of Dean vortices, characteristic of curved tubes in fluid dynamics. These patterns contribute to the non-uniformity of wall shear stress, resulting in wall shear stress being higher on the lateral wall and lower on the inner and outer walls. On the arterial side of the fistula, the oscillatory shear index and relative residence time, indicative of disturbed flow, were higher on the anastomosis floor and on the lateral wall of the distal artery, suggesting that in end-to-side AVF, the distal artery may be at increased risk for stenosis.[12]

In 2013, Ene-Iordache et al. studied the anastomotic angle in the end-to-side AVF. Using similar computational modeling, the authors compared angles of 30°, 45°, 60° and 90° between the arterial and the venous limbs of the AVF. As determined by the area of relative residence time and peak absolute value of the blood volume flow, areas of low and oscillating wall shear stress increased between the acute and the 90° angle. These data suggest that for the same hemodynamic conditions, e.g. velocity, volume, and diameter, an acute angle of 30° minimizes the zones of disturbed flow that are prone to the development of stenosis, in end-to-side AVF.[13]

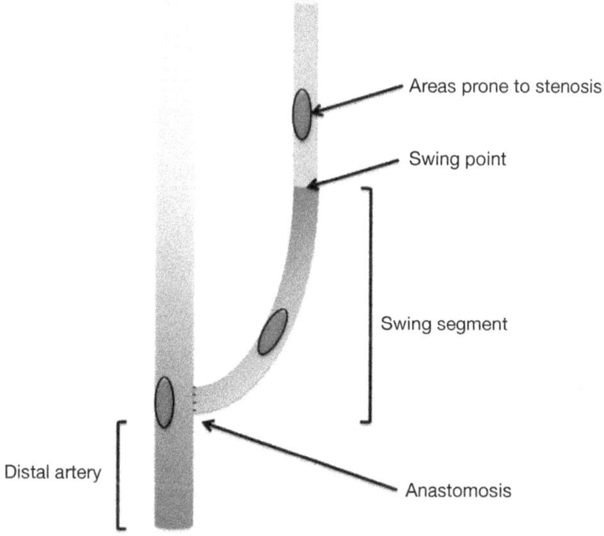

Figure 5-1. Typical configuration of an end-to-side radial-cephalic arteriovenous fistula. The swing segment, e.g. the dissected and deviated venous segment, is indicated in purple. Areas prone to stenosis are indicated in grey.

In 2015, Iori et al., a team of bioengineers and physicists, used advanced computational modeling to correlate flow and oxygen transport in end-to-side AVF. Their innovative hypothesis was that the natural curvature of the donor artery would be a key determinant of shear stress and oxygen flux to the venous wall. Combining flow and oxygen transport calculations, they concluded that an anastomosis performed on the outer curvature of a curved artery may have worse outcome, owing to low wall shear stress and low lumen-to-wall oxygen flux that leads to wall hypoxia.[14]

These computational models show that the anastomotic angle of the artery with the vein in the fistula influences the pattern of shear stress and blood flow both at and downstream from the anastomosis, determining areas prone to hemodynamic disturbance and turbulence that frequently lead to localized development of intimal hyperplasia. It has also been proposed that the swing segment of the vein, so-called because of the mobilization and vibrations within this segment, is more likely to develop intimal hyperplasia (Figure 5-1).

HEMODYNAMICS AND VESSEL WALL REMODELING

Multiple research groups have studied how hemodynamic conditions are "sensed" by the cells of the vessel wall and translated these forces into molecular pathways that lead to vessel wall remodeling, atherosclerosis or neointimal hyperplasia.[15] However there are very few specific analyses of the phenomena occurring during AVF remodeling.[16,17]

The effects of shear stress magnitude on endothelial cells are well described. Arterial endothelial cells are exposed to arterial magnitudes of shear stress *in vivo*, and these forces promote endothelial cell quiescence and confer protection from atherosclerosis; conversely, lower magnitudes of shear stress promote an activated endothelial cell phenotype as well as confer susceptibility to atherosclerosis.[18] During vessel remodeling in the arterial environment, arterial magnitudes of shear stress are typically associated with outward remodeling, whereas lower magnitudes of shear stress are typically associated with inward remodeling. The molecular pathways that are involved are not well understood but include endothelial nitric oxide synthase (eNOS), PECAM-1, and VEGFR-3.[19,20] However, the effects of shear stress magnitude on venous endothelial cells are also not as well described as the effects on arterial endothelial cells. For example, BMP signaling preferentially activates venous endothelial cells without affecting arterial endothelial cells.[21] Understanding the effects of shear stress magnitude changes on venous endothelial cells remains a critical issue to understand how venous conduits mature successfully or not.[22]

Shear stress is a vector, with both magnitude and direction. Since the direction component of wall shear stress is typically either laminar or disturbed, it is not surprising that the effects of flow on endothelial cells also depends on the flow direction. Laminar flow promotes endothelial cell quiescence, with reorganization of stress fibers within the cell body that align with the direction of flow.[23, 24] Laminar flow also induces profound changes in the expression of several vasoprotective genes, with antioxidant, anti-inflammatory, anticoagulant and anti-apoptotic activity. One of the best characterized endothelial cell transcription factors that is regulated by wall shear stress is Krüppel-like factor-2 (KLF2).[25] Pulsatile laminar flow increases KLF2 expression, which in turn induces eNOS expression to promote anti-inflammatory and anti-coagulant effects, and inhibits VCAM-1 and E-selectin expression to prevent leucocyte adhesion and extravasation. Other vasoprotective mechanisms involve inhibition of pro-inflammatory cytokines, suppression of endothelial cell proliferation, and maintenance of smooth muscle cells in a quiescent state.

In contrast, disturbed flow, typically present as low magnitude and/or oscillatory direction of wall shear stress, induces expression of pro-oxidant, pro-inflammatory, pro-coagulant and pro-apoptotic genes in endothelial cells, whereas protective genes like KLF2 are not induced.[24] Dai et al. showed an important effect of low magnitude and oscillating wall shear stress on the endothelial cell cytoskeleton, interleukin production, and nuclear translocation of transcription factor NF-κB that is related to enhanced expression of adhesion molecules.[26]

These differences between laminar and disturbed flow tend to explain why certain zones of the anastomosis are more prone to the development of intimal hyperplasia and stenosis, according to the particular types of wall shear stress that colocalize to these zones.[27]

IMPLICATIONS FOR HEMODIALYSIS PATIENTS

Computational modeling studies as well as basic science studies suggest that the configuration of the anastomosis is critical for AVF remodeling, the development of juxta-anastomotic stenoses, as well as the potential for AVF failure. However, these data are the results of idealized configurations coupled with boundary conditions; although they give an important insight into the mechanisms that govern hemodynamics and vessel remodeling in AVF, they cannot model all of the variables present in patients with vascular accesses for hemodialysis. Some of the variables that are frequently difficult to model, but are critical for AVF remodeling and outcome of the access, include pre-operative vessel quality and elasticity, vessel diameters that evolve during maturation, unintentional torsion, and variations of blood pressure and cardiac output; all of these variables and others are difficult to control in models and make each patient and each AVF unique.

To bridge the gap between the bench and bedside, we performed a clinical study to examine how anastomotic angle between the artery and the vein influences primary and secondary patency, as well as rate of reinterventions for juxta-anastomotic stenosis, in radial-cephalic fistulae.[28]

Patients and Design

Between February 2013 and September 2014, patients who received a radial-cephalic fistula in a single university hospital were retrospectively reviewed using prospectively maintained records. Among other baseline parameters, we prospectively collected anastomotic angle and vessel diameters in the operating room.

Surgical Procedures

The decision to create a distal radial-cephalic fistula was made upon clinical and duplex ultrasound examination, whenever the forearm cephalic vein was ≥ 2 mm in diameter and ≥ 10 cm in length was available for puncture, and the radial artery was ≥ 2 mm. A traditional end-to-side technique was used by a single experienced surgeon to construct the fistula under local anesthesia. The angle of the anastomosis was not decided *a priori* but was performed according to the patient's anatomy, depending on the angle between artery and vein.[8] In our practice the anastomosis is usually 9-10 mm in length; a tension-free anastomosis was performed with a continuous suture of 7-0 Prolene starting in the center of the back wall. When the anastomosis was complete and hemostatic, a sterile ruler was used to measure vessel diameters; the ruler was cut to reproduce the angle between the centerline of the artery and the centerline of the vein, and then the angled ruler was measured with a protractor to precisely measure the anastomotic angle (Figure 5-2).

Follow-up

The first Duplex ultrasound examination was performed at 4-6 weeks after AVF creation with the measurement of vessel diameters and access flow, then typically every three months or earlier in cases of access dysfunction or suspicion of stenosis. The patient was referred to the vascular surgeon for a fistulogram if any of the dialysis parameters were abnormal and/or a symptomatic stenosis was diagnosed by Duplex ultrasound examination. Reinterventions on a symptomatic stenosis were performed by an endovascular approach when feasible.

OUTCOMES AND DEFINITIONS

The primary endpoint was the cumulative rate of reintervention on the juxta-anastomotic segment, e.g. the cephalic vein within 4 cm of the anastomosis. This definition was based on reported patterns of shear stress and includes both the dissected

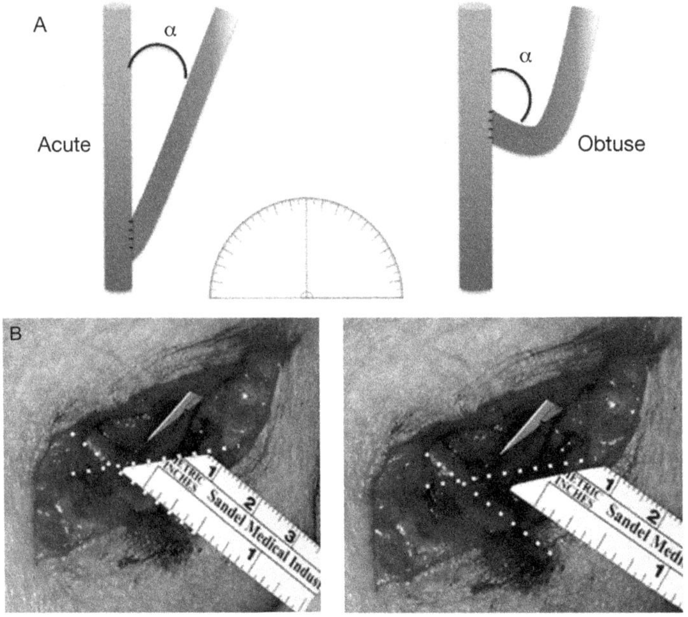

Figure 5-2. Measurement of the AVF anastomotic angle. (A) Geometry of the anastomotic angle. (B) Immediately after surgical creation of the AVF, a sterile ruler was cut to fit the anastomotic angle, and then measured using a protractor.

segment and the swing-point.[29,30] The time to reintervention was defined as the interval from the date of fistula creation until the first endovascular or surgical revision on the juxta-anastomotic segment. Secondary endpoints included primary and secondary patency of the fistula. The access was defined as functional when able to deliver a flow rate of 400 ml/min without access recirculation to maintain a treatment time of less than 4 h.[31]

RESULTS

During the 20-month study period, 73 fistulae were constructed in 73 patients. The mean patient age was 70.2 ± 13.2 years, 74% were male, and 34% were diabetic. The median follow-up was 7 months (range, 1-22 m). Overall patient survival at 12 months was 92% ± 5%.

The angle of the AVF anastomosis was directly measured in the operating room. The median anastomotic angle was 30°; 34 fistulae had an angle < 30°, and 39 had an angle ≥ 30°. Mean arterial diameters were significantly larger in patients with an angle ≥ 30° (2.8 ± 0.7 mm) compared with patients having an angle < 30° (2.5 ± 0.5 mm; p=0.03), although venous diameters were similar (3.7 ± 1.1 mm vs. 3.4 ± 0.8 mm, p=0.23).

Fistulae with an angle < 30° had significantly lower primary patency (p= 0.003, log rank test) and secondary patency (p=0.02), and a higher cumulative rate of reintervention for juxta-anastomotic stenosis (p=0.001), compared to fistulae with an angle ≥ 30°

(**Table 5-1**). There were 21 reinterventions for juxta-anastomotic stenosis that consisted of 14 balloon angioplasties and 7 surgical revisions; 4 fistulae were abandoned after failure of these interventions. Besides these 21 reinterventions, 8 more were performed in the outflow vein, 3 balloon angioplasties and 5 surgical revisions. No early thrombosis occurred.

A multivariable Cox model was performed to determine factors predictive of primary patency, secondary patency, and freedom from reintervention. Anastomotic angle was an independent factor predictive of primary patency (p=0.09), secondary patency (p=0.03) and freedom from reintervention for juxta-anastomotic stenosis (p=0.004) in patients with a radial-cephalic fistula.

We show that radial-cephalic fistulae with anastomotic angles < 30° have reduced primary and secondary patency and increased numbers of reinterventions compared to radial-cephalic fistulae with angles > 30°. These data suggest that radial-cephalic fistulae with acute anastomotic angles are prone to developing neointimal hyperplasia and juxta-anastomotic stenosis, requiring increased numbers of reinterventions.

CONCLUSIONS

Arteriovenous fistulae are non-physiological vascular constructs prone to intimal hyperplasia and characterized by high rates failure. Several in vitro studies have examined hemodynamic conditions in AVF and have colocalized zones of low magnitude and oscillatory patterns of shear stress with development of intimal hyperplasia. In addition, limiting the anastomotic angle to approximately 30–45° may limit these zones of disturbed flow. We report a clinical study in patients with a radial-cephalic AVF that shows that anastomotic angles below 30° are associated with diminished patency and increased numbers of reinterventions, and therefore should be avoided if possible. Additional clinical studies are needed to determine the optimal AVF anastomotic angle or perhaps other geometrical parameters that improve AVF outcome.

TABLE 5-1. PRIMARY PATENCY, SECONDARY PATENCY AND FREEDOM FROM JUXTA-ANASTOMOTIC PROCEDURES IN RADIAL-CEPHALIC FISTULAE WITH AN ANASTOMOTIC ANGLE < 30° OR ≥ 30°

	Primary patency		Secondary patency		Freedom from juxta-anastomotic procedures	
Anastomotic angle	<30°	≥30°	<30°	≥30°	<30°	≥30°
1 month	91%	97%	100%	100%	94%	98%
3 months	61%	90%	91%	100%	64%	92%
5 months	38%	76%	84%	97%	47%	84%
7 months	38%	63%	84%	93%	43%	74%
9 months	38%	56%	77%	93%	35%	67%
11 months	38%	56%	77%	93%	35%	67%

REFERENCES

1. Huber TS, Carter JW, Carter RL, Seeger JM. Patency of autogenous and polytetrafluoroethylene upper extremity arteriovenous hemodialysis accesses: a systematic review. *J Vasc Surg*. 2003;38(5):1005-11.
2. Sawant A, Mills PK, Dhingra H. Increased length of stay and costs associated with inpatient management of vascular access failures. *Semin Dial*. 2013;26(1):106-10.
3. Al-Jaishi AA, Oliver MJ, Thomas SM, et al. Patency rates of the arteriovenous fistula for hemodialysis: a systematic review and meta-analysis. *Am J Kidney Dis*. 2014;63(3):464-78.
4. System USRD. *2015 USRDS annual data report: Epidemiology of kidney disease in the United States*. Bethesda, MD: National Institutes of Health, Diseases NIoDaDaK; 2015.
5. Badero OJ, Salifu MO, Wasse H, Work J. Frequency of swing-segment stenosis in referred dialysis patients with angiographically documented lesions. *Am J Kidney Dis*. 2008;51(1):93-8.
6. Vassalotti JA. Arteriovenous fistula stenosis: new terminology. *Semin Dial*. 2004;17(3):243.
7. Corpataux JM, Haesler E, Silacci P, et al. Low-pressure environment and remodelling of the forearm vein in Brescia-Cimino haemodialysis access. *Nephrol Dial Transplant*. 2002;17(6):1057-62.
8. Konner K. The anastomosis of the arteriovenous fistula–common errors and their avoidance. *Nephrol Dial Transplant*. 2002;17(3):376-9.
9. Brescia MJ, Cimino JE, Appel K, Hurwich BJ. Chronic hemodialysis using venipuncture and a surgically created arteriovenous fistula. *N Engl J Med*. 1966;275(20):1089-92.
10. Sivanesan S, How TV, Bakran A. Sites of stenosis in AV fistulae for haemodialysis access. *Nephrol Dial Transplant*. 1999;14(1):118-20.
11. Van Canneyt K, Pourchez T, Eloot S, et al. Hemodynamic impact of anastomosis size and angle in side-to-end arteriovenous fistulae: a computer analysis. *J Vasc Access*. 2010;11(1):52-8.
12. Ene-Iordache B, Remuzzi A. Disturbed flow in radial-cephalic arteriovenous fistulae for haemodialysis: low and oscillating shear stress locates the sites of stenosis. *Nephrol Dial Transplant*. 2012;27(1):358-68.
13. Ene-Iordache B, Cattaneo L, Dubini G, Remuzzi A. Effect of anastomosis angle on the localization of disturbed flow in 'side-to-end' fistulae for haemodialysis access. *Nephrol Dial Transplant*. 2013;28(4):997-1005.
14. Iori F, Grechy L, Corbett RW, et al. The effect of in-plane arterial curvature on blood flow and oxygen transport in arterio-venous fistulae. *Phys Fluids. (1994)*. 2015;27(3):031903.
15. Paszkowiak JJ, Dardik A. Arterial wall shear stress: observations from the bench to the bedside. *Vasc Endovasc Surg*. 2003;37(1):47-57.
16. Haruguchi H, Teraoka S. Intimal hyperplasia and hemodynamic factors in arterial bypass and arteriovenous grafts: a review. *J Artif Organs*. 2003;6(4):227-35.
17. Lu DY, Chen EY, Wong DJ, et al. Vein graft adaptation and fistula maturation in the arterial environment. *J Surg Res*. 2014;188(1):162-73.
18. Kwak BR, Back M, Bochaton-Piallat ML, et al. Biomechanical factors in atherosclerosis: mechanisms and clinical implications. *Eur Heart J*. 2014;35(43):3013-20, 20a-20d.
19. Baeyens N, Schwartz MA. Biomechanics of vascular mechanosensation and remodeling. *Mol Biol Cell*. 2016;27(1):7-11.
20. Bryan MT, Duckles H, Feng S, et al. Mechanoresponsive networks controlling vascular inflammation. *Arterioscler Thromb Vasc Biol*. 2014;34(10):2199-205.
21. Kim JD, Lee HW, Jin SW. Diversity is in my veins: role of bone morphogenetic protein signaling during venous morphogenesis in zebrafish illustrates the heterogeneity within endothelial cells. *Arterioscler Thromb Vasc Biol*. 2014;34(9):1838-45.
22. Wan S, George SJ, Berry C, Baker AH. Vein graft failure: current clinical practice and potential for gene therapeutics. *Gene Ther*. 2012;19(6):630-6.

23. Chiu JJ, Chien S. Effects of disturbed flow on vascular endothelium: pathophysiological basis and clinical perspectives. *Physiol Rev.* 2011;91(1):327-87.
24. Franzoni M, Cattaneo I, Longaretti L, et al. Endothelial cell activation by hemodynamic shear stress derived from arteriovenous fistula for hemodialysis access. *Am J Physiol Heart Circ Physiol.* 2016;310(1):H49-59.
25. Wang N, Miao H, Li YS, et al. Shear stress regulation of Kruppel-like factor 2 expression is flow pattern-specific. *Biochem Biophys Res Commun.* 2006;341(4):1244-51.
26. Dai G, Kaazempur-Mofrad MR, Natarajan S, et al. Distinct endothelial phenotypes evoked by arterial waveforms derived from atherosclerosis-susceptible and -resistant regions of human vasculature. *Proc Natl Acad Sci U S A.* 2004;101(41):14871-6.
27. Browne LD, Bashar K, Griffin P, et al. The Role of Shear Stress in Arteriovenous Fistula Maturation and Failure: A Systematic Review. *PLoS One.* 2015;10(12):e0145795.
28. Sadaghianloo N, Jean-Baptiste E, Rajhi K, et al. Increased reintervention in radial-cephalic arteriovenous fistulas with anastomotic angles of less than 30 degrees. *J Vasc Surg.* 2015;62(6):1583-9.
29. Wang Y, Krishnamoorthy M, Banerjee R, et al. Venous stenosis in a pig arteriovenous fistula model–anatomy, mechanisms and cellular phenotypes. *Nephrol Dial Transplant.* 2008;23(2):525-33.
30. Bharat A, Jaenicke M, Shenoy S. A novel technique of vascular anastomosis to prevent juxta-anastomotic stenosis following arteriovenous fistula creation. *J Vasc Surg.* 2012;55(1):274-80.
31. Sidawy AN, Gray R, Besarab A, et al. Recommended standards for reports dealing with arteriovenous hemodialysis accesses. *J Vasc Surg.* 2002;35(3):603-10.

6

Rethinking Arteriovenous Anastomoses: Interrupted Suturing and Nonpenetrating Clips

Karl A. Illig, MD

Perhaps the most fundamental maneuver in vascular surgery is connecting two conduits together, for arterial repair, arterial bypass, or construction of arteriovenous access for hemodialysis. In turn, such conduits can be native artery, native vein, or prosthetic, in any combination. Finally, three general categories of anastomoses are most commonly constructed: Large anastomoses between an artery and prosthetic (for aneurysm repair or aortic bypass), small anastomoses between an artery and either a vein or prosthetic (for extremity arterial bypass), and small anastomoses between an artery and an outflow vein (for arteriovenous dialysis access). Empirically the first does not seem to be a problem; it is very rare for an aortic anastomosis to become significantly narrowed over time. This chapter will thus consider relatively small (generally, 8mm or less) anastomoses in the extremities.

Such anastomoses are most commonly end-to-side. Over time (months to a year or two), intimal hyperplasia develops in certain well-defined regions, depending on the direction of flow (Figure 6-1). In addition to molecular and cellular effects, hemodynamic issues play an important role in this situation. Three general processes seem to be at work: Increased particle residence times at areas of low shear stress, endothelial damage at areas of high shear stress, and abnormal activation of endothelium at areas of oscillating shear stress. In addition, the *difference* in compliance between the two materials (compliance mismatch) seems to provoke intimal hyperplasia in and of itself .[1,2] This mismatch is greatest when a prosthetic graft is anastomosed to an artery or vein, but is also important when a vein is anastomosed to an artery. All of these factors combine to produce intimal hyperplasia of varying degrees at any anastomosis in the extremities. Unfortunately, in the setting of an arteriovenous (AV) anastomosis, the abrupt transition from high to low pressure and resulting high flow, high Reynold's number, and

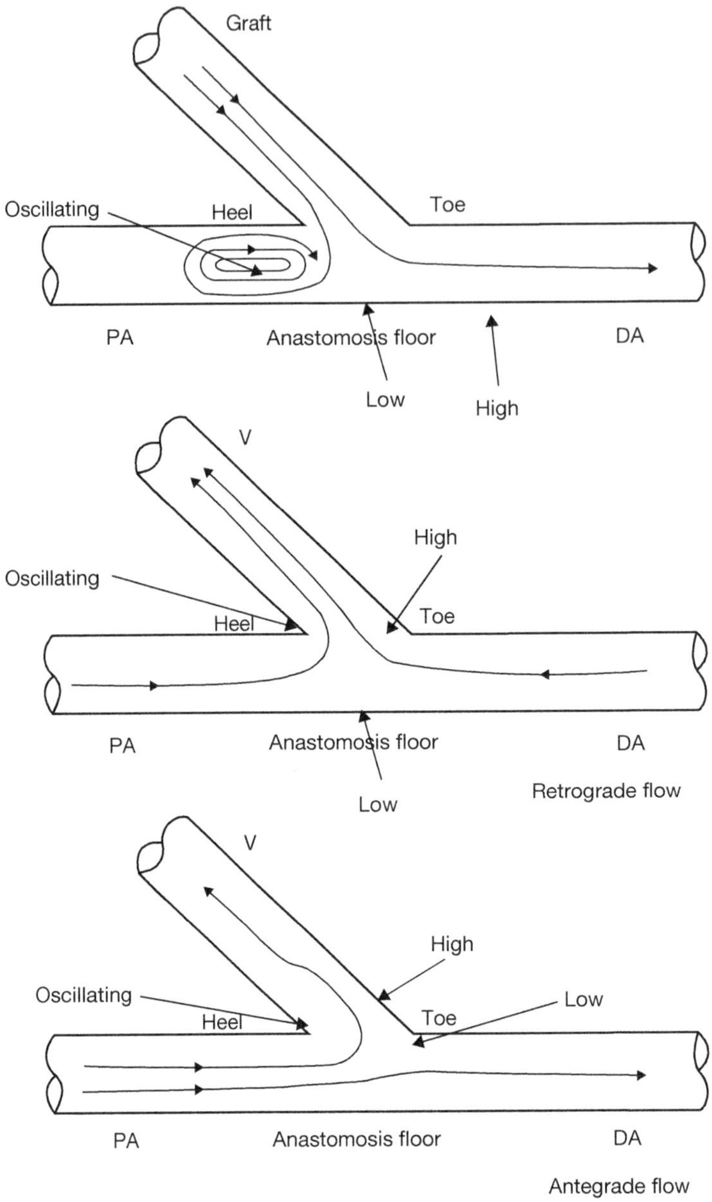

Figure 6-1. End-to-side anastomoses showing areas of high, low, and oscillating shear stress in anastomoses of varying configurations. Top: converging end-to-side anastomosis between a graft and an artery. Middle: diverging anastomosis between an artery and vein constructed for an arteriovenous anastomosis with retrograde flow. Bottom: diverging anastomosis between an artery and vein constructed for an arteriovenous anastomosis with antegrade flow. PA = proximal artery; DA = distal artery. Modified from Bogdan E, Cattaneo L, Dubini G, Remuzzi A: Effect of anastomosis angle on the localization of disturbed flow in "side-to-end" fistulae for haemodialysis access. *Nephrol Dial Transplant*. 2013;28(4):997–1005; used with permission.

resulting turbulence, the problem is hugely magnified. Empirically, AV anastomoses perform unusually poorly in this regard, with high early rates of intimal hyperplasia at any anastomosis that contribute substantially to failure. This situation thus creates a perfect "laboratory" for investigation of alternative anastomotic techniques.

BIOMECHANICS OF INTIMAL HYPERPLASIA AT AN AV ANASTOMOSIS

When an arteriovenous anastomosis is constructed for hemodialysis, two general situations are created: an anastomosis of a nearby vein to the artery, creating an AV fistula, or anastomosis of a prosthetic graft to an artery at one end and a vein at the other, creating an AV graft. There are three basic mechanical factors contributing to intimal hyperplasia: The anatomy of the anastomosis, intimal injury due to the sutures needed to connect the vessels, and the constrictive effects of a continuous suture.

The anatomy of the anastomosis is usually a topologic end-to-side connection, although flow patterns will vary according to the location of the anastomosis. An end-to-end anastomosis (usually the venous anastomosis of an AVG), can be created surgically or by means of an integrated PTFE/stent combination (Gore Hybrid Graft, Gore, Flagstaff AZ) but this strategy has not been convincingly shown to reduce IH or improve patency. The vast majority of data presented below is derived from end-to-side anastomoses, so this situation will not be further addressed in this chapter.

Intimal injury is created by any method that interferes with the integrity of the endothelium. Obviously, any technique that penetrates this layer will create some degree of injury. The degree to which this occurs with sutures used in AV anastomoses (6-0 or occasionally 5-0 non-absorbable suture) is unclear, but it seems intuitively beneficial to reduce this as much as possible. While absorbable suture, interestingly enough, seems to work as well as (or better than) non-absorbable;[3] the latter has become standard of care, at least in America. The continued presence of this foreign body, as well as the insult of initial suturing, contributes to intimal activation.

The third effect, constriction of the anastomosis by a continuous length of suture, also plays a role in the development of IH. It is very rare that the anastomosis is actually constricted by a suture line that is "too tight," but the resulting continuous length of non-stretchable suture essentially fixes the circumference of the resulting anastomosis, and as a result affects the compliance matching of the anastomosis forever.

There are thus two general strategies to address these two issues: The use of nonpenetrating techniques to avoid any insult at all to the endothelium, and the use of interrupted techniques to avoid creation of a fixed circumference at an anastomosis.

THEORETICAL AND ANIMAL DATA

The easiest intervention to make in this regard is simply to construct the anastomosis using interrupted sutures or other devices. This primarily addresses the issue of compliance mismatch, by allowing all components of the anastomosis to expand according to their intrinsic compliance, eliminating the constriction imposed by what ends up being a continuous circle of monofilament suture. An extensive review of this concept, incorporating both theoretical analysis and review of the literature up to that point, was published by Tiwari and colleagues in 2003.[4] They concluded that interrupted techniques produce clear improvement in anastomotic compliance mismatch.

Unfortunately, the effects of nonpenetrating versus penetrating interrupted technique is much harder to differentiate when reviewing basic and animal data. Virtually all such models have used one of two nonpenetrating clip techniques as a comparison to continuous suturing. Stansby and colleagues joined human veins, bovine arteries, and PTFE in a benchtop model of end-to-end anastomoses.[5] While results varied, they documented a decrease in postanastomotic compliance in arteriovenous anastomoses created using interrupted, nonpenetrating clips. Zeebregts documented some improvement in endothelial function after venous patch angioplasty using nonpenetrating clips in sheep,[6] while others have documented reduced IH[7] and improved compliance[8] in more conventional anastomoses. Interestingly, there does seem to be at least one animal model comparing *penetrating* clips to continuous sutures, also showing a reduction in IH and other beneficial effects in the interrupted group in two different reports.[9,10] Taken together, both theoretical and animal data available seem to support the concept that interrupted techniques yield better compliance and less IH than do continuous. There is very little data regarding the effects of intimal penetration versus non-penetration, however, but no data to suggest non-penetration is any worse.

EMPIRIC AND HUMAN DATA

Ultimately, of course, the critical issue is what works in humans. It is useful to review the two basic types of clips that have been used to compare against sutured anastomosis. U-clips (Medtronic, Minneapolis MN) are essentially a loop of nitinol that is "activated" by releasing it from a length of suture. This suture, in turn, is attached to a conventional needle which is passed through the materials being anastomosed.[9] These clips are thus *penetrating*. Unfortunately, they are also no longer available in the United States. The second type of clip, available since the late 1990s, was originally marketed as VCS (US Surgical Corporation, Norwalk CT) but is now known as AnastoClip (LeMaitre, Burlington MA).[11] These are, in effect, miniature staples with short, blunt ends, and are thus (theoretically) *nonpenetrating*.

There are thus two different approaches to each of two different variables to modify, identified as follows:

- Penetrating continuous: conventional suturing
- Penetrating interrupted: U-clips or interrupted suturing
- Nonpenetrating continuous: there does not seem to be such a technique
- Nonpenetrating interrupted: VCS/AnastoClips

Since there are thus three techniques to compare, our task is as follows:

- Compare penetrating continuous to penetrating interrupted techniques (isolating the issue of compliance only),
- Compare penetrating interrupted to nonpenetrating interrupted techniques (isolating the issue of endothelial penetration only), and
- Compare penetrating continuous to nonpenetrating interrupted techniques (looking at both compliance and penetration together)

Penetrating Continuous versus Penetrating Interrupted Techniques

This issue has been well studied in microvascular surgery, but little data exist exploring this comparison in AV anastomoses. Three prospective studies could be found examining U-clips versus conventional suturing. Lin and colleagues compared the two techniques in 132 patients with forearm AVFs, and found that while maturation rates did not vary, in those who did the primary patency was better in the U-clip group up to three years out.[12] By contrast, two other studies, both smaller, showed no differences between the two.[13,14] One prospective randomized trial exists comparing conventional sutured anastomoses versus partially interrupted anastomoses (three interrupted sutures near the heel on each side with a continuous suture for the remainder of the anastomosis). The authors found that primary patency at 6 weeks was better in the interrupted group (71% versus 47%), but found no differences in functional patency.[15] Overall, data are sparse, but when differences exist they lean in the direction supporting the concept that improving compliance by means of interrupting the connection between materials, by using either sutures or penetrating clips, is beneficial.

Penetrating Interrupted versus Nonpenetrating Interrupted Techniques

Unfortunately, no data exist at all. This would require a head-to-head comparison of U-clips or interrupted sutures versus nonpenetrating clips, and no such studies could be found (other than three anastomoses in Varcoe's most recent animal model).[10] We cannot thus isolate out the effects of penetration alone, controlling for compliance.

Penetrating Continuous versus Nonpenetrating Interrupted Techniques

The third and final comparison, however, yields a wealth of data. While this comparison creates differences in both compliance and endothelial penetration, it does reveal "real world" outcomes which are quite helpful.

Cooper and colleagues published an early comparison of nonpenetrating clips versus continuously sutured anastomoses in 2001, and found no differences.[16] However, the N was small in this study, 48 clips versus 34 sutures, only AV grafts were compared, and the study was retrospective. The first two prospective randomized trials were also published in 2001. Cook and colleagues were unable to show any differences between groups, but again the N was small (86 patients) and grafts only were compared.[17]. Schild and colleagues published a larger series that same year ($N = 173$) comparing both fistulas and grafts, showing benefit in the latter and trends toward benefit in the former.[18] The largest prospective randomized trial to date was published in 2004. In this trial, Zeegbregts and colleagues compared 56 continuously sutured versus 51 clipped radiocephalic AV fistulas. Primary patency at 6 months was not different (61 vs 69%, respectively), but mean secondary patency was better in the clipped group (344 vs 435 days, $P = 0.009$).[19] We thus have three prospective randomized trials to compare – while one was negative, the two largest ones (and the only two to include fistulas) showed benefit, albeit inconsistent, to the nonpenetrating interrupted technique.

There have been two fairly large retrospective reviews looking at this issue. Most recent is a review by Nguyen and colleagues, who looked at their experience over 6 years at a single VA hospital. After comparing 237 clipped and 97 sutured anastomoses, they found no differences in outcome measures.[20] However, the clipped group seemed to be different from the sutured group – more patients receiving clips had veins smaller than 3mm, more needed operative dilation, and more were undergoing radiocephalic fistulas. The largest review, by far, was published in 2003. Shenoy and colleagues performed a multicenter retrospective review, looking at 1385 anastomoses (827 AVG, 518 AVF) created over 3½ years using either continuous or clipped (VCS) techniques. Overall primary patency at 24 months was better in the clipped group

(AVF: 54% vs 34%; AVG 36% vs 17%), and interventions needed to maintain patency significantly better (Figures 6-2 and 6-3)[21]. Again, while the two retrospective reviews differ in their conclusions, the larger one (and the only one that included more than one center) showed a benefit to nonpenetrating interrupted clips over conventional suturing.

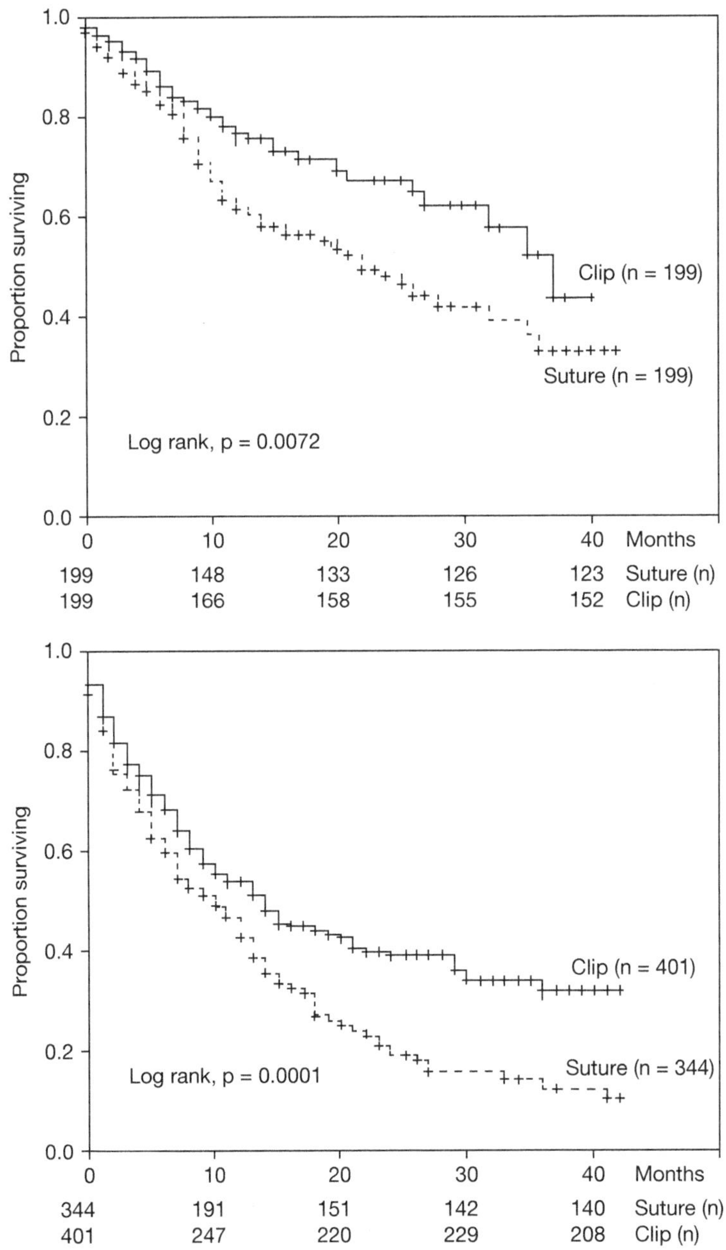

Figure 6-2. Life table curves showing primary patency rates in patients undergoing AV fistula (top) and AV graft (bottom) creation. From Shenoy S, Miller A, Petersen F, et al. A multicenter study of permanent hemodialysis access patency: Beneficial effect of clipped vascular anastomotic technique. *J Vasc Surg*. 2003;38:229–35; used with permission.

We began using AnastoClips in late December 2015. From then until June, 2016, we have performed 19 fistulas and 4 grafts (27 anastomoses) using this technique, with an additional 4 anastomoses performed using clips on the anterior wall (essentially an interrupted technique with intimal penetration along one wall and the heel and toe). Although it is cautioned that these results are both preliminary and non-peer reviewed, we have had only one fistula in this group fail so far (one graft was ligated in the recovery room due to severe steal. Operative time is shortened and we have had no excessive bleeding or other complications.

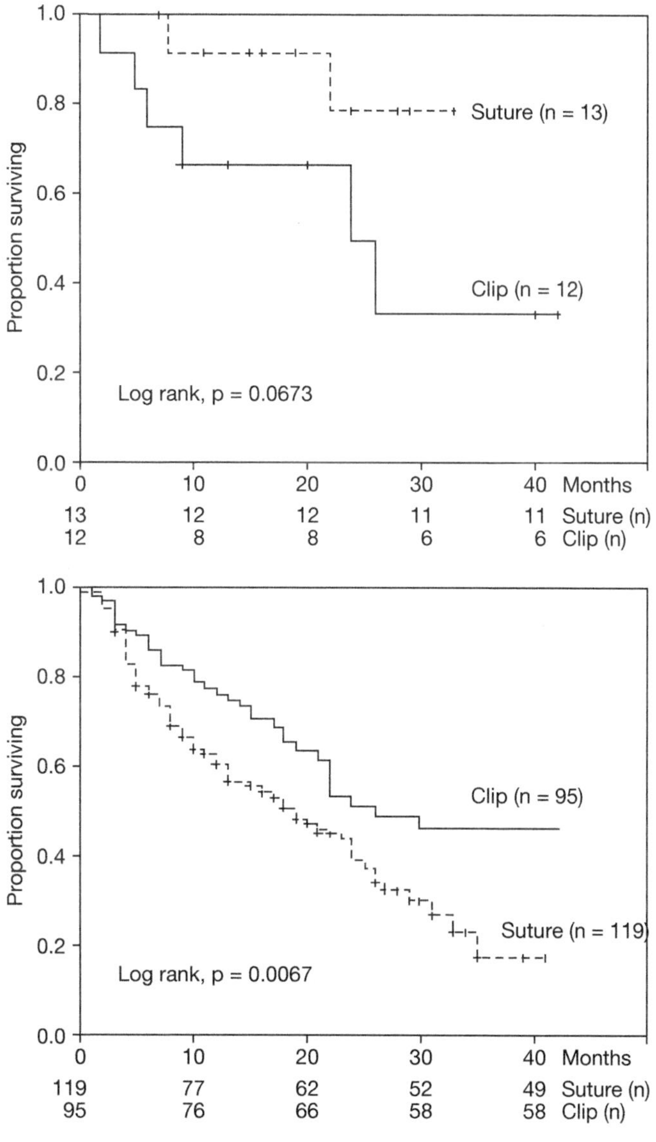

Figure 6-3. Life table curves showing secondary patency rates in patients undergoing AV fistula (top) and AV graft (bottom) creation. From Shenoy S, Miller A, Petersen F, et al. A multicenter study of permanent hemodialysis access patency: Beneficial effect of clipped vascular anastomotic technique. *J Vasc Surg*. 2003;38:229–35; used with permission.

PUTTING IT ALL TOGETHER

Intimal hyperplasia remains an unsolved problem following any small anastomosis, and an anastomosis for AV access in general creates perhaps the most fertile environment for this effect to arise.

A wealth of experimental data support the concept that any interrupted technique (suturing or either penetrating or nonpenetrating clips) offers benefit over a conventional, continuous suture. Empiric human data are sparse, but the largest prospective randomized trial does suggest some degree of benefit from an interrupted technique. There are no data to isolate out the concept of endothelial penetration or non-penetration as an isolated factor, but the largest retrospective review and prospective trials exploring the combination of both endothelial non-penetration and interruption (nonpenetrating clips versus conventional suturing) all suggest benefit. All available data suffer, however, from relatively small comparison groups, inconsistent endpoints, heterogeneous populations, and the use of somewhat old technology.

We have instituted a prospective randomized trial comparing AnastoClips to conventional sutured anastomoses in patients undergoing brachiocephalic AV fistula creation, to begin in the fall of 2016. Based on available literature we feel the differences in initial maturation rates will be modest, but we feel there is fairly suggestive data to support a 10% primary patency rate at one year. Based on this, a sample size of 165 patients per group will have an 80% chance of showing this difference. We perform approximately 100 brachiocephalic fistulas each year, and thus hope to be able to complete enrollment in 4 or 5 years. In addition, we hope to be able to enlist other interested centers, if we can ensure consistent data collection, to create a larger sample size, and hope to be able to continue the study beyond minimal numbers to acquire as much additional data (and statistical power) as possible.

REFERENCES

1. Loth F, Fischer PF, Bassiouny HS. Blood flow in end-to-side anastomoses. *Ann Rev Fluid Mechanics*. 2008;40:367.
2. Davies MG.: Intimal Hyperplasia. In Cronenwett JL, Johnston KW (eds): *Rutherford's Vascular Surgery (7th ed)*. Philadelphia; Saunders/Elsevier 2010:69–88.
3. Schmitz-Rixen T, Storck M, Erasmi H, Schmiegelow P, Horsch S. Vascular anastomoses with absorbable suture material: an experimental study. *Ann Vasc Surg*. 1991;5(3):257–64.
4. Tiwari A, Cheng KS, Salacinski H, Hamilton G, Siefalian AM. Improving the patency of vascular bypass grafts: the role of suture materials and surgical techniques on reducing anastomotic compliance mismatch. *Eur J Vasc Endovasc Surg*. 2003;25:287–95.
5. Stansby G, Knez P, Berwanger CS, et al. Does vascular stapling improve compliance of vascular anastomoses? *Vasc Surg*. 2001:35(2):115–21.
6. Zeebregts C, van den Dungen J, Buikema H, et al. Preservation of endothelial integrity and function in experimental vascular anastomoses with non-penetrating clips. *Br J Surg*. 2001;88:1201–8.
7. Komori K, Shoji T, Furuyhama T, et al. Non-penetrating vascular clips anastomosis inhibited intimal thickening under poor runoff conditions in canine autogenous vein grafts. *Eur J Vasc Endovasc Surg*. 2001;21:241–7.
8. Baguneid MS, Goldner S. Fulford PE, et al. A comparison of para-anastomotic compliance profiles after vascular anastomosis: Non-penetrating clips versus standard sutures. *J Vasc Surg*. 2001;33(4):812–20.

9. Varcoe RL, Teo AB, et al. An arteriovenous fistula model of intimal hyperplasia for evaluation of a nitinol U-clip anastomosis. *Eur J Vasc Endovasc Surg*. 2012:43(2):224–31.
10. Varcoe RL, Teo ABP, Pelletier MH, et al. A nitinol "U-clip" versus sutured arteriovenous anastomosis: Local tissue response and intimal hyperplasia development in a sheep model. *Eur J Vasc Endovasc Surg*. 2015;49:344–352.
11. Zeegbregts CJ, Kirsch WM, van den Dungen JJ. Five years' world experience with non-penetrating clips for vascular anastomoses. *Am J Surg*. 2004;187:751–60.
12. Lin PH, Bush RL, Nelson JC, et al. A prospective evaluation of interrupted nitinol surgical clips in arteriovenous fistula for hemodialysis. *Am J Surg*. 2003;186(6):625–30.
13. Bigdeli AR, Kaczmarek I, Eifert S, et al. Interrupted nitinol U-clips versus standard running suture for the central arterial T-graft anastomosis: A prospective randomized study. *Eur J Cardiothorac Surg*. 2011;40:e93–7.
14. Walker SR. U clips for arteriovenous anastomosis: a pilot randomized study. *ANZ J Surg*. 2012:82:630–2.
15. Aitken E, Jeans E, Aitken M, Kingsmore D. A randomized controlled trial of interrupted versus continuous suturing techniques for radiocephalic fistulas. *J Vasc Surg*. 2015;62:1575–82.
16. Cooper BZ, Flores L, Ramirez JA, et al. Analysis of nonpenetrating clips versus sutures for arterial venous graft anastomosis. *Ann Vasc Surg*. 2001;15:7–12.
17. Cook JW, Schuman ES, Standage BA, Heinl P: Patency and flow characteristics using stapled vascular anastomoses in dialysis grafts. *Am J Surg*. 2001;181:24–7.
18. Schild AF, Pruett CS, Martin I, et al: The utility of the VCS clip for creation of vascular access for hemodialysis: long-term results and intraoperative benefits. *Cardiovasc Surg*. 2001;9:526–30.
19. Zeegbregts C, van den Dungen JJ, van Det RJ, et al. Randomized clinical trial of continuous sutures or non-penetrating clips for radiocephalic arteriovenous fistula. *Br J Surg*. 2004;91:1438–42.
20. Nguyen KP, Teruya T, Alabi O, et al. Comparison of non-penetrating titanium clips versus continuous polypropylene suture in dialysis access creation. *Ann Vasc Surg*. 2016;32:15–9.
21. Shenoy S, Miller A, Petersen F, et al. A multicenter study of permanent hemodialysis access patency: Beneficial effect of clipped vascular anastomotic technique. *J Vasc Surg*. 2003;38:229–35.

7

Forearm versus Upper Arm Arteriovenous Graft for Dialysis Access: Which is Preferred?

Alik Farber, MD and Steven Pike, MD

INTRODUCTION

The use of artificial grafts for hemodialysis is an important and necessary component of the overall management of the patient with end-stage renal disease (ESRD). Both the National Kidney Foundation (NKF) Disease Outcomes Quality Initiative (DOQI) guidelines[1] and the Fistula First Initiative[2] are resolute on the matter of superiority of native arteriovenous fistula (AVF) access over the use of prosthetic arteriovenous grafts (AVG) and on the advantage of either over dialysis catheters. In spite of these guidelines and associated evidence, in 2010, catheters were used as the initial access for hemodialysis in 81% of cases, while hemodialysis was initiated through autologous AVF and prosthetic AVG in only 16% and 3%, respectively.[3]

Patients with ESRD are fragile, as the one-year life expectancy of a hemodialysis patient in the United states is 22% while the overall ESRD mean life expectancy is 5.8 years.[3] Factors that most commonly contribute to death in this patient population are cardiovascular disease and infection. In addition, ESRD management is costly, as the share of Medicare expenditure for chronic kidney disease (CKD) has grown from 4.2% in 1995 to 7.7% in 2003 and most recently to 20.8% in 2014.[4] The yearly expense to Medicare for a patient dialyzing through a catheter or AVG is $77,093 and $71,616, respectively.[3]

Recent evidence suggests that increased utilization of native AVF, given sub-optimal maturation rates, is a significant cause of increased dialysis catheter use. Maturation of a native AVF can take from six weeks to as long as six months, and 20%–54% of autologous access will not result in a mature fistula. In one study evaluating this association, the authors found that AVGs required more secondary procedures over the course of a year, but resulted in an average of 70 catheter days as opposed to 155 catheter days for patients dialyzed through AVFs.[5] In fact, debate exists regarding the superiority of AVF over AVG in that it is argued that data supporting improved AVF outcomes are skewed because some studies that show such superiority frequently exclude fistulae which fail to mature.[6]

Therefore, prosthetic AVG have a definitive role in the management of patients with ESRD. In cases for which an AVG is the preferred or the only access, questions exist as to the best prosthetic conduit to use, the best location in the upper extremity for AVG placement and the best configuration of the access graft. The intricacies of these decisions will be discussed in the paragraphs below.

GUIDELINES AND INDICATIONS FOR GRAFT PLACEMENT

Indications for placement of an AVG in the "Fistula First" era include exhausted or previously harvested superficial veins, unsuitable veins secondary to repeat venipuncture or phlebitis, requirement for swift initiation of dialysis with need for immediate cannulation, and inability to successfully place a dialysis catheter. Elderly patients tend to be considered better candidates for initial placement of an AVG rather than AVF due to diminished life expectancy and high risk for perioperative systemic morbidity. Important considerations include the time frame for initiation of dialysis and the patient's life expectancy, bearing in mind the functional time gained from access that is created.[7]

AVGs have a series of advantages including the presence of a large surface area and ease of cannulation. Many prosthetic AVGs can be ready for direct access 10–14 days from placement and this could lead to a significantly shorter duration of catheter use. Some types of graft conduit can even be accessed within hours of implantation, obviating the need for a catheter in patients who are being initiated on dialysis. Other advantages of AVGs include ease of surgical placement and relative simplicity of open and endovascular thrombectomy.[1]

The NKF DOQI guidelines, last published in 2006, state that "(AVG) . . . patency is independent of manufacturer, unaffected by an external wrap around the graft, and is not affected by wall thickness". Restricting the size of the arterial anastomosis or increasing the diameter of the outflow of the graft into the vein with a vein cuff have similarly yielded less than impressive results, and may negatively affect patency.[1]

As such, the general importance of autogenous AVFs as primary access for dialysis is clear. However, it is also evident that AVGs may be best in certain clinical scenarios. Woo et al.[8] conducted a study using the RAND/UCLA Appropriateness Method. An exhaustive literature review of the risks and benefits of various access options was performed by a group of experts. Next, 3816 distinct, clinically relevant, dialysis access scenarios were developed. The experts, then, reviewed each case individually and as a whole group rating them according to the appropriateness of the proposed interventions, which included AVFs and AVGs. AVG placement was agreed to be most appropriate in the case of older age, dialysis dependence, and smaller vein size. Upper arm AVGs (uAVG) were favored to forearm AVG (fAVG) in the setting of smaller forearm outflow veins. Woo et al. found that in certain scenarios, AVGs may be favored over AVF, despite nationally driven efforts to increase AVF utilization.[8]

CONDUITS

Polytetrafluoroethylene Grafts

The most frequently used material in AVG creation is expanded Polytetrafluoroethylene (ePTFE), originally marketed as Teflon. This graft is manufactured by drawing the polymer resin through a die, rather than weaving fibers together to create a fabric such as is the case with other implantable materials such as Dacron. The resulting ePTFE material is porous, thin, hydrophobic, chemically inert, and durable.[3]

Outcomes of ePTFE grafts may be dependent on a number of factors including degree of external support, diameter, and heparin bonding. Grafts may be supported with rings or unsupported. In a study of 4402 patients, investigators found 20.2% and 10.8% three-year patency rates for supported and unsupported AVGs, respectively ($P < 0.05$).[9] Another factor that may affect graft patency is the size of the graft. If the proximal anastomosis, or inflow of the graft, is too large, symptoms of steal can develop. If the venous outflow of the graft is too small, the resulting hemodynamics may lead to the development of intimal hyperplasia at the distal anastomosis resulting in graft thrombosis. A randomized multicenter study of 109 patients receiving either a 6 mm graft or 4–7 mm tapered graft placed in the brachial-antecubital loop configuration found that there was no difference in patency rates between these two grafts.[10] Another series of 507 patients in which straight brachial-axillary 6–8-mm tapered grafts were compared with 6-mm grafts found that the tapered grafts resulted in better patency rates and a better complication profile than the 6-mm nontapered grafts. In diabetic and elderly patients, however, use of tapered grafts resulted in a greater incidence of steal syndrome.[11] In a similar study comparing 6-mm straight grafts to 6–8 mm tapered grafts placed in the brachial-axillary position in nondiabetic patients younger than 70 years of age, investigators found that in order to achieve an equivalent secondary patency rate, 6-mm grafts required twice the number of rescue procedures.[12]

The most common graft-related complication is stenosis secondary to neointimal hyperplasia at the venous anastomosis. This often leads to thrombosis of the graft due to decreased flow. Attempts have been made to diminish the rates of graft thrombosis using anticoagulation or antiplatelet therapy, changes in graft configuration, or graft makeup, all without significant benefit. Bonding heparin to PTFE has also been investigated as a solution to this problem. Early comparison studies of heparin-bonded PTFE AVGs and standard PTFE AVG noted significantly improved patency,[13] however, follow-up studies found a trend toward improved patency, but no statistically significant difference.[14] In one such study involving 160 patients, secondary patency at 36 months was 81% and 68% for bonded and standard AVG, respectively, and this difference did not reach significance.[14] In 2016, a study of 483 patients found no significant difference in the patency rates of heparin-bonded and standard PTFE grafts.[14,15]

Early Access Grafts

Early access grafts have been developed out of the need to cannulate a given access before the 10–14 days necessary for an ePTFE graft to adequately incorporate into surrounding tissue. Such grafts are made of multiple layers, including an outer ePTFE layer, a middle layer of an elastomer that acts as a sealant and an inner ePTFE layer that allows immediate access without the requirement for the graft to become incorporated into the surrounding tissue. They can be implanted as primary access, or as a bridging device to maturation of an autologous AV fistula. Often, use of early access grafts can obviate the need for catheter-based dialysis.[16]

In one study comparing early access grafts to tunneled dialysis catheters, a significant reduction in the rate of bacteremia and mortality was found in patients requiring urgent dialysis access via early access grafts without incurring additional cost. In another investigation, primary and secondary patency of early access grafts was reported to be 46% and 61% at one year and this was comparable to other prosthetic access grafts. Few cannulation-related complications were identified.[17] Although advantages of early access grafts are compelling, their routine adoption has been hampered by their stiffness and associated technical difficulty in surgical placement.

Bovine Carotid Artery

Bovine carotid artery (BCA) xenografts have been used as a conduit for dialysis access but have had early difficulties with aneurysmal degeneration. Newer techniques for preparation of the graft have resulted in improved collagen cross-linking with some evidence that the risk of aneurysm formation has greatly decreased.[18]

Early studies suggested greatly improved primary patency rates of these grafts over PTFE. More recent reviews, however, suggest that this may not be accurate. In 2016, one review of 134 BCA grafts found primary and secondary patency rates to be similar to PTFE grafts. Infection rates were less with BCA grafts, although this difference did not reach statistical significance.[19] In one series, a comparison of 52 BCA grafts with 68 ePTFE grafts revealed, no significant difference between the two cohorts with respect to primary or primary-assisted patency, though the trend favored the BCA grafts. Secondary patency, however, was significantly higher for BCA grafts.[20] Unfortunately, the cost of BCA grafts is almost twice that of ePTFE grafts, but comparable in price to a heparin-bonded ePTFE grafts.[18] Therefore, consideration of potential benefits of BCA evidenced in these studies must be weighed against increased cost.

Cryopreserved Femoral Vein

Given that ESRD patients are living longer on dialysis many will require a greater number of total access procedures than in the past. ESRD patients are at increased risk for access infection and such risk is increased among those dialyzed via ePTFE AVGs. Cryopreserved femoral vein has been touted as having lower risk of access infection. A study of 48 cryopreserved femoral vein AVGs, most often placed as a replacement for graft infection to preserve an access site, had a primary one-year patency of 49% and a secondary patency rate of 75% with no infections reported.[21] In contrast, another review of 20 patients dialyzed via femoral vein AVGs found that infection occurred in 11 patients, six of whom experienced graft rupture and hemorrhage with one death. These complications occurred most frequently with placement in the thigh, and the authors concluded that use of this graft in cases of infection should be limited.[22]

Bovine Mesenteric Vein

Another option in the surgeon's arsenal of biologic grafts is bovine mesenteric vein (BMV). It has been described as an option for rescue of native AVF with replacement of either an arterial segment or the proximal venous segment of the AVF.[23] BMV grafts have been reported to have 12-month primary patency of 35.6% and 24-month secondary patency of 60.3% compared to 28.4% and 42.9% for ePTFE, respectively.[24] As a biologic alternative, available data would not preclude the use of this graft, especially in cases of failed prosthetic access or infection.

CONFIGURATION AND LOCATION

Configuration and location of AVGs may be important in access outcomes. Although AVGs can be placed in many locations in the body, they are most commonly constructed in the upper extremity, either in the fAVG or the uAVG. In the forearm, arterial inflow is derived from either the brachial or, less often, the radial artery, while the venous outflow is usually the cephalic, basilic, or median antecubital vein. In the upper arm, arterial inflow is either from the brachial, or axillary artery and venous outflow is usually through the brachial, basilic, or axillary veins. With regard to configuration, AVGs can be placed either in the straight or looped configurations. Multiple factors are considered in the choice of position and configuration including location and adequacy of donor artery and outflow vein, prior access attempts in the ipsilateral upper extremity and personal bias.[25]

In a small series of six fAVGs, the use of deep forearm veins was reviewed. In these cases, forearm veins were unusable because of small size or stricture due to repeat venipuncture. The deep veins are not subject to this trauma and tend to be larger outflow options, thus allowing for an access site that would otherwise be unavailable. During the follow up of these grafts, one failed at six months secondary to clot formation in the mid graft, while the others were patent without need for secondary intervention for 3–24 months. All grafts were used for dialysis two to three weeks after implantation.[26] In light of high primary failure rates of radiocephalic AVF reported to be as high as 24%, a multicenter trial comparing radiocephalic AVF and prosthetic fAVG was conducted. In all, 182 patients were randomized to each group. Grafts were constructed of PTFE and placed in a forearm loop configuration. Patients with arterial diameter <1 mm or an absent cephalic vein was not randomized, instead receiving a prosthetic AVG. Patients with radial arteries >2 mm and a cephalic vein of at least 1.6 mm received a radiocephalic AVF. Patients were randomized when the radial artery was between 1 and 2 mm and the cephalic vein was present, but measured less than 1.6 mm. Primary-assisted patency for AVF and AVG at one year was 44% and 63%, respectively. Required interventions included 43 in the AVF group and 79 in the AVG group. The authors concluded that in patients with poor forearm vessels, a benefit is derived from implantation of PTFE grafts, despite a higher need for interventions.[27] Of significant interest, radial artery as the graft inflow was noted to be an independent predictor of long-term graft patency.[28] When considering the type of graft used, tapering of the PTFE, as discussed previously, does not appear to improve the patency of forearm loop grafts.[10]

In another series evaluating upper arm access transposed brachiobasilic AVFs, uAVGs, and brachiocephalic AVFs were compared. AVGs were 6 mm PTFE based on the brachial artery and axillary vein. They were more likely to occlude or become infected than transposed brachiobasilic AVFs. Interestingly, transposed brachiobasilic AVFs took about a month longer than the grafts to be usable and a 9% per month risk of catheter-related bacteremia was described among those dialyzing via catheters. The authors concluded that use of brachiobasilic AVFs was preferred to the use of uAVG because of less perioperative morbidity.[29] To provide access in patients with poor venous outflow, a series of 27 patients who received upper arm looped uAVG was reviewed. Primary patency at 12 months was 51% and secondary patency at 18 months was 80%. Five patients developed irreversible occlusion, and 10 patients required secondary procedures to maintain patency. The conclusion to this case series was that arteriovenous axillary loop AVGs can be used in patients who develop steal or in patients with poor venous access sites.[30] In another study, 168 patients who received transposed basilic or cephalic vein AVFs were compared with patients who received upper arm PTFE AVGs. Cohorts were matched for age, gender, race, diabetes, and history of previously failed access. Primary patency was 48% in the AVF group and 14% in the AVG group. Five-year secondary patency was 57% and 19%, respectively. AVGs required more revisions to maintain patency and were significantly more likely to develop infection. Based on these criteria, transposed AVF was recommended over creation of a uAVG as long as anatomic criteria were met.[31]

In identifying factors related to graft failure, the Dialysis Access Consortium (DAC) evaluated the effect of dipyridamole plus aspirin therapy to prolong primary patency. In a randomized, double-blind, placebo controlled trial, 649 patients were randomized to dipyridamole plus aspirin (321 patients) or placebo (328 patients). Patients were followed for 4.5 years. In this study, 49% of grafts were in the forearm, 44% in the upper arm, 6% in the leg, and 1% in the chest. Primary-unassisted patency was found to be 23% in the placebo group and 28% in the treated group. While this difference was statistically significant, it becomes less significant clinically with the requirement to treat 20 patients for one year in order to reduce the total number of patients with primary graft failure by one patient.[32]

In a subset analysis of the DAC Graft study, 508 patients received 255 fAVG, and 253 uAVG. Recipients of fAVG were more likely to have a higher body mass index (BMI) and a greater degree of hypertension. They were also more likely to have a looped configuration to their grafts. Meanwhile, recipients of uAVG were more likely to be African American, on dialysis for a longer period of time and to have had a failed ipsilateral graft. Important measures such as rate of steal syndrome, infection, and graft patency were unaffected by either graft location or configuration (looped versus straight). Patients who received uAVG more often had failed grafts in the ipsilateral arm and have been on dialysis for a longer period of time, while patients who received fAVG were of a higher BMI and were more likely to have their outflow into superficial veins. In looking at the differences between fAVG and uAVG, it was noted that the outflow of fAVG could allow maturation of a native upper arm native fistula at a later date due to the increased flow through the utilized vein. To attempt assessment of the importance of deep versus superficial outflow vein choice, variations for both upper and lower grafts were reviewed, however no difference in patency was identified to suggest any benefits to a particular outflow vessel.[33]

Preservation of access sites is key to the longevity of the dialysis patient. Per NKF-DOQI guidelines, access is created distally first in order to maximize the number of sites available for access.[1] To that end, it would seem reasonable to always place a fAVG before moving to an upper arm access. Among the benefits of creating a forearm graft is the increased flow through the upper arm venous system. This may encourage arterialization of these veins and allow for increase in diameter of previously small upper arm veins which could be used to construct an upper arm access in the future. Although this observation may be true, this concept has not been scientifically proven.

Advantages of placing a uAVG over fAVG include the concern that patency rates in uAVG, usually sewn to larger axillary or brachial veins, are higher than those of fAVG.

The 30-day primary failure rate of a fAVG approaches 10%.[33] One comparison of fAVG and uAVG found a 6- and 18-month primary patency of 51% and 69%, and 8% and 49%, respectively.[34] The DAC subgroup analysis found that after adjustment for graft configuration, outflow vein, and history of previous access, there was no difference between fAVG and uAVG in primary and secondary failure rates.[33]

uAVG placed as a second ipsilateral access, when compared to native upper arm AVF placed as a second ipsilateral access, have been shown to have shorter catheter dependence and, as a result, less catheter-related bacteremia. In addition, they require fewer interventions to achieve maturation.[35] While comparing 71 transposed brachiobasilic AVF and 114 brachioaxillary AVG, the AVFs were only able to be used for dialysis 69% of the time as compared to 89.4% for AVGs. Primary one- and two-year patency were 45.3% and 40% for the AVFs and 56.4% and 43.2% for the AVGs, respectively.[36]

SECONDARY INTERVENTIONS

The major cause of loss of patency, or graft failure, in an AVG is thrombosis secondary to development of neointimal hyperplasia at the distal anastomosis. Angioplasty alone does not appear to be the optimal strategy to relieve the stenosis of this site because of the fibrous nature of the stenosis. A review was conducted of 23 fAVGs and 38 uAVGs with stenosis at the venous anastomosis. Stent grafts were placed in cases for which balloon angioplasty alone was found to be inadequate to relieve the stenotic outflow. Stents were found to improve patency better in forearm grafts than in upper arm grafts with secondary patency rates of 30.7% for uAVG and 19.7% for fAVG at 12 months. The authors concluded that in cases for which open repair of stenotic anastomoses is prohibited by anatomic location, such as an anastomosis high in the axilla, stenting is a viable alternative.[37]

In a prospective, randomized, multicenter trial examining the efficacy of stent graft placement versus balloon angioplasty in 190 patients, the 6-month patency of the treated area was significantly greater in the stent graft group at 51% than in the balloon angioplasty alone group at 23%. Freedom from intervention within a 6-month period was also significantly improved in the stent graft group at 32% as compared to 16% in the balloon angioplasty group. The authors noted that multiple other modalities for treatment of intimal hyperplasia at the venous anastomosis have been evaluated, but none have been found to be effective over standard balloon angioplasty. They concluded that patency and freedom from repeat intervention are improved when a stent graft is used for endovascular revision of the venous anastomosis of a prosthetic dialysis access when compared to balloon angioplasty.[38]

CONCLUSION

Despite the general consideration of autologous AVF as preferred access, AVGs are an important, and perhaps an underutilized, access type in the care of the patient with ESRD. Early intervention to create AVFs prior to dialysis initiation may result in a native fistula that requires multiple interventions to mature, thus necessitating placement of a dialysis catheter with attendant increased risk of infection and death. Hemodialysis access with the use of an AVG could, in some cases, obviate the need for catheter placement by allowing use within a significantly shorter time frame. The benefit of this type of intervention must be weighed against the loss of that site for autologous fistula creation.

The most common prosthetic material, ePTFE has patency rates similar to other prosthetic materials, though less than a fully mature native fistula. When considering the lack of need for maturation time with an AVG, primary placement in lieu of AVF creation may be indicated in certain cases, including among infirm or elderly populations. In cases of infections, biologic grafts may be used to decrease the risk of repeat infection of the graft, though repeat infection may still occur.

In accordance with published guidelines, the forearm should be the first choice for AVG placement. This allows preservation of the upper arm as a future access site, and may even be a bridge to prepare the upper arm for creation of an autologous AVF in the future. After forearm sites are exhausted, upper arm access may be deemed appropriate. Evidence from published studies does not support the practice of skipping a viable forearm site for a uAVG site. With respect to configuration, in the forearm, loop grafts are often created because the brachial artery is more commonly used as inflow over the radial artery. In the upper arm, straight grafts are more common than the looped alternatives. To date, no evidence exists to support benefit of straight over looped grafts. Of more importance is to create grafts that are based on adequately sized arteries and have good venous outflow. Configuration and placement should maximize the surface area for cannulation during hemodialysis.'

REFERENCES

1. KDOQI guidelines 2006 updates. https://www.kidney.org/professionals/guidelines/guidelines_commentaries/vascular-access (accessed 10/22/2017).
2. Fistula First. [cited 2017]. http://fistulafirst.esrdncc.org/ffcl/.
3. Cronenwett JL, Johnston KW. Rutherford's Vascular Surgery. 8th ed. Philadelphia, PA: Saunders/Elsevier; 2014.
4. Saran R, Robinson B, Abbott KC, et al. US Renal Data System 2016 Annual Data Report: Epidemiology of Kidney Disease in the United States. *Am J Kidney Dis*. 2017;69 (3 supp 1):A4.
5. Leake AE, Yuo TH, Wu T, et al. Arteriovenous grafts are associated with earlier catheter removal and fewer catheter days in the United States Renal Data System population. *J Vasc Surg*. 2015;62(1):123–127.
6. Lok CE. Fistula first initiative: advantages and pitfalls. *Clin J Am Soc Nephrol*. 2007;2(5):1043–1053.
7. Akoh, JA. Prosthetic arteriovenous grafts for hemodialysis. *J Vasc Access*. 2009;10(3):137–147.
8. Woo K, Ulloa J, Allon M, et al. Establishing patient-specific criteria for selecting the optimal upper extremity vascular access procedure. *J Vasc Surg*. 2017;65(4):1089–1103 e1.
9. Hung YN, Ko PJ, Ng YY, Wu SC. The longevity of arteriovenous graft for hemodialysis patients–externally supported or nonsupported. *Clin J Am Soc Nephrol*. 2010;5(6):1029–1035.
10. Dammers R, Planken RN, Pouls KP, et al. Evaluation of 4-mm to 7-mm versus 6-mm prosthetic brachial-antecubital forearm loop access for hemodialysis: results of a randomized multicenter clinical trial. *J Vasc Surg*. 2003;37(1):143–148.

11. Garcia-Pajares R, Polo JR, Flores A, Gonzalez-Tabares E, Solís JV. Upper arm polytetrafluoroethylene grafts for dialysis access. Analysis of two different graft sizes: 6 mm and 6-8 mm. *Vasc Endovasc Surg*. 2003;37(5):335–343.
12. Polo JR, Ligero JM, Diaz-Cartelle J, Garcia-Pajares R, Cervera T, Reparaz L. Randomized comparison of 6-mm straight grafts versus 6- to 8-mm tapered grafts for brachial-axillary dialysis access. *J Vasc Surg*. 2004;40(2):319–324.
13. Davidson I, Hackerman C, Kapadia A, Minhajuddib A. Heparin bonded hemodialysis e-PTFE grafts result in 20% clot free survival benefit. *J Vasc Access*. 2009;10(3):153–156.
14. Shemesh D, Goldin I, Hijazi J, et al. A prospective randomized study of heparin-bonded graft (Propaten) versus standard graft in prosthetic arteriovenous access. *J Vasc Surg*. 2015;62(1):115–122.
15. Davies MG, Anaya-Ayala JE, El-Sayed HF. Equivalent outcomes with standard and heparin-bonded expanded polytetrafluoroethylene grafts used as conduits for hemodialysis access. *J Vasc Surg*. 2016;64(3):715–718.
16. Glickman MH, Burgess J, Cull D, Roy-Chaudhury P, Schanzer H. Prospective multicenter study with a 1-year analysis of a new vascular graft used for early cannulation in patients undergoing hemodialysis. *J Vasc Surg*. 2015;62(2):434–441.
17. Aitken E, Thomson P, Bainbridge L, Kasthuri R, Mohr B, Kingsmore D. A randomized controlled trial and cost-effectiveness analysis of early cannulation arteriovenous grafts versus tunneled central venous catheters in patients requiring urgent vascular access for hemodialysis. *J Vasc Surg*. 2017;65(3):766–774.
18. Harlander-Locke M, Jimenez JC, Lawrence PF, et al. Bovine carotid artery (Artegraft) as a hemodialysis access conduit in patients who are poor candidates for native arteriovenous fistulae. *Vasc Endovasc Surg*. 2014;48(7-8):497–502.
19. Pineda DM, Dougherty MJ, Wismer MC, et al. Bovine carotid artery xenografts for hemodialysis access. *J Vasc Surg*. 2017;65(6):1729–1734.
20. Arhuidese I, Reifsnyder T, Islam T, et al. Bovine carotid artery biologic graft outperforms expanded polytetrafluoroethylene for hemodialysis access. *J Vasc Surg*, 2017;65(3):775–782.
21. Matsuura JH, Johansen KH, Rosenthal D, Clark MD, Clarke KA, Kirby LB. Cryopreserved femoral vein grafts for difficult hemodialysis access. *Ann Vasc Surg*. 2000;14(1):50–55.
22. Bolton WD, Cull DL, Taylor SM, et al. The use of cryopreserved femoral vein grafts for hemodialysis access in patients at high risk for infection: a word of caution. *J Vasc Surg*. 2002;36(3):464–468.
23. Benedetto F, Carella G, Lentini S, et al. Use of bovine mesenteric vein in rescue vascular access surgery. *J Vasc Access*. 2010;11(2):112–114.
24. Katzman HE, Glickman MH, Schild AF, Fujitani RM, Lawson JH. Multicenter evaluation of the bovine mesenteric vein bioprostheses for hemodialysis access in patients with an earlier failed prosthetic graft. *J Am Coll Surg*. 2005;201(2):223–230.
25. Sequeira A, Naljayan M, Vachharajani TJ. Vascular access guidelines: summary, rationale, and controversies. *Tech Vasc Interv Radiol*. 2017;20(1):2–8.
26. Skandalos I, Chatzibaloglou A, Tsalis K, et al. Prosthetic graft placement using the deep forearm veins in hemodialysis patients: a preliminary report. *Nephron*. 2000;85(4):346–347.
27. Rooijens PP, Burgmans JP, Yo TI, et al. Autogenous radial-cephalic or prosthetic brachial-antecubital forearm loop AVF in patients with compromised vessels? A randomized, multicenter study of the patency of primary hemodialysis access. *J Vasc Surg*. 2005;42(3):481–486; discussions 487.
28. Suemitsu K, Iida O, Shiraki T, et al. Predicting loss of patency after forearm loop arteriovenous graft. *J Vasc Surg*. 2016;64(2):395–401.
29. Oliver MJ, McCann RL, Indridason OS, Butterly DW, Schwab SJ. Comparison of transposed brachiobasilic fistulas to upper arm grafts and brachiocephalic fistulas. *Kidney Int*. 2001;60(4):1532–1539.
30. Jean-Baptiste E, Hassen-Khodja R, Haudebourg P, Declemy S, Batt M, Bouillanne PJ. Axillary loop grafts for hemodialysis access: midterm results from a single-center study. *J Vasc Surg*. 2008;47(1):138–143.

31. Woo K, Doros G, Ng T, Farber A. Comparison of the efficacy of upper arm transposed arteriovenous fistulae and upper arm prosthetic grafts. *J Vasc Surg*. 2009;50(6):1405-1411 e1–2.
32. Dixon BS, Beck GJ, Vazquez MA, et al. Effect of dipyridamole plus aspirin on hemodialysis graft patency. *N Engl J Med*. 2009;360(21):2191–2201.
33. Farber A, Tan TW, Hu B, et al. The effect of location and configuration on forearm and upper arm hemodialysis arteriovenous grafts. *J Vasc Surg*. 2015;62(5):1258–1264.
34. Huber TS, Carter JW, Carter RL, Seeger JM. Patency of autogenous and polytetrafluoroethylene upper extremity arteriovenous hemodialysis accesses: a systematic review. *J Vasc Surg*. 2003;38(5):1005–1011.
35. Lee T, Barker J, Allon M. Comparison of survival of upper arm arteriovenous fistulas and grafts after failed forearm fistula. *J Am Soc Nephrol*. 2007;18(6):1936–1941.
36. Weale AR, Bevis P, Neary WD, Lear PA, Mitchell DC. A comparison between transposed brachiobasilic arteriovenous fistulas and prosthetic brachioaxillary access grafts for vascular access for hemodialysis. *J Vasc Surg*. 2007;46(5):997–1004.
37. Kolakowski S Jr, Dougherty MJ, Calligaro KD. Salvaging prosthetic dialysis fistulas with stents: forearm versus upper arm grafts. *J Vasc Surg*, 2003;38(4):719–723.
38. Haskal ZJ, Trerotola S, Dolmatch B, et al. Stent graft versus balloon angioplasty for failing dialysis-access grafts. *N Engl J Med*. 2010;362(6):494–503.

8

Advances in the Biology of Prosthetic Graft for Dialysis Access

Mark G. Davies, MD, PhD, MBA

INTRODUCTION

In the United States, approximately 300,000 patients currently undergo long-term hemodialysis (HD) for end-stage renal disease annually (ESRD).[1] Functional vascular access is vital for efficient dialysis therapy but an estimated 25% of all patients starting hemodialysis will die because of inadequate vascular access or complications related to vascular access.[2] Recent trends in hemodialysis include an increase in elderly patients requiring dialysis, prevalence of clinically significant obesity, prevalence of diabetes mellitus, increasing proportion of long-term dialysis patients and use of high-efficiency dialysis. This changing demography of the dialysis population has led to an increase in the proportion of patients requiring more complex vascular access modalities for long-term hemodialysis.[3–5]

The national guidelines recommend initiation of access with autogenous arteriovenous (AV) fistulae because of their durability and their resistance to infection.[1] However, the choice of dialysis access should be individualized and based on which the patient will be provide lifetime maximal utilization. While guidelines, such as Kidney Disease Outcomes Quality Initiative (KDOQI), have succeeded in increasing the use of native AV fistulas (AVF), many hemodialysis patients in the United States continue to be dialyzed through AV grafts. (AVG).[6] Some patients have no autogenous options at initial presentation and need an AV graft. Over time, AV fistulae fail to mature, AV fistulae occlude and patients run out of autogenous alternatives. These patients need AV grafts because an AV graft is a better alternative than a tunneled central venous catheter. The most commonly used synthetic graft is Polytetrafluoroethylene (PTFE), a fluorocarbon polymer.[7] Stretch expanded PTFE (ePTFE) is preferable to standard ePTFE. Current data supports PTFE over other biologic and synthetic materials based on a lower risk of disintegration with infection, low thrombogenicity, low tissue reactivity, prolonged patency and improved surgical handling.[7] K-DOQI [1] recommends that the primary failure rate (failure within 30 days or before use for dialysis) should not be more than 15% for forearm straight grafts, 10% for forearm loop grafts, and 5% for upper arm grafts (90). Primary failure of dialysis AV graft is often caused by technical problems influenced by surgical access construction, patient demographics, comorbidity, and graft loss due to premature cannulation and hematoma formation.

The use of prosthetic material as an AV graft carries both distinct advantages and notable drawbacks. The advantages of AV grafts are short lag-time from insertion to maturation (early cannulation: 24–72 h), a large surface area available for cannulation, technically ease of cannulation, multiple insertion sites available, ability to create a variety of shapes and configurations at each insertion site, technical ease of placement for the surgeon and a belief that thrombosed AV grafts have longer patency rates after revision than do revised AV fistulas.[8] In a meta-analysis of AV fistulae compared to AV grafts, Huber et al. found 34 studies that satisfied the inclusion criteria were composed predominantly of case series or nonrandomized controlled studies; no randomized, controlled studies comparing autogenous and PTFE accesses were identified. The primary patency rate for autogenous accesses and PTFE grafts was 51% (95% CI, 48%–53%) and 33% (95% CI, 31%–36%), respectively at 18 months. The secondary patency rates were 77% (95% CI, 74%–79%) and 55% (95% CI, 51%–59%), at 18 months, for autogenous accesses and PTFE grafts, respectively. The authors concluded that the patency rate for autogenous upper extremity AV hemodialysis accesses in adults is superior to that for PTFE counterparts.[9] There is no significant difference in AV graft patency between upper arm, lower arm, and thigh sites.[8] The drawback of AV grafts include higher rates of infection and the increased rate of intervention.[10] The infection rate is reported to be 10-fold higher in AV grafts compared to AV fistulae and the presence of infection is associated with a significant decrease in long-term patency. However, while thrombosis of AV grafts is common (25%of AV grafts compared to 9% of AV fistulas), salvage of a thrombosed grafts is superior to an AV fistula. Although grafts have a higher incidence of thrombosis, postrevision grafts have a significantly longer patency than do revised fistulas.

PATHOPHYSIOLOGY

A newly placed PTFE AV graft requires a period of wound healing and incorporation of fibrous tissue before use. This period is generally 2–4 weeks. Flow increases to a maximum in a few weeks. The absolute flow is limited by the diameter of the graft at its distal anastomosis or by the size of the draining vein. Stenosis predominantly occurs in the draining vein and results in a reciprocal drop in flow through the access. Serial measurements of intra-access pressure or flow can provide an indication of the development of venous stenosis. AV grafts begin to thrombose at flow rates less than 600 mL/min—well above the level required for adequate dialysis (300 mL/min).[11] In a prospective randomized comparison of two grafts of different diameter—6 mm straight versus 8 mm tapered to 6 mm—at the arterial site, placed in the upper limb for HD, Polo et al. [12] demonstrated superior patency and lower complication rates with the larger diameter graft. Their results showed that the larger diameter graft produced a higher access flow rate (1397 vs. 975 mL/min) and better primary and secondary patency rates.

The high failure rate of PTFE dialysis grafts is ascribed to problems in the venous distal outflow tract. The majority of stenoses occur at the venous anastomoses and within 1 cm of the anastomosis.[13] A greater initial mismatch in elastic properties between the vein and the graft and elevated local peak systolic velocity at the venous PTFE anastomoses correlate with the occurrence of anastomotic stenosis within the first two years.[14,15] Graft geometry will also have a significant impact on internal hemodynamics and the development of venous intimal hyperplasia. The volume of the vibration signal set up by blood flowing through the relatively rigid PTFE graft has a better correlation with venous anastomotic intimal-medial thickness than either pressure or flow velocity.[16] An end-to-end or end-to-side anastomosis has no impact on the intimal hyperplastic response in the recipient vein as flow stability, turbulence, and kinetic energy transfer are equivalent.[16] Venous anastomotic intimal hyperplasia develops in unbanded grafts where flow is 100% greater than a banded equivalent and there is a direct correlation between the Reynolds number and subsequent intimal hyperplasia development in the outflow vein.[17] There is no good predictor of the time for first prosthetic graft failure, however, time on dialysis prior to graft placement does correlate well with early graft failure.[18] There is no correlation between raised fibrinogen levels and fistula failure.[19]

AV grafts experience a luminal response and a perigraft response. Perigraft tissue infiltration and tissue encapsulation occurs mainly in the external region of the prosthetic graft and increases with duration of implantation. Fibrous tissue penetrates the wall and partitions off the outer layer. The presence of external reinforcement does not effect this tissue infiltration.[20] On the luminal surface, studies of retrieved human PTFE grafts have shown that between 5 and 24 days after implantation, red blood cells and fibrin cover the anastomotic lines and some of the luminal surface while the remainder remains bare. Macrophages can be found scattered throughout these early thrombi on the surface. Between 11 and 48 months, a single layer of endothelial cells or a thin layer of fibrin covering the anastomotic segments is found. At this time, vascular smooth muscle cells and collagen are identified at the anastomoses as intimal hyperplasia develops. Samples from 94 to 149 months after implantation show that the anastomotic intimal hyperplasia is relatively unchanged with the same thickness and length as that seen in grafts retrieved between 11 to 36 months. Evidence of chronic inflammation can be seen with macrophages, lymphocytes, monocytes, and giant cells identifiable along the incorporated ePTFE grafts.[21] Luminal surfaces of graft explanted between 94 to 149 months are covered by a connective tissue matrix with superposed scattered thrombi.[22] No current evidence exists that prosthetic grafts inserted into the human circulation are able to fully develop an endothelialized intima along the entire flow surface.[20] Rather, endothelial cells manage to populate the luminal surface in just the few centimeters near the anastomoses. The remainder of the graft is usually covered with a thin irregular layer of organized fibrin, containing platelets and leukocytes, interspersed with areas of exposed PTFE.[20,23]

Formation of the neo-endothelium in a PTFE graft can occur through two processes, transmural endothelialization by capillary ingrowth and endothelialization by migration from the anastomoses. Capillary ingrowth through the graft wall depends upon the porosity of the graft. In low-porosity grafts (10 and 30 μm internodal distance), luminal endothelial coverage is limited to small areas near the anastomoses.[24] In higher porosity grafts (60 and 90 μm internodal distance), luminal endothelial coverage is complete.[25,26] A second process whereby endothelialization of PTFE grafts occurs is ingrowth from the anastomoses. Transmural fibrocapillary incorporation of PTFE vascular grafts provides a key supporting structure essential to the progression and attachment of endothelial cell ingrowth from the anastomoses. Porosity of the graft is important as nonporous grafts have a ragged and friable endothelial advancement zone.[27] New experimental evidence also supports fallout endothelialization from the blood stream as a third possible mode of graft healing.[28] The process of neoendothelial healing can be divided into six stages: platelet aggregation phase (Stage I), fibrin network phase (Stage II), bridging phase (Stage III), progression phase (Stage IV-A), transmural migration phase (Stage IV-B in thin wall-long fibril length) intimal closure phase (Stage V), endothelial thromboresistance phase (Stage VI).[29] In the ovine model, mural thrombosis is a prominent feature extending several centimeters from the venous anastomosis for up to three months after PTFE fistula placement. Over this three-month period, the thrombus is actively organized by invasion of macrophages and capillaries from adjacent areas of neointima and in places becomes covered by endothelial cells.[30] In experimental grafts, vascular smooth muscle cells accompany the capillary endothelium into the graft lumen, exhibit vascular smooth muscle cell immunostaining, and proliferate under the luminal endothelium to form an intima.[31] At the anastomoses, vascular endothelial and vascular smooth muscle cells derived from the incised ends of the adjacent artery appear to form the intima and migrate together along the luminal surface of the graft at approximately 0.2 mm/day. Both cell types proliferate in association with the growing edge.[31] Despite completion of the endothelial coverage, the vascular endothelial and smooth muscle cells located over the anastomoses continue to proliferate and intimal cross-sectional areas in these regions are always greater than within the adjacent graft. Increased vascular endothelial cell growth factor (VEGF) expression is detected at the venous anastomosis of PTFE grafts.[32] The neointima of a prosthetic graft is composed of a greater extracellular matrix component than an equivalent arterial lesion.[33] Although fibroblasts are invariably found in the graft matrix and in the adventitia, they do not appear to contribute to the formation of neointima.[31] Studies have demonstrated flow-dependent formation of mature neointimal hyperplasia in PTFE grafts.[34,35] Grafts under high-flow conditions (created by placement of a distal fistula) form smaller intimal layers than those that heal under normal flow.[35] If normal flow is returned to an ePTFE graft previously allowed to heal during high-flow conditions, the neointima undergoes accelerated thickening within 28 days with a striking increase in proteoglycan deposition.[34,36,37] Conversely, creation of a high-flow environment in an ePTFE graft that healed under normal flow conditions will induce regression of the neointimal layer.[38]

In an attempt to reduce the development of neointimal hyperplasia in ePTFE grafts, seeding of endothelial cells onto the PTFE has received considerable attention. Initial clinical reports on seeding microvascular cells onto the PTFE used for peripheral bypass surgery have met with promising results. Endothelial cells seeded onto the PTFE surface in vitro retain the ability to inhibit thrombin coagulant activity.[39] In vitro ePTFE impregnated with fibrin glue containing FGF-1 and heparin retain more seeded endothelial cells than fibrin glue with fibronectin.[40,41]

There is insufficient evidence to determine if pharmacological therapy with aspirin, fish oil, ticlopidine, clopidogrel, PRT-201, dipyridamole, dipyridamole plus aspirin, warfarin will improve AV graft patency compared to untreated AV grafts.

BIOLOGY OF HEPARIN

The choice of heparin as a surface modulator in ePTFE grafts is based on its vascular biology. Heparin is a linear, polydisperse polysaccharide consisting of repeating units of 134-linked pyranosyluronic acid and 2-amino- 2-deoxyglucopyranose (glucosamine) residues.[42] Heparin binds to the enzyme inhibitor antithrombin III, causing a conformational change that results in its activation through an increase in the flexibility of its reactive site loop.[43] The activated antithrombin III then inactivates thrombin, factor Xa, and other proteases. The rate of inactivation of these proteases by antithrombin III can increase by up to 1000-fold due to the binding of Heparin.[44] Heparin binds to antithrombin III via a specific pentasaccharide sulfation sequence contained within the heparin polymer: GlcNAc/NS(6S)-GlcA-GlcNS(3S,6S)-IdoA(2S)-GlcNS(6S). The conformational change in antithrombin III on heparin binding mediates its inhibition of factor Xa. For thrombin inhibition, however, thrombin must also bind to the heparin polymer at a site proximal to the pentasaccharide. The highly negative charge density of heparin contributes to its very strong electrostatic interaction with thrombin. The formation of a ternary complex between antithrombin III, thrombin, and heparin results in the inactivation of thrombin. For this reason, heparin's activity against thrombin is size-dependent, with the ternary complex requiring at least 18 saccharide units for efficient formation.[45] In contrast, antifactor Xa activity requires only the pentasaccharide-binding site of the heparin molecule. Heparin has a potent antiproliferative effect on vascular smooth muscle cells, and this effect is independent of its anticoagulant activity.[46,47] Its inhibitory effect on vascular smooth muscle cells is mediated in part through interactions with cell receptors, growth factors, adhesion molecules, and proteinase inhibitors. Smooth muscle cells possess specific high-affinity receptors for heparin/heparan sulfates. Heparin also decreases thrombospondin synthesis and the decreased concentrations of thrombospondin results in decreased DNA synthesis.[48] This may be due to the fact that thrombospondin and epidermal growth factor act synergistically to stimulate DNA synthesis. In addition, heparin decreases the number of epidermal growth factor receptors on smooth muscle cells thus decreasing the ability of the cells to respond to growth stimulation. Heparin decreases the affinity of basic Fibroblast Growth Factor (FGF) binding to FGF receptors but increases the ability of acidic FGF to stimulate endothelial cell proliferation by 100-fold.[49,50] Heparan sulfates derived from postconfluent endothelial cells and smooth muscle cells inhibit the migration and proliferation of vascular smooth muscle cells and this inhibitory activity is highly dependent on the presence of heparanases, which can generate heparan sulfate fragments that in turn act as growth inhibitors.[51–54]

Heparin-bonded ePTFE graft

In an effort to counter the high failure rates of AV grafts, several modified prosthetic grafts have been introduced into the clinical arena with limited successes.[55] ePTFE remains the most widely used graft for hemodialysis access and thus the most appropriate graft material to modify. Experimental studies have shown that heparin-coating of ePTFE grafts results in reduced platelet deposition compared with noncoated standard ePTFE grafts.[56,57] Similar thromboresistant benefits of heparin surface coating in reducing platelet activation and deposition have been demonstrated in various clinical devices, including hemodialysis filters and intravascular stents, and cardiopulmonary bypass circuitry.[58–60] The rationale for the use of heparin bonding was that it would reduce thrombotic risk in both early and late stages and modulate intimal hyperplasia at the graft-vessel interface, thus providing resistance to thrombosis and stenosis and thereby prolonging patency.[55, 61] Utilizing the Carmeda BioActive Surface (CBAS), the most clinically effective hemocompatible heparin sulfate surface, the bonded surface actively reduces thrombus formation.[62,63] This heparin binding technology is based upon covalent endpoint attachment of heparin to a biomaterial surface, enabling maintenance of functional heparin bioactivity. CBAS-ePTFE grafts have uniform heparinization and sustained in vivo heparin bioactivity. Reduced platelet deposition is correlated with heparin activity as low as 7 pmol/cm^2 and under sustained exposure to blood constituents, heparin activities persisted in vivo for three months at levels between 15 and 25 pmol/cm^2, which is well above the activity needed to reduce platelet deposition. A HB-ePTFE graft (CBAS-ePTFE, Propaten©, WL Gore, Flagstaff, AZ) was introduced in 1996 and made commercially available in 2007 as a hemodialysis conduit.

Clinical Outcomes of HB-ePTFE Graft

Nine reports on the outcomes of standard and HB-ePTFE AV grafts have been published. Eight of nine are retrospective studies and one is a prospective study (Table 8-1). Davidson et al. reported a retrospective analysis of 83 grafts and showed that HB-PTFE grafts had significantly improved 6- and 12-month "clot-free survival" when compared to S-PTFE grafts.[64] Charlton-Ouw et al. compared brachiocephalic AVF to both HB-AV grafts and standard brachio-axillary AV grafts.[65] In their study, heparin bonding was associated with a loss of primary (HR: 2.69), assisted primary (HR: 3.8), and secondary patency (HR: 4.1) on multivariable Cox regression analysis. Allemang et al., Cox et al., Belczak et al., and Zea et al. demonstrated that HB-AV grafts failed to improve patency or decrease secondary interventions when compared to standard AV grafts.[66–69] Most recently, in a prospective randomized study to compare the patency of standard AV grafts with HB-AV grafts, Schemesh et al. demonstrated no significant difference in patency of standard ePTFE AV grafts or a HB-AV grafts.[70] Schemesh et al. did note that the HB-AV grafts had a significantly less thrombosis in first 5 months after implantation compared to the standard ePTFE graft.[70] Davies et al. demonstrated that the two-year primary, assisted primary, and secondary patency rates were 20 ± 7% versus 18 ± 8% (P = 0.85), 35 ± 8% versus 28 ± 7%(P = 0.51), and 38 ± 6% versus 36 ± 7%(P = 0.83) for HB-AV grafts versus standard AV grafts, respectively.[71] The number of secondary interventions was similar in the both groups with 2.1 and 1.9 interventions per person-year of follow-up for HB-AV grafts versus standard AV grafts, respectively (P = 0.87). There were no significant differences in pseudo aneurysm formation (5% vs. 6%; P = 1.00) or in infection (11% vs. 12%, P = 1.00) between HB-AV and standard AV grafts. Functional dialysis durations in this study were equivalent between HB-AV grafts and standard AV grafts.[71]

From the literature, the cost of HB-PTFE grafts has been reported to 18% more than that of S-PTFE grafts.[65] One study estimated that the difference was $650 for equivalent graft lengths and in their hands if no heparin grafts were used over period of their study, the total institutional cost savings would translate to $39,404 in 2013 dollars (approximately $938 per month).[66] Our institutional costs reflect a similar difference in the two materials. Two recent literature reviews and meta-analyses have

TABLE 8-1. OUTCOMES OF STANDARD AND HEPARIN-BONDED EPTFE AV GRAFTS

			Standard		Heparin-Bonded (HB)		
Authors	Year	Number	1 year Primary Patency	1 year Secondary Patency	1 year Primary Patency	1 year Secondary Patency	Result
Davidson et al.[64]	2008	150	–	58%	–	78%	HB Superior
Thermann et al.[72]	2010	40	–	75%	–	75%	Equivalence
Charlton-Ouw et al.[65]	2011	138	67%	–	44%	–	Equivalence
Cox et al.[67]	2014	93	23%	49%	25%	42%	Equivalence
Allemang et al.[66]	2014	223	37%	75%	29%	70%	Equivalence
Belczak et al.[68]	2015	45	–	68%	–	80%	HB Superior
Shemesh et al.[70]	2015	160	12%	81%	14%	82%	Equivalence
Zea et al.[69]	2016	301	30%	90%	40%	90%	Equivalence
Davies et al.[71]	2016	483	35%	66%	54%	70%	Equivalence

determined that based on the current data, HB-AV grafts offer no distinct advantage over standard AV grafts and their preferential use in access surgery cannot be recommended based on the available evidence.[73,74]

CONCLUSION

As the dialysis access population increases and survival of those on dialysis lengthens, the need for an alternative to autogenous access will increase. ePTFE grafts remain the most common alternative but suffer from lower patency rates and increased maintenance. Modulation of the surface of these grafts represents an attractive proposition and the introduction of HB-ePTFE was intended to enhance the longevity of ePTFE AV grafts. Based on the available data, HB-AV grafts offer no distinct advantage over standard AV grafts. While modulating the surface of the grafts alters the biology of the graft surface, it does not address the biology of the outflow tracts, which remain the Achilles heel for the longitudinal success of AV grafts.

REFERENCES

1. KDOQI. KDOQI clinical practice guidelines and clinical practice recommendations for diabetes and chronic kidney disease. *Am J Kidney Dis*. 2007;49(suppl 2):S12–S154.
2. Foley RN, Collins AJ. End-stage renal disease in the United States: an update from the United States Renal Data System. *J Am Soc Nephrol*. 2007;18(10):2644–2648.

3. Enzler M, Rajmon T, Lachat M, Largiader F. Long-term function of vascular access for hemodialysis. *Clin Transplant*. 1996;10(6 pt 1):511–515.
4. Gibson KD, Caps MT, Kohler TR, et al. Assessment of a policy to reduce placement of prosthetic hemodialysis access. *Kidney Int*. 2001;59(6):2335–2345.
5. Collins AJ, Hanson G, Umen A, Kjellstrand C, Keshaviah P. Changing risk factor demographics in end-stage renal disease patients entering hemodialysis and the impact on long-term mortality. *Am J Kidney Dis*. 1990;15(5):422–432.
6. Navuluri R, Regalado S. The KDOQI 2006 vascular access update and fistula first program synopsis. *Sem Intervent Radiol*. 2009;26(2):122–124.
7. Rodriguez A, Shalhub S. Hemodialysis access: fundamentals and advanced management. In: Shalhub S, Dua A, Shin S, eds. *Hemodialysis Access*. Cham: Springer; 2017:281–288.
8. Schild AF, Perez E, Gillaspie E, Seaver C, Livingstone J, Thibonnier A. Arteriovenous fistulae vs. arteriovenous grafts: a retrospective review of 1,700 consecutive vascular access cases. *J Vasc Access*. 2007;9(4):231–235.
9. Huber TS, Carter JW, Carter RL, Seeger JM. Patency of autogenous and polytetrafluoroethylene upper extremity arteriovenous hemodialysis accesses: a systematic review. *J Vasc Surg*. 2003;38(5):1005–1011.
10. Akoh JA. Prosthetic arteriovenous grafts for hemodialysis. *J Vasc Access*. 2009;10(3):137–147.
11. Sullivan KL, Eschelman DJ, eds. Hemodynamics of failing dialysis grafts. *Seminars in Interventional Radiology*. Copyright© 1997 by Thieme Medical Publishers; 1997;14(1):5–13.
12. Polo JR, Ligero JM, Diaz-Cartelle J, Garcia-Pajares R, Cervera T, Reparaz L. Randomized comparison of 6-mm straight grafts versus 6-to 8-mm tapered grafts for brachial-axillary dialysis access. *J Vasc Surg*. 2004;40(2):319–324.
13. Kanterman RY, Vesely TM, Pilgram TR, Guy BW, Windus DW, Picus D. Dialysis access grafts: anatomic location of venous stenosis and results of angioplasty. *Radiology*. 1995;195:135–139.
14. Hofstra L, Bergmans DC, Leunissen KM, Hoeks AP, Kitslaar PJ, Tordoir JH. Prosthetic arteriovenous fistula and venous anastomotic stenosis: influence of a hoigh velocity on development of intimal hyperplasia. *Blood Purif*. 1996;14:345–349.
15. Hofstra L, Bergmans DC, Leunissen KM, et al. Anastomotic intimal hyperplasia in prosthetic arteriovenous fistulas for hemodialysis is associated with initial high flow velocity and not with mismatch in elastic properties. *J Am Soc Nephrol*. 1995;6:1625–1633.
16. Fillinger MF, Reinitz ER, Schwartz RA, et al. Graft geometry and venous intimal-medial hyperplasia in arteriovenous loop grafts. *J Vasc Surg*. 1990;11:556–566.
17. Fillinger MF, Reinitz ER, Schwartz RA, et al. Beneficial effects of banding on venous intimal-medial hyperplasia in arteriovenous loop grafts. *Am J Surg*. 1989;158:87–94.
18. Taber TE, Maikranz PS, Haag BW, et al. Maintanence of adequate hemodialysis access prevention of neointimal hyperplasia. *ASAIO J*. 1995;41:842–846.
19. Louridas C, Botha JR, Levien L, Milno FJ, Meyers AM, Myburgh JA. Vascular access for hemodialysis experience at Johannesburg Hospital. *S Afr Med J*. 1984;66:637–640.
20. Guidoin R, Chakf'e N, Maurel S, et al. ePTFE arterial prostheses in humans: histopathological study of 298 surgically excised grafts. *Biomaterials*. 1993;14:678–693.
21. Olofason P, Rabahie GN, Matsumoto K, et al. Histopathological characterization of explanted human prosthetic arterial grafts: implications for the prevention and management of graft infection. *Eur J Vasc Endovasc*. 1995;9:143–151.
22. Swedberg SH, Brown BC, Sigley R, Wight TN, Gordon D, Nicholls SC. Intimal fibromuscular hyperplasia at the venous anstomosis of PTFE grafts in hemodialysis patients clinical immunocytochemical light and electron microscopic assessment. *Circulation*. 1989;80:1726–1736.
23. Cho JS, Ouriel K, DeWeese JA, Green RM, Chen GY, Stoughton J. Thrombus formation on PTFE surfaces: The importance of vWF. *Cardiovasc Surg*. 1995;3:645–691.
24. Golden MA, Hanson SR, Kirkman TR, Schneider PA, Clowes AW. Healing of polytetrafluoroethylene arterial grafts is influenced by graft porosity. *J Vasc Surg*. 1990;11:838–844.

25. Golden MA, Au YPT, Kenagy RD, Clowes AW. Growth factor gene expression by intimal cells in healing polytetrafluoroethylene grafts. *J Vasc Surg*. 1990;11:580–585.
26. Reidy M, Chao S, Kirkman. T.R., Clowes AW. Endothelial regeneration VI: chronic nondenuding injury in baboon vascular grafts. *Am J Pathol*. 1986;123:432–439.
27. Tsuchida H, Wilson SE, Ishimaru S. Healing mechanisms of high porosity PTFE grafts significance of transmural structure. *J Surg Res*. 1997;71:187–195.
28. Shi Q, Hong-De Wu M, Hayashida N, et al. Proof of fallout endothelialization of impervious Dacron grafts in the aorta and inferior vena cava of the dog. *J Vasc Surg*. 1994;20:546–556.
29. Lanzetta M, Owen ER. Neoendothelialisation of PTFE microvascular grafts: a five year experience. *Microsurgery*. 1995;16:404–411.
30. Kohler TR, Ferguson MS, Kirkman TR. Thrombosis contributes to intimal hyperplasia in a sheep model of dialysis access fistula. *J Vasc Res*. 1996;33(suppl 1):51 (abstract).
31. Clowes AW, Kirkman TR, Reidy MA. Mechanisms of arterial graft healing. Rapid transmural capillary ingrowth provides a source of intimal endothelium and smooth muscle in porous PTFE prostheses. *Am J Pathol*. 1986;123:220–230.
32. Cordero JA, Quist M, LoGerfo FW. VEGF expression in healing PTFE vascular grafts. *J Vasc Res*. 1996;33(suppl 1):44 (abstract).
33. Mesh CL, Majors A, Mistele D, Graham LM, Ehrhart LA. Graft smooth muscle cells specifically synthesize increased collagen. *J Vasc Surg*. 1995;22:142–149.
34. Geary RL, Kohler TR, Vergal S, Kirkman TR, Clowes AW. Time course of flow-induced smooth muscle cell proliferation and intimal thickening in endothelialized baboon vascular grafts. *Circ Res*. 1993;74:14–23.
35. Kohler TR, Kirkman TR, Kraiss LW, Zierler BK, Clowes AW. Increased blood flow inhibits neointimal hyperplasia in endothelialized vascular grafts. *Circ Res*. 1991;69:1557–1565.
36. Kraiss LW, Kirkman TR, Kohler TR, Zierler B, Clowes AW. Shear stress regulates smooth muscle proliferation and neointimal thickening in porous PTFE grafts. *Arterioscler Thromb*. 1991;11:1844–1852.
37. Kraiss LW, Geary RL, Mattsson EJR, Vergel S, Au YPT, Clowes AW. Acute reductions in blood flow and shear stress induce platelet-derived growth factor-A expression in baboon prosthetic grafts. *Circ Res*. 1996;79:45–53.
38. Mattsson EJR, Kohler TR, Vergel SM, Clowes AW. Increased blood flow induces regression of intimal hyperplasia. *Arterioscler Thromb Vasc Biol*. 1997;17:2245–2249.
39. Gillis-Haegerstrand C, Frebelius S, Haegerstrand A, Swedenborg J. Cultured human endothelial cells seeded on ePTFE support thrombin-mediated activation of protein C. *J Vasc Surg*. 1996;24:226–234.
40. Greisler HP, Cziperle DJ, Kim DU, et al. Enhanced endothelialization of ePTFE grafts by FGF-1 pretreatment. *Surgery*. 1992;112:244–254.
41. Gray JL, Kang SS, Zenni GC, et al. FGF-1 affixation stimulates ePTFE endothelialization without intimal hyperplasia. *J Surg Res*. 1994;57:596–612.
42. Muñoz EM, Linhardt RJ. Heparin-binding domains in vascular biology. *Arterioscler Thromb Vasc Biol*. 2004;24(9):1549–1557.
43. Chuang Y-J, Swanson R, Raja SM, Olson ST. Heparin enhances the specificity of antithrombin for thrombin and factor Xa independent of the reactive center loop sequence evidence for an exosite determinant of factor Xa specificity in heparin-activated antithrombin. *J Biol Chem*. 2001;276(18):14961–14971.
44. Björk I, Lindahl U. Mechanism of the anticoagulant action of heparin. *Mol Cell Biochem*. 1982;48(3):161–182.
45. Petitou M, Hérault J-P, Bernat A, et al. Synthesis of thrombin-inhibiting heparin mimetics without side effects. *Nature*. 1999;398(6726):417–422.
46. Guyton JR, Rosenberg RD, Clowes AW, Karnovsky MJ. Inhibition of rat arterial smooth muscle cell proliferation by heparin. In vivo studies with anticoagulant and nonanticoagulant heparin. *Circ Res*. 1980;46(5):625–634.
47. Clowes AW, Karnowsky MJ. Suppression by heparin of smooth muscle cell proliferation in injured arteries. *Nature*. 1977;265(5595):625–626.

48. Majack RA, Coates-Cook S, Bernstein P. Platelet derived growth factor and heparin-like glycosaminoglycans regulate thrombospodin synthesis and deposition in the matrix by smooth muscle cells. *J Cell Biol.* 1985;105:1059–1070.
49. Klagsbrun M, Edelman ER. Biological and biochemical properties of fibroblast growth factors. *Arteriosclerosis.* 1989;9:269–278.
50. Gospodarowicz D, Ferrara N, Schweigerer L, Neufeld G. Structural characterization and biological functions of fibroblast growth factor. *Endocr Rev.* 1987;8:95–114.
51. Clowes AW, Karnovsky MJ. Suppression by heparin of smooth muscle cell proliferation in injured arteries. *Nature.* 1979;265:625–627.
52. Castellot JI, Favreau LV, Karnovsky MJ, Rosenberg RD. Inhibition of vascular smooth muscle cell growth by endothelium cell-derived heparin. *J Biol Chem.* 1982;257:11256–11260.
53. Majack RA, Clowes AW. Inhibition of vascular smooth muscle cell migration by heparin-like glycosaminoglycans. *J Cell Physiol.* 1984;118:253–256.
54. Majesky MW, Schwartz SM, Clowes MM, Clowes AW. Heparin regulates smooth muscle S phase entry in the injured rat carotid artery. *Circ Res.* 1987;61:296–300.
55. Scott EC, Glickman MH. Conduits for hemodialysis access. *Semin Vasc Surg.* 2007;20(3):158–163.
56. Heyligers JM, Verhagen HJ, Rotmans JI, et al. Heparin immobilization reduces thrombogenicity of small-caliber expanded polytetrafluoroethylene grafts. *J Vasc Surg.* 2006;43(3):587–591.
57. Lin PH, Chen C, Bush RL, Yao Q, Lumsden AB, Hanson SR. Small-caliber heparin-coated ePTFE grafts reduce platelet deposition and neointimal hyperplasia in a baboon model. *J Vasc Surg.* 2004;39(6):1322–1328.
58. Tayama E, Hayashida N, Akasu K, et al. Biocompatibility of heparin coated extracorporeal bypass circuits: New heparin bonded bioline system. *Artif Organs.* 2000;24(8):618–623.
59. Dewanjee MK, Palatianos GN, Kapadvanjwala M, et al. Neutrophil dynamics and retention in lung, oxygenator, and arterial filter during cardiopulmonary bypass in a pig model. *ASAIO J.* 1994;40(3):M547–M553.
60. Serruys PW, Emanuelsson H, Van Der Giessen W, et al. Heparin-coated Palmaz-Schatz stents in human coronary arteries. *Circulation.* 1996;93(3):412–422.
61. Clowes AW. Regulation of smooth muscle cell function by heparin. *J Vasc Surg.* 1992;15:911–913.
62. Begovac P, Thomson R, Fisher J, Hughson A, Gällhagen A. Improvements in GORE-TEX® vascular graft performance by Carmeda® bioactive surface heparin immobilization. *Eur J Vasc Endovasc Surg.* 2003;25(5):432–437.
63. Jordan SW, Chaikof EL. Novel thromboresistant materials. *J Vasc Surg.* 2007;45(6): A104–A115.
64. Davidson I, Hackerman C, Kapadia A, Minhajuddib A. Heparin bonded hemodialysis e-PTFE grafts result in 20% clot free survival benefit. *J Vasc Access.* 2008;10(3):153–156.
65. Charlton-Ouw KM, Nosrati N, Miller 3rd C, Coogan SM, Safi HJ, Azizzadeh A. Outcomes of arteriovenous fistulae compared with heparin-bonded and conventional grafts for hemodialysis access. *J Vasc Access.* 2011;13(2):163–167.
66. Allemang MT, Schmotzer B, Wong VL, et al. Heparin bonding does not improve patency of polytetrafluoroethylene arteriovenous grafts. *Ann Vasc Surg.* 2014;28:28–34.
67. Cox SR, Moawad JA, Marshall LA, et al. Patency rates among heparin-bonded and conventional polytetrafluoroethylene grafts for upper extremity hemodialysis access. *J Vasc Access.* 2014;19(3):153–157.
68. Belczak SQ, Abrão SR, Bertoldi V, et al. Alternative grafts for brachioaxillary hemodialysis access: 1-year comparative results. *J Vasc Brasil.* 2015;14(2):133–138.
69. Zea N, Menard G, Le L, et al. Heparin-bonded polytetrafluorethylene does not improve hemodialysis arteriovenous graft function. *Ann Vasc Surg.* 2016;30:28–33.
70. Shemesh D, Goldin I, Hijazi J, et al. A prospective randomized study of heparin-bonded graft (Propaten) versus standard graft in prosthetic arteriovenous access. *J Vasc Surg.* 2015;62:115–122.

71. Davies MG, Anaya-Ayala JE, El-Sayed HF. Equivalent outcomes with standard and heparin-bonded expanded polytetrafluoroethylene grafts used as conduits for hemodialysis access. *J Vasc Surg*. 2016;64(3):715–718.
72. Thermann F, Sollert U, Ukkat J, Dralle H. Rroximalization of the arterial inflow (PAI) in patients with dialysis access-induced ischemic syndrome: first report on long-term clinical results. *J Vasc Access*. 2010;11:143–149.
73. Lazarides M, Argyriou C, Antoniou G, Georgakarakos E, Georgiadis G, eds. Lack of evidence for use of heparin-bonded grafts in access surgery: a meta-analysis. *Semin Vasc Surg*. 2016;24:192–197.
74. Olsha O, Goldin I, Shemesh D. Heparin-bonded expanded polytetrafluorethylene grafts in hemodialysis access. *J Vasc Access*. 2016;17:S79–S84.

9

Bioengineered Vascular Access Grafts

Ehsan Benrashid, MD; David N. Ranney, MD; and Jeffrey H. Lawson MD, PhD

Patients with end-stage renal disease (ESRD), of which the most common form of renal replacement therapy (RRT) is hemodialysis (HD), account for a large proportion of healthcare expenditures. Unfortunately, because of the restricted availability of kidneys for transplantation, many patients spend years on the transplant waiting list, or are simply ineligible for renal transplantation due to advanced age or other exclusion criteria. In the meanwhile, many ESRD patients are maintained on HD, with well-established guidelines stating that, provided adequate anatomy, initial vascular access should be through upper extremity arteriovenous fistula (AVF).[1] This landmark surgical technique, as first described by Drs. Brescia, Cimino, and Appel, revolutionized the care of patients with ESRD.[2] Along with the development of the first true access method/"device" several years prior—the Scribner shunt[3]—these two medico surgical advances were directly responsible for the establishment and rapid advances in the fields of nephrology and vascular access. However, owing to limitations in individual anatomy, prior access procedures, and a host of other factors, placement of AVF is not always a realistic option for patients with ESRD. Hence, other strategies and materials for vascular access have been developed in the past 50 years, such as the tunneled dialysis catheter or arteriovenous graft (AVG).

Unfortunately, these "alternative" or "non-preferential" vascular access options are not without complications—such as thrombosis, central venous stenosis, poor patency when compared to AVF, and infection. As such, numerous attempts have been made, especially in the case of AVG, to create less thrombotic blood-contacting surfaces and materials more resistant to infection. With the advent of the field of bioengineering, along with the rapid development of tissue engineering techniques, alternative *biologic* graft materials to the more conventional *synthetic* polytetrafluoroethylene (PTFE) and expanded PTFE (ePTFE) have been developed. Additionally, it is becoming apparent that these bioprosthetic devices are emerging as potential options for readily available "off the shelf" access.[4] Given the rapidly growing interest in bioengineered vascular grafts (BEVGs) for HD access—with potential extension to other cardiovascular indications—and our institutional experience as one of the first groups in the United States to implant these devices for dialysis access in patients, we set as our objective for this chapter to describe the historical context, development, and potential clinical application of BEVGs.

HISTORICAL CONTEXT OF BEVGs

The historical context and setting for BEVG development and use in the modern era is important to understand, as many prior attempts at creation of vascular conduits concerned the utilization and creation of heterografts or allografts through various modification techniques of pre-existing, or "native," artery or vein. As such, our aim for this section is to briefly discuss the initial tissue engineering attempts for vascular tissue of heterologous origin—or what is oftentimes termed as a "bioprosthetic vascular conduit."[5]

Heterograft Dialysis Access Conduit Development and Utilization

The initial creation of a truly bioengineered blood vessel can be considered as that described by Rosenberg et al. in the 1960s,[6] with enzymatic degradation of what was assumed to be antigenic components ("muscle and elastica") in bovine carotid artery grafts. In their initial experience, implantation of these devices as thoracic or thoracoabdominal aortic replacement in canine models yielded acceptable patency results, with further microscopic examination showing almost complete lining of the graft with a native intimal layer and a relative paucity of inflammatory infiltrate in the vessel layers.[6] Shortly thereafter, enzymatically-treated bovine carotid artery became commercially available for use as vascular conduit as the Artegraft® (Artegraft, North Brunswick, NJ). Importantly, it should be noted that this bioprosthetic device was available several years before the first widely accepted synthetic vascular conduits, in the form of PTFE and ePTFE, were available off the shelf. However, several studies demonstrating limitations of the Artegraft® device, in particular its susceptibility to thrombosis and aneurysm or pseudoaneurysm formation at HD cannulation sites,[7–10] along with the eventual widespread acceptance of improved PTFE-based grafts, resulted in their decreased use.

Many subsequently postulated that aneurysmal degradation of the first iteration of the Artegraft® was largely a result of the proteolytic breakdown process in the manufacturing of these grafts. As a result of these initial studies with bovine heterografts, further interest was spurred in developing a biologic alternative to PTFE and ePTFE. For instance, additional bioprosthetic bovine collagen-based prostheses were developed in the form of the Solcograft-P® (Solco Basle Ltd., Birsfelden-Basle, Switzerland), which demonstrated adequate short-term patency, but had an astonishingly high rate of aneurysm formation over one study period and was hence abandoned.[11] More recent improvements in the manufacturing process have resulted in the most recent iteration of the Artegraft®, which by at least one study appears to be a suitable alternative for dialysis access in patients who are otherwise poor AVF candidates.[5]

Continued modifications to the manufacturing process subsequently yielded the BioPolyMeric® (BPM) graft (St. Jude Medical, Inc., Saint Paul, MN), which was a glutaraldehyde-tanned bovine carotid artery graft initially developed for infrainguinal reconstruction.[12] Reports of the utilization of this device, which was taken off the market prior to this initial publication, are however limited in regard to dialysis access applications, although patency rates when used in infrainguinal reconstruction were comparable to PTFE. A final device adjunct in the realm of bovine heterograft development, a glutaraldehyde-tanned bovine mesenteric vein graft, ProCol® (Hancock Jaffe Laboratories, Inc., Irvine CA), has been shown to demonstrate acceptable patency results in "high risk" or anatomically unfavorable (for AVF) dialysis access patients.[13,14] The authors should note that interestingly enough, given an extremely poor patency rate over the short-term, this product was deemed unacceptable for use in additional vascular surgical applications—such as infrainguinal reconstruction[15]—although ProCol® remains available as a readily available HD access conduit at this date.

ALLOGRAFT DIALYSIS ACCESS CONDUIT DEVELOPMENT AND UTILIZATION

The first true attempts at creation and widespread marketing of a readily available human-based, or allogenic, bioprosthetic graft device was through the efforts of Dardik et al., who described the use of human umbilical veins (derived from umbilical cords) treated with glutaraldehyde.[16] In this study the authors describe the creation of the graft from the chemical and structural modification of it utilizing a polyester fiber mesh, to its implantation as upper and lower extremity AVG conduit in a primate model (baboon). Notably, the authors determined that functionality was maintained in 7/9 upper extremity AVG over a four-month period, with no incidence or propensity toward aneurysm despite weekly needle punctures. Subsequent studies utilizing this so-called, but now defunct, Dardik Biograft® (Meadox Laboratories, Oakland, NJ) as vascular prosthesis in humans demonstrated comparable patency to autogenous saphenous vein in lower extremity arterial reconstruction, with apparently fewer overall infectious complications.[17,18] Notably, access-specific studies utilizing the Dardik Biograft® demonstrated a complication rate (as defined by infection, thrombosis, aneurysm, or steal) of approximately 50%, with the overwhelming majority of these complications due to thrombosis of the bioprosthetic graft.[19] Reinforcing the aforementioned work of Rubio and Farrell demonstrating a particular propensity for graft thrombosis,[19] *in vitro* studies of the Dardik Biograft® demonstrated that the graft, over the short-term (mimicking the peri-implantation period) had a particularly increased propensity toward thrombogenicity as measured by platelet aggregation studies.[20]

An additional readily available human-derived bioprosthetic dialysis access conduit is available in the form of cryopreserved femoral or saphenous vein, in its most recent iteration the CryoVein® (CryoLife, Inc., Kennesaw, GA). Initial studies demonstrated comparable patency of these devices to PTFE in dialysis access, although their placement was associated with a particular propensity for pseudoaneurysm formation, as in the initial Artegraft® studies.[21,22] The very first iteration of this bioprosthetic conduit, the Synergraft® (CryoLife, Inc., Kennesaw, GA), was not, however, supported for HD access applications relative to PTFE (in patients without suitable anatomy for upper extremity AVF). This was due to the fact that the Synergraft® demonstrated, again, a higher propensity for aneurysm formation and an almost two-times higher rate of access failure—30% failure in Synergraft® vs. 15% in PTFE.[23] Additionally, 65% of cryopreserved femoral vein grafts were found to have a major complication in one study, with a concomitant poor primary patency of 28% over 17 months in patients at high risk for access site infection.[24] Several of the very first studies with this first iteration of a readily available human bioprosthetic graft were terminated due to CryoLife's FDA-mandated recall of several vascular prostheses. It should be noted that the Synergraft®, is currently commercially available for cardiac surgical applications, and owing to CryoLife's decellularization process, purports a paucity of induction of the immune response, making it beneficial for patients with potential future requirements for transplantation. As will be discussed, this lack of induction of the immune response is a vital component in the design and implantation of BEVG, as many patients are candidates for renal transplantation.

SELECTION CRITERIA FOR BEVG

As can be demonstrated, BEVGs appear to be best served in patient populations in which the patient does not want to or cannot be subjected to the morbidity of an additional procedure (i.e., concomitant femoral or saphenous vein harvesting), or in patients that have already exhausted this option (i.e., prior saphenous vein harvest). As described above, for the indications of dialysis access, BEVGs appear to be most useful in patients with unsuitable anatomy for AVF, prior failed AVG prostheses, or in access site infection or risk of infection. Prior to the description of the development and utilization of BEVGs, it should be noted that these devices are to be considered clinically feasible only if they meet the following criteria.[4,25,26]

- Maintain a low incidence of infectious complications.
- Do not generate an antigenic response.
- Remain patent to a degree that rivals autogenous tissue as conduit.
- Withstand degradation, but are porous enough to allow for cellular migration and seeding.
- Maintain adequate suture strength and are easily suturable.
- Have the ability to remodel.
- Are responsive to physiologic stimuli.
- Have an anti-thrombotic blood-contacting interface.
- Are durable.
- Are cost-effective.
- Are readily available.

EMERGENCE AND CLINICAL USE OF BEVG

Aside from the aforementioned bioprosthetic devices, true tissue- or bio-engineered vascular grafts were initially brought into the foray by the pioneering work of Weinberg and Bell in 1986,[27] who described the creation of an *in vitro*, multilayered collagen tube from animal collagen and bovine endothelial and smooth muscle cells (SMCs), utilizing a Dacron structural scaffold upon which these cellular constituents were seeded. Subsequently, a completely de-novo human cell–based "vascular tube" was created by L'Heureux et al. in 1993, with omission of any synthetic scaffold incorporated into the graft itself—as the graft was cultured *in vitro* around a glass mandrel.[28] Unfortunately, both of these devices were plagued by poor mechanical strength and were susceptible to degeneration, and due largely to these concerns, clinical trials were not performed.[27,28]

Given the limitations in the strength and durability of these initial BEVG, a series of strategies to modify the structural characteristics have been done in the years since. These modification processes have targeted the timeframe over which the graft is degraded, as well as the strength characteristics of the bio-scaffold material itself, which is utilized as the structural framework from which the hollow vascular tube graft is created. Briefly, examples have included modification of the BEVG culture medium or thickness of the scaffold to stiffen the graft itself, or attempts to line the device with chemical moieties that stimulate extracellular matrix (ECM) production and deposition.[29–32]

Despite modifications to the manufacturing process of BEVG, the idea that the endogenous vascular remodeling process must remain intact has always remained at the forefront of the creation of these vessels. This is of utmost importance as the structural scaffold upon which many of these grafts are created, which are composed of materials that must be degraded over time, such as polyglycolic acid or polyglycerol sebacate, must allow endogenous ECM remodeling to take place for graft incorporation. Other techniques to manipulate the environment under which the graft is synthesized include creating the graft under pulsatile conditions (a "biomimetic" approach – designed to simulate neovessel formation),[33] or utilization of the body as a "bioreactor." In this latter technique, hollow synthetic tubular scaffolds were implanted into body cavities (i.e., peritoneal or pleural cavities) and subsequently seeded *in vivo* with what was later determined to be myofibroblasts, collagen, and mesothelium.[34,35] In essence, this eliminated both a large proportion of the *in vitro* process of BEVG synthesis and, theoretically, any potential future antigenicity should the device be implanted in the organism that served as the initial "bioreactor." Criticisms of the "bioreactor" approach centered over the length of time required for BEVG creation with this technique and potential for antigenicity when used as an allotransplanted, as opposed to the aforementioned autotransplanted graft, and have not been extended to human subjects to this date.

Additional work by the group of Dahl et al. in which BEVG were decellularized after their initial creation set the stage for potential "off-the-shelf" availability of these devices for use in many vascular applications.[36] In principle, the decellularization process allows for what essentially is a hollow ECM-component tube to be stored and subsequently either: 1) seeded with the patient's own endothelium as derived from a small superficial venous biopsy; or 2) implanted into subjects at a later date, with the thought that the remodeling process will result in a structure that eventually forms a three-layered blood vessel. Notably these grafts, despite the detergents utilized in the decellularization process, did not appear to be more susceptible to mechanical stress or aneurysmal degeneration in animal models, unlike prior bioprosthetic iterations.[36] Finally, additional pioneering work in the field of tissue engineering by L'Heureux and colleagues yielded the technique of "sheet-based tissue engineering," in which fibroblasts cultured in conditions promoting ECM deposition form a flat sheet, which can be layered or rolled into a cylindrical tube resembling a blood vessel.[37] Importantly, this technique avoided the utilization of any synthetic compounds (which would need to be subject to degradation) in the formation of the neovessel.

Given the excitement over the potential for these conduits to remodel and function as native vascular tissue, the group of Shinoka et al. performed what can be considered the first reported human implantation of BEVGs, in the form of a pulmonary arterial conduit into a child with single ventricle physiology and pulmonary atresia after a prior failed repair.[38] This was largely based on this group's series of experiments in which they showed the feasibility of congenital cardiac application of these devices by demonstrating both patency and durability of BEVGs when utilized as conduit in pulmonary arterial replacement in an ovine model.[39] It should be noted that the initial BEVG implanted in a human was synthesized much in the same manner as this group's ovine model, instead using the child's autogenous vein constituents as the source of cells subsequently seeded onto a biodegradable scaffold.[38] Utilizing similar BEVG manufacturing techniques, these authors have remarkably gone on to complete implantation of their BEVGs in a cohort of 42 patients, with mid-term results demonstrating acceptable patency and a relatively low rate of reintervention, with no graft loss at this mid-term time point.[40] It should be noted that any BEVG produced as described by this study must be done so in a proactive fashion, as they are seeded with autologous bone marrow constituents, and hence were not necessarily readily available for implantation.

A final technical modification to the synthesis process of BEVGs is in electrospinning, in which application of an electric field guides the formation of polymers around structures that can be crafted to resemble vascular tubes.[41] Recent modifications to the electrospinning process have resulted in the co-spinning of collagen and elastin fibers to the create a three-layered vessel—with an intact and separate intimal, medial, and adventitial layer—more closely mimicking the three-layered nature of blood vessels and hence conferring structural stability to the TEVG.[42] Despite their promise and ease of synthesis, electrospun BEVG have yet to be implanted in clinical trials.

Subsequently, interest in the realm of BEVG application as a conduit was stimulated in the vascular access device market. In part, this is due to the fact that: 1) currently available synthetic graft materials (i.e., PTFE, Dacron, Teflon) are poor options for conduit given poor patency relative to AVF and a higher incidence of infectious complications; and 2) if the BEVG should fail in its dialysis application, most patients with ESRD can be dialyzed through, at a minimum, an indwelling central venous catheter (amongst the other modalities available). This is in opposition to utilization of BEVGs as a conduit in infrainguinal bypass procedures, where the morbidity of graft loss due to thrombosis or other factors may necessitate amputation.

As such, the first application of BEVG technology was reported in the first iteration of the Cytograft® (Cytograft Tissue Engineering, Inc., Novato, CA).[43] This device, which was made utilizing autologous fibroblasts and endothelial cells from each respective patient, was implanted in 10 subjects whom had a history of failed dialysis access. Despite primary patency comparable to conventional synthetic materials over the short term (78% at 1 month, 60% at six months), with 9/10 grafts reported as being successfully cannulated following implantation, 2/9 of these grafts underwent early structural failure, with several device failures and complications thought secondary to the graft eliciting the endogenous immune response.[44] A subsequent foray into the dialysis access market by Cytograft was via the Lifeline® graft, which was created in a more proactive fashion than the Cytograft®, by isolating autologous endothelial cells and fibroblasts from a respective patient and forming the BEVG several months prior to implantation (stored at –80°C).[45] In doing so, Cytograft performed the initial attempts at producing a personalized, "off-the-shelf" conduit for HD access, which could be stored and subsequently implanted at a later time. Later work utilizing the Lifeline® graft, this time with non-self donor cells to construct an "allogenic graft," demonstrated eventual graft failure in 2/3 patients, with the last additional patient succumbing to sepsis prior to determination of any short-term patency results.[46] Despite these poor results, one insight gleaned by the authors of this study was that these allogenic BEVG did not induce a systemic immune response, through examination of human leukocyte antigen (HLA) sensitization, panel reactive antibody values, or cross-reactivity tests.[46] This remains vital to these devices being of potential use in the long-term, as induction of any immune response from antigen present on substrates utilized during graft synthesis or HLA sensitization—both from non-self BEVG constituent donors—could render future renal transplantation at risk.

Further clinical work was then performed through development of the Humacyte Acellular Vessel (HAV; Humacyte, Inc., RTP, NC), which utilizes aortic vascular smooth muscle cells to seed a biodegradable synthetic scaffold, which is then decellularized prior to implantation (hence removing antigenic cells), producing a final acellular graft which can in theory be stored for some time—again, bringing to light the importance of "off the shelf access."[47] In initial animal models, utilization of the HAV as an AVG in baboons, or as conduit for coronary or peripheral bypass in canines, resulted in the majority of conduits patent at 1, 3, and 6 months for the AVG model, and at 1 week, 1 month, and 1 year in the arterial bypass model.[47] Current studies with the HAV are being performed for both HD access and arterial reconstruction indications, with 60 grafts currently implanted in six centers worldwide for HD access, and 20 lower extremity arterial bypass grafts implanted in one center in Europe.[48] Follow-up is ongoing, but a significant number of these grafts implanted for both indications have been functioning for over two years (unpublished data, JHL).

A final clinical application of BEVG, which although extraneous to the realm of dialysis access, we would be remiss to mention was recently described in the work of Olausson et al.[49] These authors describe their utilization of decellularized donor iliac vein subsequently seeded with host stem cells to relieve extrahepatic portal venous obstruction in a child (through interposition grafting), in order to avoid transplantation and lifelong immunosuppression, with an adequate result.

LIMITATIONS, CHALLENGES, AND FUTURE DIRECTIONS OF BEVG

As mentioned, there are several limitations and challenges for BEVG that must be considered, especially when utilized in the realm of HD access. Chief among these is the lack of antigenicity of the compounds and cells utilized in synthesis of both the bio-scaffold and graft itself, as stimulation of the immune response would raise concern for rejection in any subsequent solid organ transplantation. As mentioned in the text, preliminary studies have demonstrated a lack of the immune response to grafts created from allogenic donors,[46] although mid- and long-term immune response data for both the HAV and the Lifeline® graft are incumbent on ongoing clinical trials. Additionally, as previous authors have demonstrated dramatically increased costs with bioprosthetic grafts (five to 10 times greater than that for PTFE),[24] questions remain given the potential cost for BEVG. This cost conundrum is magnified when one considers that, at baseline, each patient on HD has been shown to account for approximately $80,000 in Medicare funds alone on an annual basis,[50] although more durable access may result in average decreased costs over time.

Additional concerns remain over the durability of the graft in terms of dialysis access, and whether the endogenous remodeling process will be so robust as to cause aneurysmal degeneration of chronically needled segment of the BEVGs utilized for HD, as prior bioprosthetic graft devices have been shown prone to. Finally, one must take into account the fact that the time to creation of these BEVGs is of utmost importance, hence our highlighting of the concepts of "ready availability" and "off-the-shelf access." Studies have demonstrated that grafts such as the HAV, which can be synthesized from cadaveric donor tissue and are eventually decellularized and stored as an essentially hollow ECM tube are designed to be readily available.[47] Admittedly, aside perhaps from the acutely infected dialysis access, the ready availability of BEVG may not drastically impact the HD patient in need of access, as there remain backup modalities and access choices for RRT, however unfavorable they are. However, with the possibility that extension of BEVGs to other clinical applications such as coronary or peripheral arterial bypass is on the horizon given these pending clinical trials, the underlying urgency regarding availability and timeliness of conduit creation is further magnified.

A final but separate note must be made about a rapidly evolving field, that of three-dimensional (3D) printing of neovessels in which the printing of materials in a repetitive fashion cumulatively forms a complex object with 3D geometry.[51] Theoretically, this process can result in the formation of not only hollow vascular tubes, but also both solid and hollow organs, such as the kidney and bowel, respectively. Several groups have demonstrated *in vitro* formation of BEVGs through 3D printing,[52–54] with some utilizing endothelial cells as the precursor "bio ink." It must be mentioned, again, that similar to the other modalities as mentioned above, these techniques have yet to be validated in clinical trials. It should be noted, however, that 3D bioprinting shows some promise in the fact that it can produce vessels in a relatively rapid and customized fashion, and thus subsequently overcomes some of the aforementioned time limitations of BEVGs synthesized via "more conventional" methodology.

CONCLUSION

Vascular access technology has experienced several seminal events in its history, dating as far back as the 1950s, which have dramatically altered the course of the fields of both vascular surgery and nephrology. The recent development of BEVG, along with more modernized approaches to the synthesis and creation of these devices reflects a tremendous volume of work done by basic scientists, bioengineers, and clinicians alike. In part, this represents a reaction to the inadequacy of synthetic and bioprosthetic vascular conduits for patients with difficult access or that are not necessarily suitable for autogenous AVF, or who have expended other access options. As described, BEVGs have the capability to dramatically impact the realm of dialysis access, oncologic vascular reconstructive, and coronary or peripheral arterial bypass procedures, amongst other indications, if they display physiologic responses to endogenous vasoactive compounds, remain anti-thrombotic, resistant to infection, durable, easy to handle, and above all, are readily available. Indeed, the current utilization of dialysis access technology initially developed almost half a century ago may seem archaic when compared to other treatment alternatives afforded to vascular surgery patients by modern technical advances, such as in the case of the ever-evolving endovascular approaches to the treatment of peripheral arterial and aortic pathology. Ongoing clinical trials will allow us to determine if these BEVGs meet the minimum requisite criteria as a viable dialysis conduit for the difficult vascular access patient.

REFERENCES

1. National Kidney Foundation. K/DOQI clinical practice guidelines for chronic kidney disease: evaluation, classification, and stratification. *Am J Kidney Dis.* 2002;39:S1–266.
2. Brescia MJ CJ, Appel K, Hurwich BJ. Chronic hemodialysis using venipuncture and a surgically created arteriovenous fistula. *N Engl J Med.* 1966;275:1089–92.
3. Scribner BH CJ, Buri R, Quinton W. The technique of continuous hemodialysis. *Trans Am Soc Artif Intern Organs.* 1960;10–11:88–103.
4. Manson RJ, Unger JM, Ali A, Gage SM, Lawson JH. Tissue-engineered vascular grafts: autologous off-the-shelf vascular access? *Semin Nephrol.* 2012;32:582–91.
5. Harlander-Locke M, Jimenez JC, Lawrence PF, et al. Bovine carotid artery (Artegraft) as a hemodialysis access conduit in patients who are poor candidates for native arteriovenous fistulae. *Vasc Endovasc Surg.* 2014;48:497–502.
6. Rosenberg N, Henderson J, Lord GH, Bothwell JW. An Arterial Prosthesis of Heterologous Vascular Origin. *JAMA.* 1964;187:741–3.
7. Merickel JH, Anderson RC, Knutson R, Lipschultz ML, Hitchcock CR. Bovine carotid artery shunts in vascular access surgery. Complications in the chronic hemodialysis patient. *Arch Surg.* 1974;109:245–50.
8. Chinitz JL, Tokoyama T, Bower R, Swartz C. Self-sealing prosthesis for arteriovenous fistula in man. *Trans Am Soc Artif Intern Organs.* 1972;18:452–7.
9. Rosenberg N, Thompson JE, Keshishian JM, VanderWerf BA. The modified bovine arterial graft. *Arch Surg.* 1976;111:222–6.
10. Hertzer NR, Beven EG. Venous access using the bovine carotid heterograft: Techniques, results, and complications in 75 patients. *Arch Surg.* 1978;113:696–700.
11. Schroder A, Imig H, Peiper U, Neidel J, Petereit A. Results of a bovine collagen vascular graft (Solcograft-P) in infra-inguinal positions. *Eur J Vasc Surg.* 1988;2:315–21.
12. Holdsworth RJ, Naidu S, Gervaz P, McCollum PT. Glutaraldehyde-tanned bovine carotid artery graft for infrainguinal vascular reconstruction: 5-year follow-up. *Eur J Vasc Endovasc Surg.* 1997;14:208–11.
13. Widmer MK, Aregger F, Stauffer E, et al. Intermediate outcome and risk factor assessment of bovine vascular heterografts used as AV-fistulas for hemodialysis access. *Eur J Vasc Endovasc Surg.* 2004;27:660–5.
14. Katzman HE, Glickman MH, Schild AF, Fujitani RM, Lawson JH. Multicenter evaluation of the bovine mesenteric vein bioprostheses for hemodialysis access in patients with an earlier failed prosthetic graft. *J Am Coll Surg.* 2005;201:223–30.
15. Kovalic AJ, Beattie DK, Davies AH. Outcome of ProCol, a bovine mesenteric vein graft, in infrainguinal reconstruction. *Eur J Vasc Endovasc Surg.* 2002;24:533–4.
16. Dardik H, Ibrahim IM, Dardik I. Arteriovenous fistulas constructed with modified human umbilical cord vein graft. *Arch Surg.* 1976;111:60–2.
17. Dardik H, Ibrahim IM, Baier R, Sprayregen S, Levy M, Dardik, II. Human umbilical cord. A new source for vascular prosthesis. *JAMA.* 1976;236:2859–62.
18. Hirsch SA, Jarrett F. The use of stabilized human umbilical vein for femoropopliteal bypass. Experience with 133 operations with 5-year follow-up. *Ann Surg.* 1984;200:147–52.
19. Rubio PA, Farrell EM. Modified human umbilical vein graft arteriovenous fistulae as a source of angioaccess in maintenance hemodialysis. *Cardiovasc Dis.* 1980;7:51–7.

20. Goldman M, Gunson B, Hawker RJ, McCollum CN. Human umbilical vein and polytetrafluorethylene arterial grafts compared in an artificial circulation. *Br J Surg*. 1983;70:4–6.
21. Madden RL, Lipkowitz GS, Browne BJ, Kurbanov A. Experience with cryopreserved cadaveric femoral vein allografts used for hemodialysis access. *Ann Vasc Surg*. 2004;18:453–8.
22. Matsuura JH, Johansen KH, Rosenthal D, Clark MD, Clarke KA, Kirby LB. Cryopreserved femoral vein grafts for difficult hemodialysis access. *Ann Vasc Surg*. 2000;14:50–5.
23. Madden RL, Lipkowitz GS, Browne BJ, Kurbanov A. A comparison of cryopreserved vein allografts and prosthetic grafts for hemodialysis access. *Ann Vasc Surg*. 2005;19:686–91.
24. Bolton WD, Cull DL, Taylor SM, et al. The use of cryopreserved femoral vein grafts for hemodialysis access in patients at high risk for infection: A word of caution. *J Vasc Surg*. 2002;36:464–8.
25. Sell SA, McClure MJ, Garg K, Wolfe PS, Bowlin GL. Electrospinning of collagen/biopolymers for regenerative medicine and cardiovascular tissue engineering. *Adv Drug Deliv Rev*. 2009;61:1007–19.
26. Thomas AC, Campbell GR, Campbell JH. Advances in vascular tissue engineering. *Cardiovasc Pathol*. 2003;12:271–6.
27. Weinberg CB, Bell E. A blood vessel model constructed from collagen and cultured vascular cells. *Science* 1986;231:397–400.
28. L'Heureux NS, Germain LS, Labbe RS, Auger FA. In vitro construction of a human blood vessel from cultured vascular cells: A morphologic study. *J Vasc Surg*. 1993;17:499–509.
29. Girton T, Oegema T, Grassl E, Isenberg B, Tranquillo R. Mechanisms of stiffening and strengthening in media-equivalents fabricated using glycation. *J Biomech Eng*. 2000;122:216–23.
30. Girton T, Oegema T, Tranquillo RT. Exploiting glycation to stiffen and strengthen tissue equivalents for tissue engineering. *J Biomed Mater Res*. 1999;46:87–92.
31. L'Heureux N, Paquet S, Labbe R, Germain L, Auger F. A completely biological tissue-engineered human blood vessel. *FASEB J*. 1998;12:47–56.
32. Walles T, Herden T, Haverich A, Mertsching H. Influence of scaffold thickness and scaffold composition on bioartificial graft survival. *Biomaterials*. 2003;24:1233–39.
33. Niklason LE, Gao J, Abbott W, et al. Functional arteries grown in vitro. *Science*. 1999;284:489–93.
34. Campbell J, Efendy J, Campbell G. Novel vascular graft grown within recipient's own peritoneal cavity. *Circ Res*. 1999;85:1173–8.
35. Chue WL, Campbell GR, Caplice N, et al. Dog peritoneal and pleural cavities as bioreactors to grow autologous vascular grafts. *J Vasc Surg*. 2004;39:859–67.
36. Dahl SL, Koh J, Prabhakar V, Niklason LE. Decellularized native and engineered arterial scaffolds for transplantation. *Cell Transplant*. 2003;12:659–66.
37. L'Heureux N, Dusserre N, Konig G, et al. Human tissue-engineered blood vessels for adult arterial revascularization. *Nat Med*. 2006;12:361–5.
38. Shin'oka T, Imai Y, Ikada Y. Transplantation of a tissue-engineered pulmonary artery. *N Engl J Med*. 2001;344:532–3.
39. Shinoka T, Shum-Tim D, Ma P, et al. Creation of viable pulmonary artery autografts through tissue engineering. *J Thorac Cardiovasc Surg*. 1998;115:536–46.
40. Shin'oka T, Matsumura G, Hibino N, et al. Midterm clinical result of tissue-engineered vascular autografts seeded with autologous bone marrow cells. *J Thorac Cardiovasc Surg*. 2005;129:1330–8.
41. Matthews JA, Wnek GE, Simpson DG, Bowlin GL. Electrospinning of collagen nanofibers. *Biomacromolecules*. 2002;3:232–8.
42. Boland ED, Matthews JA, Pawlowski KJ, Simpson DG, Wnek GE, Bowlin GL. Electrospinning collagen and elastin: preliminary vascular tissue engineering. *Front Biosci*. 2004;9:1422–32.
43. L'Heureux N, McAllister TN, de la Fuente LM. Tissue-engineered blood vessel for adult arterial revascularization. *N Engl J Med*. 2007;357:1451–3.

44. McAllister T, Maruszewski M, Garrido S, et al. Effectiveness of haemodialysis access with an autologous tissue-engineered vascular graft: A multicentre cohort study. *Lancet.* 2009;373:1440–46.
45. Wystrychowski W, Cierpka L, Zagalski K, et al. Case study: First implantation of a frozen, devitalized tissue-engineered vascular graft for urgent hemodialysis access. *J Vasc Access.* 2011;12:67–70.
46. Wystrychowski W, McAllister TN, Zagalski K, Dusserre N, Cierpka L, L'Heureux N. First human use of an allogeneic tissue-engineered vascular graft for hemodialysis access. *J Vasc Surg.* 2014;60:1353–7.
47. Dahl S, Kypson A, Lawson J, et al. Readily available tissue-engineered vascular grafts. *Sci Transl Med.* 2011;3:68ra9.
48. Benrashid E, McCoy CC, Youngwirth LM, et al. Tissue Engineered Vascular Grafts: Origins, Development, and Current Strategies for Clinical Application. *Methods.* 2015. http://dx.doi.org/10.1016/j.ymeth.2015.07.014. [Epub ahead of print.]
49. Olausson M, Patil PB, Kuna VK, et al. Transplantation of an allogeneic vein bioengineered with autologous stem cells: A proof-of-concept study. *Lancet.* 2012;380:230–7.
50. USRDS. Atlas of chronic kidney diesase and end-stage renal disease in the United States. United States Renal Data System (2013). Available from htttp://www.usrds.org/atlas.aspx. Accessed 31 July 2015.
51. Murphy SV, Atala A. 3D bioprinting of tissues and organs. *Nat Biotechnol.*2014;32:773–85.
52. Cui X, Boland T. Human microvasculature fabrication using thermal inkjet printing technology. *Biomaterials.* 2009;30:6221–7.
53. Lee VK, Kim DY, Ngo H, et al. Creating perfused functional vascular channels using 3D bioprinting technology. *Biomaterials.* 2014;35:8092–102.
54. Zhao L, Lee VK, Yoo SS, Dai G, Intes X. The integration of 3-D cell printing and mesoscopic fluorescence molecular tomography of vascular constructs within thick hydrogel scaffolds. *Biomaterials.* 2012;33:5325–32.

10

Dialysis Access Coding: New and Upcoming Changes

Matthew J. Sideman, MD and Francesco A. Aiello, MD

January 2017 will bring about dramatic changes in coding for the endovascular maintenance of the dialysis access circuit. These changes are the results of ongoing concerted efforts on the parts of both the Center for Medicare and Medicaid Services (CMS) and the American Medical Association (AMA) to identify potentially misvalued services. The AMA RVU Update Committee (RUC) and CMS have established screens for potentially misvalued services. One of these screens is for any two codes billed together more than 75% of the time. When services are captured in a billed together screen, the codes must be sent back to the Current Procedural Terminology (CPT) panel to be bundled into one all-inclusive new code. These rules and screens have been created to both simplify the coding structure and to correct any misvalued services. In January 2015, CPT codes 35475, 35476, 36147, 36148, 37236, 37238, 75791, 75962, and 75968 were identified as being frequently reported together in various combinations. CMS and RUC convention also now mandate valuing codes in the context of the whole "family" of related codes instead of valuing individual codes to maintain relativity of values within the code set.

It is against this backdrop that a new family of codes to describe the work to maintain a dialysis circuit was created by a joint workgroup of members from the Society for Vascular Surgery, the Society for Interventional Radiology, the Renal Physicians Association, and the American College of Radiology. The new family consists of nine codes to describe all endovascular maintenance and treatment of the dialysis circuit. This "family" of codes includes imaging, angioplasty, stenting, coil embolization and thrombectomy of the peripheral dialysis circuit as well as any additional angioplasty and stenting of central venous stenosis/occlusions. The family of codes was created in collaboration with the above mentioned societies, presented and subsequently approved at the CPT Editorial Panel meeting in September 2015 with only minor changes.[1] After approval by the CPT panel meeting, the codes were then presented at the January 2016 RUC meeting and the final RUC recommendations were submitted to CMS for final valuation.[2] The new codes and values will go into effect on January 1, 2017. At the time of writing of this chapter, the new values for these codes have only been published in the Medicare Physician Fee Schedule (MPFS) Proposed Rule and will not be final until the Final Rule is published sometime in November 2016.[3]

PREVIOUS CODING CONVENTION

Prior to January 2017, imaging of the dialysis circuit was described with CPT code 36147 (Introduction of needle and/or catheter, arteriovenous shunt created for dialysis (graft/ fistula); initial access with complete radiological evaluation of dialysis access, including fluoroscopy, image documentation and report (includes access of shunt, injection[s] of contrast, and all necessary imaging from the arterial anastomosis and adjacent artery through entire venous outflow including the inferior or superior vena cava)). Alternatively, if the fistulogram was performed from a remote site without direct access to the dialysis circuit, CPT code 75791 (Angiography, arteriovenous shunt (eg, dialysis patient fistula/graft), complete evaluation of dialysis access, including fluoroscopy, image documentation and report (includes injections of contrast and all necessary imaging from the arterial anastomosis and adjacent artery through entire venous outflow including the inferior or superior vena cava), radiological supervision and interpretation) can be used to report diagnostic imaging.

If angioplasty was performed within the venous side of the dialysis circuit, CPT code 35476 (Transluminal balloon angioplasty, percutaneous; venous) with its corresponding supervision and interpretation (S&I) CPT code 75978 (Transluminal balloon angioplasty, venous (eg, subclavian stenosis), radiological supervision and interpretation) were used to report angioplasty within the circuit and/or within the central venous outflow. However, if the angioplasty involved the arterial anastomosis (including the juxta-anastomotic segment) then CPT codes 35475 (Transluminal balloon angioplasty, percutaneous; brachiocephalic trunk or branches, each vessel) and its corresponding S&I code 75862 (Transluminal balloon angioplasty, peripheral artery other than renal, or other visceral artery, iliac or lower extremity, radiological supervision and interpretation) or 75964 (Transluminal balloon angioplasty, each additional peripheral artery other than renal or other visceral artery, iliac or lower extremity, radiological supervision and interpretation (List separately in addition to code for primary procedure)) were reported.

Stent placement within a dialysis circuit and/or within the central venous system was reported with CPT code 37238 (Transcatheter placement of an intravascular stent(s), open or percutaneous, including radiological supervision and interpretation and including angioplasty within the same vessel, when performed; initial vein). This code was introduced into the CPT manual in 2014 after the original stent and S&I code were bundled into one due to the billed together >75% of the time rule. Percutaneous thrombectomy was reported with CPT code 36870 (Thrombectomy, percutaneous, arteriovenous fistula, autogenous or nonautogenous graft (includes mechanical thrombus extraction and intra-graft thrombolysis)). In contra-distinction to the other listed codes, 36870 is a 90-day global code while the other codes are 0-day global codes. If an additional access to the dialysis circuit was required to perform any intervention, CPT code 36148 (Introduction of needle and/or catheter, arteriovenous shunt created for dialysis (graft/fistula); additional access for therapeutic intervention (List separately in addition to code for primary procedure)) was reported to capture this additional work.

Additional adjunctive procedures for maintenance of the dialysis access circuit include embolization of significant side branches and atherectomy of the circuit. Embolization was coded with CPT code 37241 (Vascular embolization or occlusion, inclusive of all radiological supervision and interpretation, intraprocedural roadmapping, and imaging guidance necessary to complete the intervention; venous, other than hemorrhage (eg, congenital or acquired venous malformations, venous and capillary hemangiomas, varices, varicoceles)) which is a newly bundled code combining the procedure and the radiologic S&I first published in the 2014 CPT manual. Atherectomy of the dialysis circuit is considered experimental. If atherectomy is performed in the arterial inflow of the circuit, it would be reported with a temporary or Category III CPT Code (0237T - Transluminal peripheral atherectomy, open or percutaneous, including radiological supervision and interpretation; brachiocephalic trunk and branches, each vessel). There is no code to describe atherectomy in the venous system or dialysis circuit and CPT Code 37799 (Unlisted procedure, vascular surgery) would be used.

A summary of the previous coding convention with their 2016 existing work relative value units (wRVUs) is provided in Table 10-1.

TABLE 10-1. SUMMARY OF THE PREVIOUS CODING CONVENTION WITH 2016 EXISTING WORK RELATIVE VALUE UNITS

CPT Code	Description	2016 wRVU
35475	Angioplasty arterial anastomosis	6.60
35476	Angioplasty dialysis circuit (and central veins)	5.10
36147	Fistulogram	3.72
36148	Second access of dialysis circuit	1.00
36870	Percutaneous thrombectomy	5.20
37238	Venous stent; initial vein	6.29
37241	Embolization; venous	9.00
37799	Unlisted vascular procedure	0.00*
75791	Fistulogram through existing needle access	1.71
75962	Arterial angioplasty S&I; initial vessel	0.54
75964	Arterial angioplasty S&I; each additional vessel	0.36
75978	Venous angioplasty S&I	0.54
0237T	Atherectomy; brachiocephalic arteries and branches	0.00*

*Category III and unlisted procedures have no RVU values. Payments have to be negotiated individually

NEW CODING FAMILY

The new family of codes to report maintenance of the dialysis access circuit consists of nine bundled codes in 3 subsets. The first subset describes imaging and/or intervention and includes codes to describe a fistulogram (36901), fistulogram with angioplasty (36902), fistulogram with angioplasty and stent placement including all S&I (36903). The second subset describes thrombectomy with or without additional intervention and includes codes to describe percutaneous thrombectomy (36904), thrombectomy with angioplasty (36905), and thrombectomy with angioplasty and stent placement (36906). The third "subset" is a group of three add on codes to describe central venous angioplasty done through the hemodialysis access (+36907), central venous stent through the hemodialysis access (+36908), and coil embolization of the hemodialysis access (+36909). The 90 day global for thrombectomy has been removed and all codes are either 0 day globals or add on codes; add on codes do not have their own global period designation.

CPT code 36901 (Introduction of needle(s) and/or catheter(s), dialysis circuit, with diagnostic angiography of the dialysis circuit, including all direct puncture(s) and catheter placement(s), injection(s) of contrast, all necessary imaging from the arterial anastomosis and adjacent artery through entire venous outflow including the inferior or superior vena cava, fluoroscopic guidance, radiologic supervision and interpretation and image documentation and report;) will replace the work of 36147.

CPT code 36902 (Introduction of needle(s) and/or catheter(s), dialysis circuit, with diagnostic angiography of the dialysis circuit, including all direct puncture(s) and catheter placement(s), injection(s) of contrast, all necessary imaging from the arterial anastomosis and adjacent artery through entire venous outflow including the inferior or superior vena cava, fluoroscopic guidance, radiologic supervision and interpretation and image documentation and report; with transluminal balloon angioplasty, peripheral dialysis segment, including all imaging and radiological supervision and interpretation necessary to perform the angioplasty) will replace the work of 36147, 35476 and 75978. It will also replace the work of 35475, 75962 and 75964 as the new coding convention does not differentiate between an angioplasty performed within the body of a dialysis circuit and an angioplasty performed at the arterial anastomosis.

CPT code 36903 (Introduction of needle(s) and/or catheter(s), dialysis circuit, with diagnostic angiography of the dialysis circuit, including all direct puncture(s) and catheter placement(s), injection(s) of contrast, all necessary imaging from the arterial anastomosis and adjacent artery through entire venous outflow including the inferior or superior vena cava, fluoroscopic guidance, radiologic supervision and interpretation and image documentation and report; with transcatheter placement of intravascular stent(s) peripheral dialysis segment, including all imaging and radiological supervision and interpretation necessary to perform the stenting, and all angioplasty within the peripheral dialysis segment) will replace the work of 36147 and 37238.

CPT code 36904 (Percutaneous transluminal mechanical thrombectomy and/or infusion for thrombolysis, dialysis circuit, any method, including all imaging and radiological supervision and interpretation, diagnostic angiography, fluoroscopic guidance, catheter placement(s), and intraprocedural pharmacological thrombolytic injection(s);) will replace the work of 36147, 36148, and 36870. Again, the 90 day global has been removed and the code is now a 0 day global like the other codes in the family.

CPT code 36905 (Percutaneous transluminal mechanical thrombectomy and/or infusion for thrombolysis, dialysis circuit, any method, including all imaging and radiological supervision and interpretation, diagnostic angiography, fluoroscopic guidance, catheter placement(s), and intraprocedural pharmacological thrombolytic injection(s); with transluminal balloon angioplasty, peripheral dialysis segment, including all imaging and radiological supervision and interpretation necessary to perform the angioplasty) will replace the work of 36147, 36148, 36870, 35476 and 75798. It also potentially replaces the work of 35475, 75962, and 75964 for the reasons stated above.

CPT code 36906 (Percutaneous transluminal mechanical thrombectomy and/ or infusion for thrombolysis, dialysis circuit, any method, including all imaging and radiological supervision and interpretation, diagnostic angiography, fluoroscopic guidance, catheter placement(s), and intraprocedural pharmacological thrombolytic injection(s); with transcatheter placement of an intravascular stent(s), peripheral dialysis segment, including all imaging and radiological supervision and interpretation to perform the stenting and all angioplasty within the peripheral dialysis circuit) will replace the work of 36147, 36148, 36870, and 37238.

CPT code +36907 (Transluminal balloon angioplasty, central dialysis segment, performed through dialysis circuit, including all imaging and radiological supervision and interpretation required to perform the angioplasty) is a new add on code that will be used to report angioplasty of central venous lesions when approached through the dialysis access circuit. It will replace the work of 35476 and 75978.

CPT code +36908 (Transcatheter placement of an intravascular stent(s), central dialysis segment, performed through dialysis circuit, including all imaging and radiological supervision and interpretation required to perform the stenting, and all angioplasty in the central dialysis segment) is a new add on code that will be used to report stent placement within central venous lesions when approached through the dialysis access circuit. It will replace the work of 37238.

CPT code +36909 (Dialysis circuit permanent vascular embolization or occlusion (including main circuit or any accessory veins), endovascular, including all imaging and radiological supervision and interpretation necessary to complete the intervention) is a new add on code that will be used to report embolization of significant side branches off of a dialysis circuit. It will replace the work of 37241.

At the time of writing of this chapter, the new family of codes has been valued at the RUC and sent to CMS for final valuation.[2] The 2017 MPFS (Medicare Physician Fee Schedule) Proposed Rule was published at the beginning of July 2016.[3] Multiple stakeholders including the Society for Vascular Surgery will submit comments about the values in the Proposed Rule. Final valuation will be set when the 2017 MPFS Final Rule is published likely some time in November. Table 10-2 summarizes the new codes, RUC recommended values, and the CMS proposed values from the 2017 MPFS Proposed Rule.

TABLE 10-2. RUC AND CMS PROPOSED VALUES

CPT Code	Description	RUC Recommended wRVU	CMS Proposed wRVU
36901	Fistulogram	3.36	2.82
36902	Fistulogram with angioplasty	4.83	4.24
36903	Fistulogram with stent	6.39	5.85
36904	Thrombectomy	7.50	6.73
36905	Thrombectomy with angioplasty	9.00	8.46
36906	Thrombectomy with stent	10.42	9.88
+36907	Central venous angioplasty	3.00	2.48
+36908	Central venous stent	4.25	3.73
+36909	Embolization of access	4.12	3.48

IMPLICATIONS OF NEW CODES

It is easy to see that these new codes will result in a devaluation of work provided for the maintenance of the dialysis circuit. Even when taking into consideration the multiple procedure reduction when reporting more than one code under the previous coding convention, the new codes and CMS proposed values will result in a reduction of 16–61% of work RVUs. With the proposed conversion factor for 2017 decreasing from $35.8043 to $35.7751 each RVU will generate less dollars than they did in 2016. There are also reductions in non-facility practice expense RVUs, facility practice expense RVUs, and liability insurance RVUs for all of the new codes compared to the previous codes. While a direct one to one comparison between the new and old dialysis codes is difficult due to bundling, CPT codes 36147 and 36901 are candidates from direct comparison. (see Table 10-3) Using Medicare claims utilization data, breakdown on site of service, and the 2016 conversion factor, CMS spent an estimated $201,434,023.88 in 2016 for CPT code 36147. Assuming the same claims data and site of service distribution for 2017 and assuming the proposed values become final for the new codes, CMS will spend $137,575,783.36 for CPT code 36901 in 2017. This represents a savings of $63,858,240.52 or 31.70% for the Medicare program.

SUMMARY

There will be new CPT codes for reporting the maintenance of the dialysis circuit beginning in January 2017. These nine new codes will simplify coding and billing but will also represent a significant decrease in reimbursement for physician services, both professional fees and office based practices. The significance of these changes will vary and be dependent on the site of service, office versus facility, as well as the volume or percentage of a practice spent providing these services. This drastic decline in reimbursement for some of these procedures could possibly effect the practice patterns and potentially shift patients back into the hospital setting from physician offices. This may also lead to delays in access to care for many dialysis patients. We would strongly recommend that each physician perform a careful analysis of the effects of these upcoming changes upon their practice and change their practice patterns accordingly.

TABLE 10-3. FISTULOGRAM EXPENTITURE COMPARISON

CPT	Descriptor	Tot NF RVU	Tot Fac RVU	Utilization	Physician Office	Outpt Hospital	Inpt Hospital	Dollars
36147	Fistulogram	23.90	5.43	338,353	61.04%	30.39%	7.16%	$201,434,023.88
36901	Fistulogram	16.03	4.21	338,353	61.04%	30.39%	7.16%	$137,575,783.36

REFERENCES

1. CPT® Editorial Summary of Panel Actions October 2015. http://www.ama-assn.org/ama/pub/physician-resources/solutions-managing-your-practice/coding-billing-insurance/cpt/cpt-summary-panel-actions.page. (Accessed July 16, 2016.)
2. RUC Recommendations, Minutes and Voting, February 2016 RUC Recommendations. http://www.ama-assn.org/ama/no-index/physician-resources/ruc-recommendations.page. (Accessed July 24, 2016.)
3. Medicare Program; Revisions to Payment Policies Under the Physician Fee Schedule and Other Revisions to Part B for CY 2017; Medicare Advantage Pricing Data Release; Medicare Advantage and Part D Medical Low Ratio Data Release; Medicare Advantage Provider Network Requirements; Expansion of Medicare Diabetes Prevention Program Model. https://www.federalregister.gov/articles/2016/07/15/2016-16097/medicare-program-revisions-to-payment-policies-under-the-physician-fee-schedule-and-other-revisions. Updated July 15, 2016. (Accessed July 24, 2016.)

11

Dialysis Vascular Access and Transvenous Cardiac Devices

Haimanot Wasse, MD, MPH and Dirk Hentschel, MD

Cardiac implantable electronic devices (CIED) are implanted for the treatment of cardiac rhythm disturbances and include pacemakers (PMs) and implantable cardioverter-defibrillators (ICDs). Their placement in U.S. chronic kidney disease (CKD) and end-stage renal disease (ESRD) patients has increased over time, and it is estimated that 10% of U.S. hemodialysis patients have a CIED.[1]

CKD and ESRD patients commonly experience cardiac rhythm disorders in which a pacemaker is indicated. Further, while an ICD significantly improves survival in CKD and ESRD patients with underlying ischemic heart disease, cardiomyopathy and congestive heart failure who experience ventricular tachycardia or fibrillation (secondary prevention), the survival benefit is not as significant as that attributed to ICD placement in the general population.[2] Specifically, a meta-analysis found a nearly three-fold higher mortality in ESRD patients with ICD than non-ESRD patient with ICD.[3] ICD placement for primary prevention shows survival benefit in patients with CKD-3a and b; however, overall mortality in CKD-4 patients is such that no survival benefit after ICD placement is observed.[4] This may reflect higher mortality of the device placement procedure and subsequent clinical events such as infection or device exchange and competing mortality from comorbid conditions. Alternatively, benefits of ICD placement may be attenuated by noncardiovertable rhythms such as bradycardia and asystole.

CIED AND CENTRAL VENOUS STENOSIS

CIED-related central venous stenosis can occur in non-ESRD and ESRD patients, and stenosis can develop from the venotomy site to any portion of the vessel wall that is in contact with the CIED leads and extend to the superior vena cava.[5] Among a series of non-ESRD patients evaluated six months following transvenous pacemaker placement,

64% were noted to have developed central venous stenosis, however only 2.6% were clinically symptomatic.[6] The presence of an ipsilateral upper extremity arteriovenous access, however, can significantly increase venous return by adding 1000–2000 mL/min mean blood flow, unmasking clinically significant stenosis with venous hypertension manifesting as arm swelling and development of collateral veins. While arm swelling is not universal after ipsilateral CIED and dialysis access placement, the majority of published case studies and case series report the onset of complications due to venous hypertension within 6 months of concurrent access and device presence.

CIED AND VASCULAR ACCESS PATENCY

Reports from limited case series have examined whether the presence of a CIED influences arteriovenous (AV) access patency. In one report, the outcomes of AV access creation were compared between patients with ipsilateral (n = 19) versus contralateral (N = 17) CIED placement.[7] Patients with ipsilateral CIED placement experienced a primary AV access failure rate of 78.9% versus 35.3% in patients with contralateral placement (P = 0.02).[7]

CENTRAL VEIN STENOSIS AFTER CIED LEAD PLACEMENT

Implantation of cardiac devices is associated with stenosis and occlusion of the central veins, ranging from between 3.6 and 33% for occlusion and between 10 and 65% for stenosis.[8–10] In 7–14% of patients, there are pre-existing stenoses of the central veins.[8,9] It is unclear if this is due to cannulation of the veins at a prior point in time or truly a natural occurrence. Lead entry through the subclavian or cutdown to the cephalic vein does not appear to make a difference,[9,11–14] neither does left versus right-sided insertion.[13,14] However, clinical symptoms occur only in a minority of patients with documented central venous stenosis (1-5%). Symptomatic cases can be treated with angioplasty and stent placement,[15–23] but long-term success is not well documented. In the largest retrospective study, 50% of stenoses had recurred after 26 months.[15] While these reports describe placement of stents across the central venous stenosis with CRMD leads in place, more recently lead extraction prior to angioplasty and stent placement with subsequent insertion of new CRMD leads has been performed.[24,25] Recent expert consensus guidelines of the Heart Rhythm society recommend lead extraction prior to stent placement to avoid lead entrapment complications and future lead extractions.[26] There is concern that bacteremia is more common in dialysis patients necessitating lead removal more frequently, such that lead entrapment would pose a great difficulty. The only available retrospective study addressing the question of increased complication rates for CRMDs in ESRD patients documents a higher rate of device related complications such as lead dislodgement and elevated defibrillator thresholds, hematoma formation at the insertion site, and a non-significant trend to higher incidence of pocket infections[27]; in total, major complications were reported in 29% of dialysis patients compared to 5% in non-ESRD patients. On the other hand, presence of renal failure (OR = 1.76) and older age (OR = 1.63 per 20 years) are risk factors for in-hospital mortality in patients admitted with CRMD infections.[28]

Available data on central vein stenosis in dialysis patients with autogenous AV or prosthetic accesses and ipsilateral cardiac device leads is limited. One retrospective center analysis of 495 transvenous pacemaker insertions identified 14 patients with ipsilateral dialysis accesses.[29] Ten of these 14 patients (71%) had clinical symptoms; eight of these had a total occlusion of the subclavian vein and required ligation of the dialysis access. The four asymptomatic patients died from unrelated causes within 6 months after implantation of the cardiac device. Tourret and colleagues report a case of symptomatic subclavian vein stenosis immediately after creation of an autogenous AV access 21 months after an ipsilateral pacemaker was inserted.[30] In this case, the access had to be ligated to control symptoms. Ten other cases from the literature are reviewed in this report, with time of symptoms after AVF creation ranging from immediately to two years. In total of six AVFs were abandoned due to symptoms,[31–34] three underwent angioplasty, but eventually had to be ligated,[35] and one underwent angioplasty and placement of a stent and remained patent 8 months after the intervention.[36] Ultimately, ipsilateral dialysis accesses and CRMDs should be avoided.

CIED-INSERTION SITES: IMPLICATIONS AND OUTCOMES

1) Subclavian Vein

Since the 1980s, it has been known that subclavian vein catheters are associated with subclavian vein stenosis and thrombosis.[37] Schillinger established that three weeks after removal of a Shaldon hemodialysis catheter, stenoses were present in 42% of patients who had a subclavian vein catheter, but only in 10% who had internal jugular vein catheters.[38] A report on the natural history of subclavian vein stenoses in dialysis patients finds a stenosis in just over 50% of patients at the time of removal of subclavian vein catheters. Some of these stenoses improve, but after 3–6 months, 28% of subclavian veins had stenosis severity of greater than 30%.[39] Insertion of tunneled hemodialysis catheters into the subclavian veins should be considered a measure of last resort as ipsilateral long-term access options can be severely jeopardized.

We recommend avoiding insertion of CIEDs leads via subclavian veins ipsilateral to an existing or planned hemodialysis access. Contralateral insertion may be acceptable if life expectancy of the patient in question is limited. However, in young and middle-aged patients, alternative CIED lead insertion sites should be explored.

2) Cephalic Vein

The cephalic vein has been used for CIED lead insertion for many decades. It is typically ligated distally, thereby complicating ipsilateral forearm accesses and excluding an upper arm autologous brachial-cephalic access. When evaluated, the incidence of central venous stenosis is not different for cephalic vein versus subclavian vein insertion. Ipsilateral cephalic vein insertion of CIED leads to an existing or planned hemodialysis access is contraindicated. Contralateral insertion requires careful weighing of life expectancy and need for new vascular access.

3) Femoral Vein

Traditional indications for CIED lead placement using a femoral approach include use in children, occluded thoracic central veins, anomalies in the central thoracic veins, and the presence of a very thin anterior chest wall such that it cannot accommodate a device pocket.[40,41] The femoral route has also been demonstrated as successful in children where endovascular lead placement is often not possible due to small subclavian vein size.[42] Advantages of the femoral approach as compared to an open thoracic approach for epicardial lead placement are lower morbidity from anesthesia and surgery, as well as cost. Weinstein et al. reported on 100 consecutive cases of temporary pacing via the femoral route and found minimal complications.[43] The largest series of permanent femoral pacing systems in adults was published by Ellestad and French.[44] They described the ease of 95 pacemaker implantations via the femoral/iliac route. Atrial lead displacement was the major complication occurring in 21%. Mathur et al reported the next largest series in 27 adult patients.[41] No thromboses or lead fractures were observed but atrial lead displacement occurred in 20% in this series. The authors reported that during the last 4 years of the study, no atrial lead displacements occurred and this was attributed to increased operator experience. Two pacemaker pocket pre-erosions required the pulse generators to be repositioned. A more recent study by Garcia Guerrero et al described their experience with the transfemoral approach for 12 permanent pacemaker systems.[45] Their lead displacement rate was 0%. Furthermore, they described a modification of previous techniques in which the pocket is in the anterior thigh rather than the lower abdomen.

Clinical success with the transfemoral route appears to be supported in the literature in-spite of limited numbers. The reported disadvantages of femoral lead placement include a slightly higher risk of lead detachment and thromboembolism. Rates of such complications in earlier reports of the femoral approach have seemingly abated with more modern active fixation leads, lower device pocket location (thigh and pelvis versus abdominal), and increasing operator experience. While the ability to measure such risks is skewed given that the two largest series of the femoral approach in adults are 95 and 27 patients, we feel that known risks do not outweigh the benefits of preserving the central venous circuit of CKD patients. Therefore, we recommend adding the CKD/dialysis patient to the list of indications for this approach based on the current literature.

4) Internal Jugular Veins

The internal and external jugular veins are established as insertion sites of choice for tunneled hemodialysis catheters (KDOQI Vascular Access Guidelines 2006).[46] The catheter is tunneled in a gentle curve to avoid kinking as the catheter traverses the clavicle. Transvenous pacing using the internal jugular vein was described first with ligation of the vein,[47] and then without.[48] Brodman and Furman reported on 90 patients, 5% of the total population, in whom cephalic and external jugular vein lead insertion was not possible.[49] The internal jugular vein was ligated, in apparent follow-up, and for up to 7 years they did not report out-of-the-ordinary complications. Lead fracture rates of cephalic, external and internal jugular veins in 2226 patients with a total of 2563 leads (total of 100 lead fractures) were reported by Alt et al in 1987.[50] While fracture rates were higher for internal jugular vein insertion than for cephalic or external jugular vein, these particular rates are not annualized, nor are they differentiated by type of lead. The study spans the years 1965 to 1980, and includes three different types of lead wire (Elema, singlefilar and multifilar coil), with different length of follow-up. Since this report, there has not been a large study including the internal jugular vein as lead insertion sites.

5) Epicardial Leads

Given the risk of development of central venous stenosis from transvenous CIED lead insertion, it is useful to consider alternate routes when indicated. The central veins can be avoided completely with surgical placement of an epicardial left ventricular lead CIED, as the leads traverse through the subcutaneous tissue. Data among pediatric populations show similar complication and survival rates between endocardial versus epicardial lead placement.[51–53] Recent data from a large series of 216 adult non-ESRD patients undergoing epicardial lead CIED placement with 5-year follow-up demonstrated a decrease in epicardial LV pacing threshold during the initial 6 months following implantation, that then stabilized, and a cumulative incidence of device infection of 9.6% compared with 3%–4% reported in patients with transvenous leads.[54] The authors attribute this to a more complicated patient population that previously underwent device replacements and upgrades, risk factors for infection. De novo epicardial lead CIEDs had an infection rate of 1.6 per 100 CIED-years versus 4.7 per 100 CIED-years among patients receiving a replacement device.

Overall, epicardial systems could be considered an alternate option for patients with advanced CKD or ESRD, particularly those with limited venous access options, but require surgical expertise as placement requires a thoracotomy.

6) Subcutaneous Devices

Subcutaneous ICDs have a single lead for sensing and defibrillation and are tunneled subcutaneously without the need for imaging at the time of implantation, offering an advantage over surgically placed epicardial leads that require a cardiothoracic surgeon. They are primarily used in young patients to treat ventricular fibrillation and avoid transvenous lead placement, but lack pacing capability and are not indicated for ventricular tachycardia.[55] Although long-term subcutaneous lead survival has not yet been documented, no primary lead failures have been reported to date.[55] When compared with transvenous CIEDs, subcutaneous ICDs offer several advantages, including relative ease of extraction. To date, data is limited in the ESRD patient population, however, a series of 27 dialysis patients demonstrates that subcutaneous ICDs can be successfully placed in long-term dialysis patients with an AV access, are not associated with excess risk of implant related complications or inappropriate shocks,[56] and offer the advantage of minimization of the risk of central venous stenosis and the potential for reduced risk of infection.

MANAGEMENT OF CIED–ASSOCIATED CENTRAL VENOUS STENOSIS

Percutaneous balloon angioplasty (PTA) without stent placement is considered the standard treatment for symptomatic central vein stenosis with reported primary patency rates of up to 50% and secondary patency up to 86% at 12 months.[57] The concern with repeated PTA is long-term CIED lead stability, yet to date, there is no evidence that PTA has a negative impact on lead function.[57] In the setting of failed PTA, reports describe use of stent insertion,[58] however because this results in CIED lead entrapment, significant difficulty in patient management can arise when the leads require removal, such as in the case of sepsis or endocarditis. In accordance, the Heart Rhythm Society expert consensus on transvenous lead extraction recommends CIED lead removal prior to stent deployment at sites of CIED-lead associated stenosis.[26]

CIED AND CKD PATIENT PROGRESSING TOWARDS ESRD

In planning for hemodialysis access in the late-stage CKD patient, the primary goal is preventing central venous stenosis. To this end, the American Society of Diagnostic and Interventional Nephrology published recommendations in 2012 related to CIED placement in CKD and ESRD patients, partly summarized in Figure 11-1.[57] For patients preparing to initiate dialysis in whom a CIED is recommended, it is suggested that the cardiologist, nephrologist, and primary physician review the risks and benefits of CIED therapy, anticipated vascular access requirements, dialysis modality and prognosis. From there, thorough vessel mapping is warranted via Doppler ultrasound or venography in advance of CIED placement, and CIED leads should be placed contralateral to the side of anticipated dialysis access. Among patients with an existing CIED, new AV access should be placed contralateral to the CIED. It is recommended that epicardial leads be considered in patients requiring a new CIED, or CIED lead replacement in order to avoid central venous stenosis.

In the setting of CIED-related central stenosis, PTA without stent placement is the preferred treatment and stent-entrapment of CIED leads should be avoided. Given the high risk of catheter-related blood stream infection, concurrent CIED and central venous catheter use should be avoided. Finally, it is recommended that wearable cardioverter defibrillators should be considered for patients at risk of sudden cardiac death, particularly in the setting of an infection preventing immediate CIED placement or in those transitioning from central venous catheter to use of an arteriovenous access.

CIED-RELATED INFECTION IN END-STAGE RENAL DISEASE PATIENTS

The severity of renal dysfunction is associated with an increased risk of CIED infection.[59] The number of ESRD patients hospitalized for CIED-related infection has increased over the past decade and is most recently estimated at 300.3 versus 6.1 hospitalizations per 100,000 persons compared with nondialysis groups, respectively.[60] Moreover, ESRD patients experience twofold greater in-hospital mortality following CIED infection-related hospitalization.[60]

Surgical Management of CIED-Related Infection

In a recent retrospective analysis of patients admitted to Mayo Clinic between 1991-2008, 415 patients were identified as having CIED infection, defined as the presence of presence of a pocket infection or bacteremia.[61] Of the 415 patients, 17 (4%) were hemodialysis patients; of these, 53% had a concurrent tunneled dialysis catheter in place. All HD patients presented with positive blood cultures, while pocket infections were more likely in non-HD patients. Further, HD patients were more likely to be diagnosed with CIED-infective endocarditis compared to those in the non-HD group (41% vs. 21%, respectively). The two leading pathogens were coagulase-negative staphlococci (29%) and methicillin-resistant staphylococcus aureus (29%).

The primary surgical approach to CIED infection in the HD patients was CIED removal (82%) and the success of device removal was similar between HD and

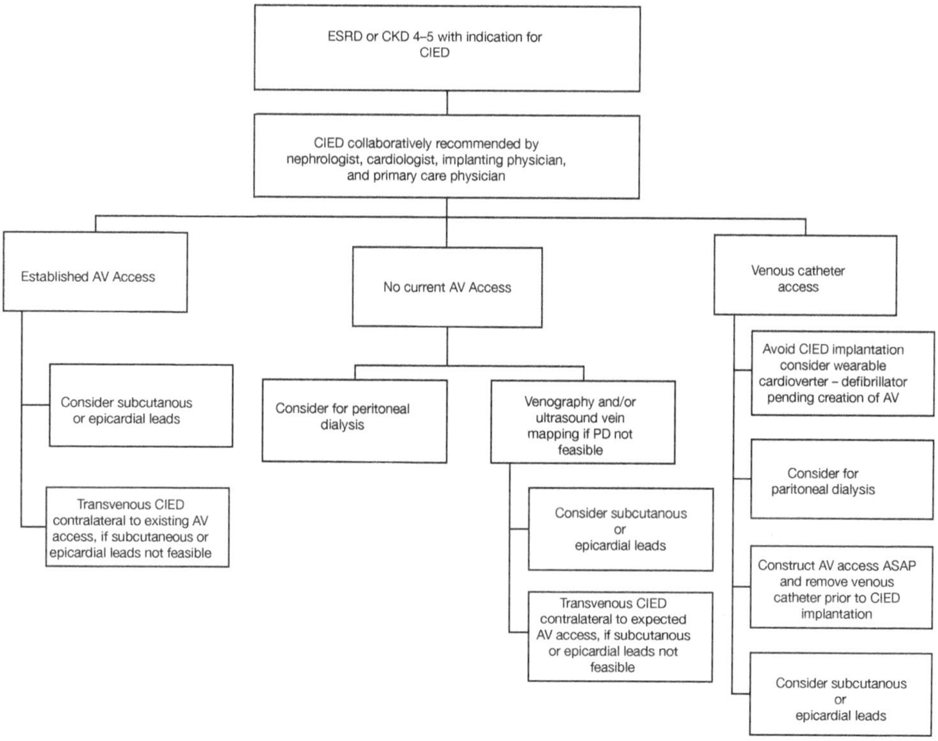

Figure 11-1. CIED Implantation in CKD stage 4–5 and ESRD patients. Modified from Figure 4 in Saad TF, Hentschel DM, Koplan B, et al.[57]

non-HD patients. By day 90 following diagnosis, 76% of HD patients survived vs. 92% non-HD patients, and by study end (average 2.2-year follow-up), 59% of HD patients died vs. 32% of non-HD patients, suggesting that mortality remains elevated in HD patients despite CIED-device removal.

CONCLUSIONS

CIED-associated central venous stenosis is best prevented through the careful selection of sites for transvenous CIED leads and ipsilateral placement to an existing or future AV access. This is best accomplished through close communication between the patient, nephrologist, cardiologist, interventionalist and access surgeon. CIED-related central stenosis may be avoided through surgical placement of subcutaneous or epicardial leads.

REFERENCES

1. Charytan DM, Patrick AR, Liu J, et al. Trends in the use and outcomes of implantable cardioverter-defibrillators in patients undergoing dialysis in the United States. *Am J Kidney Dis. The official journal of the National Kidney Foundation.* Sep 2011;58(3):409–17.

2. Herzog CA, Li S, Weinhandl ED, Strief JW, Collins AJ, Gilbertson DT. Survival of dialysis patients after cardiac arrest and the impact of implantable cardioverter defibrillators. *Kidney Int.* Aug 2005;68(2):818–25.
3. Sakhuja R, Keebler M, Lai TS, et al. Meta-analysis of mortality in dialysis patients with an implantable cardioverter defibrillator. *Am J Cardiol.* Mar 1 2009;103(5):735–41.
4. Nakhoul GN, Schold JD, Arrigain S, et al. Implantable cardioverter-defibrillators in patients with CKD: A propensity-matched mortality analysis. *Clinical journal of the American Society of Nephrology : CJASN.* Jul 7 2015;10(7):1119–27.
5. Asif A, Carrillo R, Garisto JD, et al. Epicardial cardiac rhythm devices for dialysis patients: Minimizing the risk of infection and preserving central veins. *Semin Dial.* Jan-Feb 2012;25(1):88–94.
6. da Costa SSD, Neto AS, Costa R, Caldas JG, Martinelli M. Incidence and risk factors of upper extremity deep vein lesions after permanent transvenous pacemaker implant: A 6-month follow-up prospective study. *Pace.* Sep 2002;25(9):1301–6.
7. Tan CS, Jie C, Joe J, et al. The impact of transvenous cardiac devices on vascular access patency in hemodialysis patients. *Semin Dial.* Nov-Dec 2013;26(6):728–32.
8. Oginosawa Y, Abe H, Nakashima Y. The incidence and risk factors for venous obstruction after implantation of transvenous pacing leads. *Pacing Clin Electrophysiol.* Nov 2002;25(11):1605–11.
9. Korkeila P, Nyman K, Ylitalo A, et al. Venous obstruction after pacemaker implantation. *Pacing Clin Electrophysiol.* Feb 2007;30(2):199–206.
10. Goto Y, Abe T, Sekine S, Sakurada T. Long-term thrombosis after transvenous permanent pacemaker implantation. *Pacing Clin Electrophysiol.* Jun 1998;21(6):1192–5.
11. Lickfett L, Bitzen A, Arepally A, et al. Incidence of venous obstruction following insertion of an implantable cardioverter defibrillator. A study of systematic contrast venography on patients presenting for their first elective ICD generator replacement. *Europace.* Jan 2004;6(1):25–31.
12. Sticherling C, Chough SP, Baker RL, et al. Prevalence of central venous occlusion in patients with chronic defibrillator leads. *Am Heart J.* May 2001;141(5):813–6.
13. Zuber M, Huber P, Fricker U, Buser P, Jager K. Assessment of the subclavian vein in patients with transvenous pacemaker leads. *Pacing Clin Electrophysiol.* Dec 1998;21(12):2621–30.
14. Haghjoo M, Nikoo MH, Fazelifar AF, Alizadeh A, Emkanjoo Z, Sadr-Ameli MA. Predictors of venous obstruction following pacemaker or implantable cardioverter-defibrillator implantation: A contrast venographic study on 100 patients admitted for generator change, lead revision, or device upgrade. *Europace.* May 2007;9(5):328–32.
15. Kalman PG, Lindsay TF, Clarke K, Sniderman KW, Vanderburgh L. Management of upper extremity central venous obstruction using interventional radiology. *Ann Vasc Surg.* May 1998;12(3):202–6.
16. Qanadli SD, El Hajjam M, Mignon F, et al. Subacute and chronic benign superior vena cava obstructions: Endovascular treatment with self-expanding metallic stents. *AJR Am J Roentgenol.* Jul 1999;173(1):159–64.
17. Slonim SM, Semba CP, Sze DY, Dake MD. Placement of SVC stents over pacemaker wires for the treatment of SVC syndrome. *J Vasc Interv Radiol.* Feb 2000;11(2 Pt 1):215-s9.
18. Grace AA, Sutters M, Schofield PM. Balloon dilatation of pacemaker induced stenosis of the superior vena cava. *Br Heart J.* Apr 1991;65(4):225–6.
19. Teo N, Sabharwal T, Rowland E, Curry P, Adam A. Treatment of superior vena cava obstruction secondary to pacemaker wires with balloon venoplasty and insertion of metallic stents. *Eur Heart J.* Sep 2002;23(18):1465–70.
20. Gilard M, Perennes A, Mansourati J, et al. Stent implantation for the treatment of superior vena cava syndrome related to pacemaker leads. *Europace.* Apr 2002;4(2):155–8.
21. Lanciego C, Rodriguez M, Rodriguez A, Carbonell MA, Garcia LG. Permanent pacemaker-induced superior vena cava syndrome: successful treatment by endovascular stent. *Cardiovasc Intervent Radiol.* Nov-Dec 2003;26(6):576–9.

22. Park HW, Kim W, Cho JG, Kang JC. Multiple pacing lead-induced superior vena cava syndrome: Successful treatment by balloon angioplasty. *J Cardiovasc Electrophysiol.* Feb 2005;16(2):221–3.
23. Lam YY, Chan JY. An unusual case of non-malignant superior vena cava obstruction. *Hong Kong Med J.* Jun 2006;12(3):232–4.
24. Chan AW, Bhatt DL, Wilkoff BL, et al. Percutaneous treatment for pacemaker-associated superior vena cava syndrome. *Pacing Clin Electrophysiol.* Nov 2002;25(11):1628–33.
25. Bolad I, Karanam S, Mathew D, John R, Piemonte T, Martin D. Percutaneous treatment of superior vena cava obstruction following transvenous device implantation. *Catheter Cardiovasc Interv.* May 2005;65(1):54–9.
26. Wilkoff BL, Love CJ, Byrd CL, et al. Transvenous lead extraction: Heart Rhythm Society expert consensus on facilities, training, indications, and patient management: This document was endorsed by the American Heart Association (AHA). *Heart Rhythm.* Jul 2009;6(7):1085–104.
27. Dasgupta A, Montalvo J, Medendorp S, et al. Increased complication rates of cardiac rhythm management devices in ESRD patients. *Am J Kid Dis.* 2007;49(5):656–63.
28. Voigt A, Shalaby A, Saba S. Rising rates of cardiac rhythm management device infections in the United States: 1996 through 2003. *J Am Coll Cardiol.* Aug 1 2006;48(3):590–1.
29. Teruya TH, Abou-Zamzam AM, Jr., Limm W, Wong L. Symptomatic subclavian vein stenosis and occlusion in hemodialysis patients with transvenous pacemakers. *Ann Vasc Surg.* Sep 2003;17(5):526–9.
30. Tourret J, Cluzel P, Tostivint I, Barrou B, Deray G, Bagnis CI. Central venous stenosis as a complication of ipsilateral haemodialysis fistula and pacemaker. *Nephrol Dial Transplant.* May 2005;20(5):997–1001.
31. Stone WJ, Wall MN, Powers TA. Massive upper extremity edema with arteriovenous fistula for hemodialysis. A complication of previous pacemaker insertion. *Nephron.* 1982;31(2):184–6.
32. Korzets A, Chagnac A, Ori Y, Katz M, Zevin D. Subclavian vein stenosis, permanent cardiac pacemakers and the haemodialysed patient. *Nephron.* 1991;58(1):103–5.
33. Deighan CJ, McLaughlin KJ, Simpson K, Jones JM. Unsuspected subclavian vein stenosis resulting from a permanent pacing wire. *Nephrol Dial Transplant.* Nov 1996;11(11):2333–4.
34. Cavatorta F, Campisi S, Zollo A. Subclavian vein stenosis: A potentially serious complication in chronic hemodialysis patients with permanent cardiac pacemakers. *Int J Artif Organs.* Jun 1997;20(6):316–8.
35. Chuang CL, Tarng DC, Yang WC, Huang TP. An occult cause of arteriovenous access failure: Central vein stenosis from permanent pacemaker wire. Report of three cases and review of the literature. *Am J Nephrol.* Sep-Oct 2001;21(5):406–9.
36. Konner K, Vorwerk D. Permanent pacemaker wires causing subclavian vein stenosis in presence of AV fistula—Is it ever wrong to try angioplasty and stenting? *Nephrol Dial Transplant.* Aug 1997;12(8):1735–8.
37. Bozzetti F, Scarpa D, Terno G, et al. Subclavian venous thrombosis due to indwelling catheters: A prospective study on 52 patients. *JPEN. J Parenter Enteral Nutr.* Nov-Dec 1983;7(6):560–2.
38. Schillinger F, Schillinger D, Montagnac R, Milcent T. Post catheterisation vein stenosis in haemodialysis: Comparative angiographic study of 50 subclavian and 50 internal jugular accesses. *Nephrol Dial Transplant.* 1991;6(10):722–4.
39. Hernandez D, Diaz F, Rufino M, et al. Subclavian vascular access stenosis in dialysis patients: Natural history and risk factors. *J Am Soc Nephrol.* Aug 1998;9(8):1507–10.
40. Barakat K, Hill J, Kelly P. Permanent transfemoral pacemaker implantation is the technique of choice for patients in whom the superior vena cava is inaccessible. *Pacing Clin Electrophysiol.* Apr 2000;23(4 Pt 1):446–9.
41. Mathur G, Stables RH, Heaven D, Ingram A, Sutton R. Permanent pacemaker implantation via the femoral vein: An alternative in cases with contraindications to the pectoral approach. *Europace.* Jan 2001;3(1):56–9.

42. Costa R, Filho MM, Tamaki WT, et al. Transfemoral pediatric permanent pacing: Long-term results. *Pacing Clin Electrophysiol.* Jan 2003;26(1 Pt 2):487–91.
43. Weinstein J, Gnoj J, Mazzara JT, Ayres SM, Grace WJ. Temporary transvenous pacing via the percutaneous femoral vein approach. A prospective study of 100 cases. *Am Heart J.* May 1973;85(5):695–705.
44. Ellestad MH, French J. Iliac vein approach to permanent pacemaker implantation. *Pacing Clin Electrophysiol.* Jul 1989;12(7 Pt 1):1030–3.
45. Garcia Guerrero JJ, De La Concha Castaneda JF, Fernandez Mora G, et al. Permanent transfemoral pacemaker: A single-center series performed with an easier and safer surgical technique. *Pacing Clin Electrophysiol.* Jul 2005;28(7):675–9.
46. National Kidney Foundation. KDOQI Clinical Practice Guidelines and Clinical Practice Recommendations for 2006 Updates: Hemodialysis adequacy, peritoneal dialysis adequacy and vascular access. *Am J Kid Dis.* 2006;48: S1–S322.
47. Leininger BJ, Neville WE. Use of the internal jugular vein for implantations of permanent transvenous pacemakers. Experiences with 22 patients. *Ann Thorac Surg.* Jan 1968;5(1):61–5.
48. Rao G, Zikria EA. Technique of insertion of pacing electrode through the internal jugular vein. *J Cardiovasc Surg (Torino).* May-Jun 1973;14(3):294.
49. Brodman R, Furman S. Pacemaker implantation through the internal jugular vein. *Ann Thorac Surg.* Jan 1980;29(1):63–5.
50. Alt E, Volker R, Blomer H. Lead fracture in pacemaker patients. *Thorac Cardiovasc Surg.* Apr 1987;35(2):101–4.
51. Cecchin F, Frangini PA, Brown DW, et al. Cardiac resynchronization therapy (and multisite pacing) in pediatrics and congenital heart disease: Five years experience in a single institution. *J Cardiovasc Electr.* Jan 2009;20(1):58–65.
52. Dodge-Khatami A, Johnsrude CL, Backer CL, et al. A comparison of steroid-eluting epicardial versus transvenous pacing leads in children. *J Card Surg.* Sep-Oct 2000;15(5):323–9.
53. Beaufort-Krol GC, Mulder H, Nagelkerke D, Waterbolk TW, Bink-Boelkens MT. Comparison of longevity, pacing, and sensing characteristics of steroid-eluting epicardial versus conventional endocardial pacing leads in children. *J Thorac Cardiovasc Surg.* Mar 1999;117(3):523–8.
54. Buiten MS, van der Heijden AC, Klautz RJ, Schalij MJ, van Erven L. Epicardial leads in adult cardiac resynchronization therapy recipients: A study on lead performance, durability, and safety. *Heart Rhythm.* Mar 2015;12(3):533–9.
55. Lewis GF, Gold MR. Clinical experience with subcutaneous implantable cardioverter-defibrillators. *Nature Rev Cardiol.* Jul 2015;12(7):398–405.
56. El-Chami MF, Levy M, Kelli HM, et al. Outcome of Subcutaneous Implantable Cardioverter Defibrillator Implantation in Patients with End-Stage Renal Disease on Dialysis. *J Cardiovasc Electrophysiol.* 2015;26(8):900–4.
57. Saad TF, Hentschel DM, Koplan B, et al. Cardiovascular implantable electronic device leads in CKD and ESRD patients: Review and recommendations for practice. *Semin Dial.* Jan-Feb 2013;26(1):114–23.
58. Saad TF, Myers GR, Cicone J. Central vein stenosis or occlusion associated with cardiac rhythm management device leads in hemodialysis patients with ipsilateral arteriovenous access: a retrospective study of treatment using stents or stent-grafts. *J Vasc Access.* 2010 Oct-Dec;11(4):293–302.
59. Tompkins C, McLean R, Cheng A, et al. End-stage renal disease predicts complications in pacemaker and ICD implants. *J Cardiovasc Electrophysiol.* Oct 2011;22(10):1099–104.
60. Opelami O, Sakhuja A, Liu X, et al. Outcomes of infected cardiovascular implantable devices in dialysis patients. *Am J Nephrol.* 2014;40(3):280–7.
61. Hickson LJ, Gooden JY, Le KY, et al. Clinical presentation and outcomes of cardiovascular implantable electronic device infections in hemodialysis patients. *Am J Kid Dis.* Jul 2014;64(1):104–10.

12

Drug-Coated Balloons in Dialysis Access

Syed M. Hussain, MD and Nikolous Karagiorgos, MD

End-stage renal disease (ESRD) is treated in a total of 600,000 patients in the United States annually. More than 120,000 patients are started dialysis every year. Hemodialysis and its associated procedures and interventions represent a significant burden to the healthcare system, and there is also a significant associated financial cost. The annual cost of the treatment of these ESRD patients is over $50 billion Medicare dollars.[1]

In considering all ESRD patients, 7% are on peritoneal dialysis, 30% undergo renal transplant, and 63% utilize hemodialysis. Where hemodialysis access (HD access) is concerned, 19% of patients are dialyzed with dialysis catheters, 63% utilize arteriovenous fistulas (AVFs), and 18% utilize arteriovenous grafts (AVGs). Over the past 20 years, there has been a significant shift from the use of AVGs to the use of AVSs. The primary patency of AVFs and AVGs varies and is reported at 48%–80% at 12 months, and at 50%–70% at 24 months.[2–4] Preserving the patency of the AVGs and AVFs is critical for the ESRD patient population.

In the United States, nearly 75,000 patients undergo chronic hemodialysis treatment using a prosthetic hemodialysis graft.[5] The majority of these patients develop neointimal hyperplastic stenosis at the venous outflow anastomosis and also along the vascular access circuit, often within the first year after graft placement.[6]

Balloon angioplasty remains the standard treatment for significant neointimal hyperplastic stenosis which results in clinically significant complications in both prosthetic hemodialysis grafts and autogenous AVFs.[7]

However, there is increasing clinical evidence that balloon angioplasty is not as effective as previously believed. The "reasonable goal" of 50% primary patency at six months, as stated in the 2006 Kidney Disease Outcomes Quality Initiative (KDOQI) Guidelines for Vascular Access, can oftentimes be difficult to achieve using angioplasty alone.[7] Although conventional therapies have prolonged access viability, primary patency rates leave much room for improvement. Percutaneous transluminal angioplasty (PTA) demonstrates a patency of 23%–72.8% at six months. Cutting balloon demonstrates a patency of 47.9% at six months. The placement of a bare-metal stent demonstrates a 39.3% patency at six months. The placement of a stent graft demonstrates a patency of 51%–53% at six months.

PATHOPHYSIOLOGY OF STENOSIS

When an AVF is created, a connection is made between a high-pressure arterial system and a low-pressure venous system. Vessel wall stress occurs at the outflow anastomosis and causes nitrous oxide release and venous dilation. In a favorable situation, the vein dilates and produces a usable fistula. However, high shear stress gradients and compliance mismatch can lead to endothelial cell damage and intimal hyperplasia. Traumatic balloon dilation of the venous outflow tract can contribute to this abnormal hyperplasia. Surgical injury, uremia, and traumatic needle insertion are also recognized causes and contributors to venous neointimal hyperplasia (NIH).

Histopathologists examining the juxta-anastomotic vein in the setting of AVF failure have described venous NIH and adverse vascular remodeling (venous constriction) as a likely cause of outflow stenosis.[8] It is not yet clear whether failure of maturation secondary to a juxta-anastomotic stenosis occurs secondary to adverse vascular remodeling (venous constriction) or intimal hyperplasia or a combination of both. Venous NIH is well recognized at the AVG-venous anastomosis and in mature fistulas with stenosis.

TYPES OF STENOSIS

Some lesions respond well to PTA and have relatively low restenosis rates, whereas other lesions (e.g., those at the cephalic arch, those involving surgical "swing points," or those at a polytetrafluoroethylene graft-venous anastomosis) have higher restenosis rates. Should treatment strategies for lesions with higher restenosis rates differ from lesions elsewhere?

Different appearances of AV access stenosis on ultrasound have been described. In 2012, Yamamoto et al. described three types of stenosis seen on ultrasound in the outflow vein of AVGs: a vascular constriction type, a neointimal proliferation type, and a third type that has features of both constriction and neointimal proliferation. The study involved 46 patients who underwent stent placement to treat AVG outflow vein stenosis. The primary patency rate of the treatment site at 6, 12, 18, and 24 months poststent placement for the vascular constriction type was 100.0%, 92.3%, 84.6%, and 75.2%, respectively. Those rates were 66.7%, 33.3%, 33.3%, and 25.0% for the neointimal proliferation type, and 90.5%, 52.4%, 38.1%, and 27.2% with the mixed type. Only the vascular constriction type displayed excellent primary patency rates after stent placement.[9]

Patency rates may vary depending on the type of stenosis (NIH vs. vascular constriction vs. a combination of both), but it is well recognized that patency rates vary according to the site of stenosis within the access circuit. For example, there are high recurrence rates for cephalic arch stenoses. The peri-anastomotic vein (the anastomotic and juxta-anastomotic vein) is an area that is typically treated with either PTA or surgery. A prospective study evaluating 112 PTA procedures demonstrated primary patency rates of 75%, 51%, and 41% at 6, 12, and 18 months, but secondary patency rates of 94%, 90%, and 90% at 6, 12, and 18 months, respectively.[9]

The cephalic arch is a region with both a high restenosis and rupture rate. Various treatment strategies have been applied, including PTA, cutting-balloon angioplasty, bare-metal stent placement, and stent graft placement. Higher primary patency rates have been demonstrated after stent graft implantation, but primary assisted patency rates are similar, with more intervention being noted in cases when PTA is used.[10]

High flow across the cephalic arch may determine the high stenosis rate, and flow reduction surgery is a recognized treatment of cephalic arch stenosis, reducing the number of PTA interventions.[11] The cephalic vein passes through the deltopectoral and claviculopectoral fascia, which may limit vein dilation or exert pressure. Whether these stenoses are secondary to a more fibrotic stenosis or venous intimal hyperplasia or a combination of both is unknown. The high pressure needed at inflation and the relatively higher rate of cutting-balloon use suggest a fibrotic stenosis; however, a high recurrence rate implies a process involving venous intimal hyperplasia with or without aggressive inflammation and fibrosis.[12]

WHAT HAPPENS AFTER BALLOON ANGIOPLASTY?

The main disadvantage of endovascular treatment for arterial atherosclerotic occlusive disease is clinical relapse due to NIH formation, induced mainly by barotrauma and inflammation following angioplasty. However, in dialysis access AVFs and AVGs, the pathophysiology of stenosis is different. Various mechanical and biochemical parameters contribute to continuous NIH proliferation. It is believed that ongoing NIH proliferation in AVFs and AVGs is due to nonphysiologic flow dynamics that develop when there is a direct anastomosis of a high-pressure arterial system into a low-pressure venous one. This arterial-to-venous flow circuit generates tangential wall and shear stress, compliance mismatch between arteries and veins, and flow turbulence throughout the circuit. The pathophysiology of vascular access stenosis includes smooth muscle cell (SMC) hyperplasia and angiotensin-mediated, NIH-related augmented pressure.

Studies from coronary arterial models have shown that angioplasty can cause endothelial and SMC injury, which results in migration of SMCs and myofibroblasts from the media to the intima where they proliferate, resulting in intimal hyperplasia.[13] There may be a difference in response to injury within an arterialized vein, and aggressive restenosis may be observed. There is evidence that fibroblasts migrate from the adventitia, given that adventitial-derived fibroblasts and myofibroblasts are seen in NIH at the AVG anastomosis.[14]

HOW CAN WE LOWER RESTENOSIS RATE?

Kim et al. demonstrated that venous SMCs are more sensitive to antiproliferative agents, for example, paclitaxel, when compared with arterial SMCs.[15]

A stent graft can resist elastic recoil, optimize luminal diameter, and provides a physical barrier to prevent restenosis by the offending lesion. These characteristics of stent grafts have made these appealing devices for treatment of neointimal hyperplastic stenoses. However, widespread acceptance of stent grafts has been tempered by the greater cost of the device when compared with balloon angioplasty. The use of stent grafts as the first treatment of all stenosis continues to be debated.[16]

A meta-analysis from University of Wisconsin compared the primary patency rates of stenotic vascular access treated with stent placement versus angioplasty. Ten studies with a total of 860 subjects met the inclusion criteria, including six experimental studies and four observational studies. There was significantly higher overall primary patency in those receiving stent placement than in those treated with angioplasty (pooled relative risk [RR] = 0.79; 95% confidence interval [CI]: 0.65–0.96). The estimate did not differ by study design. The effect of treatment differed significantly ($P = 0.001$) by the type of stents used, however. In studies including nitinol stents (six studies, 678 patients), six-month patency was significantly better for stent placement than angioplasty (pooled RR = 0.67; 95% CI: 0.54–0.84), whereas there was no significant differences between stent placement and angioplasty in those studies using bare-metal stents exclusively (four studies, 182 patients; pooled RR = 1.09; 95% CI: 0.91–1.32). There was significant heterogeneity between studies (I(2) = 70.6%; $P < 0.0001$). Our results suggest that stent placement may confer an advantage over balloon angioplasty in primary patency of dialysis access stenosis.[17]

A prospective, multicenter trial included 293 patients randomized (1:1) to the stent graft ($n = 145$) or balloon angioplasty ($n = 148$) group for treatment of stenosis at the venous anastomosis of dysfunctional ($n = 164$) or thrombosed ($n = 129$) hemodialysis grafts. The primary study end point was target lesion primary patency at six months; participants were followed for up to 24 months. Primary patency of the access circuit was a secondary end point. Statistical analysis of effectiveness was performed using both the intent-to-treat population and the effectiveness-per-protocol (EPP) populations for primary patency end points. The six-month target lesion primary patency was statistically greater in the stent graft group than the balloon angioplasty group (intent-to-treat, 51.6% vs. 34.2% [$P = 0.006$]; EPP, 52.9% vs. 35.5% [$P = 0.008$]). Compared with the angioplasty group, the stent graft group increased the median time from the index procedure to the next intervention on the target lesion by 95 days (203 vs. 108 days). Patients with dysfunctional (stenotic) grafts had higher target lesion primary patency compared with patients with thrombosed grafts regardless of treatment (EPP, stent graft, 64.6% vs. 36.1% and balloon angioplasty, 45.8% vs. 23.5%). When compared with angioplasty, using a stent graft for treatment of a venous anastomotic stenosis of a thrombosed graft increased the six-month target lesion primary patency by 53.6% (EPP, 36.1% vs. 23.5%).[18]

OVERVIEW OF DRUG-COATED BALLOONS

There are currently two FDA approved drug-coated balloons (DCBs) commercially available for use in the United States and worldwide. The Lutonix Balloon (BARD—Phoenix, AZ) and the IN.PACT Admiral Balloon (Medtronic—Minneapolis, MN). Both balloons use the same drug, paclitaxel, for their base. Paclitaxel is a lipophilic, cytotoxic agent that stabilizes tubulin polymers and prevents their disassembly, thereby halting the progression of mitosis from prophase to metaphase. The end result is that treated cells cannot divide. More specifically, paclitaxel halts SMC proliferation at the angioplasty site and reduces NIH.[19–20] Both balloons are 0.035 compatible systems and are available in 4–7 mm diameters and lengths ranging from 40 to 150 mm. Both are indicated for treatment in native superficial femoral and popliteal artery lesions including in stent restenosis in the lower extremities.

Although both balloons utilize paclitaxel as their drug of choice, the key difference involves the dosage of drug used and the excipient/coating on the balloon. Lutonix has a dosage of 2.0 ug/mm^2 and IN.PACT Admiral has a dosage of 3.5 ug/mm.[2] Sorbitol/polysorbate is the excipient of choice for the Lutonix balloon and urea is the excipient of choice for IN.PACT Admiral. Balloon surface excipients enable drug elution within the vessel wall, inhibiting cell proliferation and reducing NIH while avoiding the use of permanent bare metal or covered stents. Multicentered randomized trials for both balloon technologies have demonstrated efficacy in treatment of lower extremity peripheral vascular disease.[21] Outcomes have been different for the two trials which may be attributed to dosage of drug and the type of excipient utilized on the balloon. The paclitaxel from the IN.PACT balloon has been found in the media of blood vessels up to 180 days after drug delivery as compared to Lutonix which demonstrated drug concentration up to 60 days. Furthermore, the drug from the IN.PACT balloon stays in the media in the solid phase much longer than the Lutonix balloon, thus exerting its antiproliferative effects over a longer period of time as it solubilizes slowly and in a more controlled fashion. However, this discussion is beyond the scope of this chapter. Nevertheless, the outcomes from both trials have been favorable compared to conventional balloon angioplasty (CBA) in treatment of lower extremity femoral-popliteal lesions.

IS THERE A ROLE FOR DCBS IN AVF AND AVG STENOSIS?

The main disadvantage of endovascular treatment for arterial atherosclerotic occlusive disease is clinical relapse due to NIH formation, induced mainly by barotrauma and inflammation following angioplasty.[22] However, in dialysis access AVFs and AVGs, the pathophysiology of stenosis is different as discussed in an earlier section of this chapter. Mechanical and biochemical elements play a key role in this occurrence of stenosis.

Mechanical factors contribute to ongoing NIH, including repetitive needle punctures that can lead to both endothelial disruption and fibrotic wall changes. Biochemical mediators of NIH include endothelial dysfunction due to oxidative stress produced by chronic inflammation present in dialysis patients, as well as foreign body reaction (for AVGs).[23] Any or all of these factors lead to exaggerated fibromuscular neointimal proliferation—even without endothelial layer disruption. This type of NIH stenosis may have a technically satisfactory result following balloon dilation, but in general, most reports cite poor short-term plain balloon angioplasty and bare-metal stent patency rates in AV access treatment. Although the National Kidney Foundation's KDOQI guidelines suggest that angioplasty of AV access stenosis should yield at least a 50% six-month primary patency rate, reported primary patency rates from more-recent publications have found that this patency rate may be well below 50% at six months.[24]

While conventional therapies have prolonged HD access viability, primary patency rates leave much room for improvement. Plain old balloon angioplasty (POBA) patency rates can range anywhere between 23% and 72% at six months. However, average is considered to be approximately 30%. Bare-metal stents do not seem to improve this by much averaging 39.3% at six months. Cutting-balloon angioplasty yields about 47% at six months and covered stent grafts come in at 51%–53% patency at six months.[25] Based on these outcomes and the natural history of stenosis in AVF and AVG, it begs the question if DCB therapy can have an impact on the patency rates of stenotic lesions in HD access?

Multiple single center prospective experiences and single center randomized trials have shown significant benefit of treating these lesions with DCB therapy. Some have shown doubling or tripling of patency rates compared to CBA. (See Table 12-1 for all the details of the various studies.) When discussing HD access patency, patency is often measured in months as opposed to years when discussing lower extremity arterial interventions due to the nature of the stenosis involved in HD access. Katsanos et al. reported six-month patency results on a single center randomized trial comparing IN.PACT DCB to POBA in 40 patients with both AVF and AVG stenosis. Central veins were not included in the trial. Average lesion length was 5.7 cm. Patency rates at six months were 70% for DCB and 25% for POBA. Dialysis circuit rates were 65% patency for DCB and 20% for POBA. Interestingly, 55% of the patients required post-DCB high-pressure balloon angioplasty (HPBA) due to inadequate results achieved with DCB alone. Suffice it to say that DCB has showed promise over POBA.[26] Kitrou et al. also reported six-month primary patency results in a single center randomized trial comparing IN.PACT DCB to HPBA in 40 patients, 20 patients in each arm. Patency was measured in days with a median freedom from target lesion revascularization (TLR) was 308 days in DCB group and 161 days in HPBA group. Furthermore, dialysis circuit patency was 270 days in DCB group and 161 days in HPBA. Once again, 65% of patients in the DCB group required post-dilatation with a high-pressure balloon catheter due to unsatisfactory angiographic results.[27] Patane et al. performed a single center single arm trial with IN.PACT DCB on radiocephalic AVF only. Patency rates at six months were 96%, 12 months 91%, 24 months 58%.[28] Kitrou et al. most recently reported six-month patency results

TABLE 12-1. DEFINITIONS AND STATISTICAL METHODS ACROSS STUDIES MAY DIFFER

	Lutonix AV[1]	Katsanos[2,3]	Kitrou[4]	Patanè[5]	Kitrou[6]	Swinnen[7]
Study design	Multicenter, prospective, RCT (1:1)	Single center, prospective, RCT (1:1)	Single center, prospective, RCT (1:1)	Single center, prospective, single arm	Single center, retrospective	Single center, retrospective
Subject #	285	40	40	26	39	37
DCB	Lutonix™ 035 (Bard)	IN.PACT™ DCB (Medtronic)	IN.PACT™ DCB (Medtronic)	IN.PACT™ DCB (Medtronic)	Lutonix™ 035 (Bard)	IN.PACT™ DCB (Medtronic)
Lesion type	AVF	AVF/G	AVF	AVF	AVF/G	AVF ISR
Endpoints	NR	6-mo 1 Patency DCB: 70.0% PTA: 25.0%	Median FF TLR DCB: 308 days PTA: 161 days	6-mo Patency 1: 96.1% 2: 100%	6-mo 1 Patency: 72.2%	12-mo FF TLR DCB: 69% Non-DCB: 19%
Other follow-up	240-day 1 Patency DCB: 61.6% PTA: 49.4%	12-mo 1 Patency DCB: 35.0% PTA: 5.0%	Median circuit 1 Patency DCB: 270 days PTA: 161 days	12-mo Patency 1: 90.9% 2: 100% 24-mo Patency 1: 57.8% 2: 94.7%	Median access survival AVF:311 days AVG: 237 days	

NR = endpoint not reported; primary patency = 1; secondary patency = 2.

using the Lutonix DCB on AVF and AVG. This was a single center retrospective trial involving 39 patients. Results were favorable with 72% patency rates with DCB at six months favoring AVF versus AVG.[29] Clearly, these trials, albeit single center studies, demonstrated very encouraging results for use of DCB over CBA for treatment of HD access stenosis. Although AVG had less favorable results compared with AVF, they still showed significant improvement over CBA for the same types of lesions. Swinnen et al. went a step further to evaluate the use of DCB technology in in-stent restenosis of HD access. A total of 37 AVFs were evaluated of which none had any previous treatment with a DCB catheter. The IN.PACT DCB was utilized to look at 12-month outcomes free from reintervention on these restenotic stents. The patency rates were 69% for DCB arm versus 19% for non-DCB treatment. Thus, demonstrating superiority with DCB over CBA techniques.[30] These trials produced a platform demanding a more controlled and larger trial to see if there truly was a benefit in utilizing DCB technology in AV access stenosis.

The first prospective multicenter randomized study for AV access was performed most recently utilizing the Lutonix DCB catheter. Results of this study were presented in January 2017 at the LINC meeting in Leipzig, Germany. The study involved 23 global sites with 285 subjects enrolled with 1:1 randomization to PTA. Primary endpoints were six-month patency of target lesion and 30 day freedom from serious adverse events. Follow-up was conducted at 1, 3, 6, 9, 12, 18, and 24 months. Inclusion criteria consisted of fistula created greater than 30 days with more than one HD session, six needles utilized, and catheter removed for more than 30 days, lesion length of less than 10 cm and at least 50% stenosis, must have successful predilatation with HPBA, and vessel diameter between 4 and 12 mm. Exclusion criteria consisted of lower extremity access, access thrombosis, central vein involvement, greater than two lesions in a circuit, secondary nontarget lesion that cannot be treated, or presence of a bare or covered stent in the target lesion or secondary nontarget lesion. De novo lesions comprised 30% in the DCB arm and 27% in the PTA arm. Tandem lesion accounted for 2.8% in DCB and 7% in PTA. Target lesion length was 2.8 cm and 2.9 cm, respectively. Results at 240 days demonstrated favorable safety and efficacy for Lutonix DCB. The trial showed that DCB was noninferior to PTA. Target lesion primary patency was 61.6% for DCB versus 49.4% for CBA ($P = 0.02$). There were 29.8% fewer interventions needed to keep the HD access patent in the DCB arm versus the PTA arm.[31] The conclusion one can draw from this trial is that DCB shows significant promise for overcoming an Achilles heel in treatment of HD access stenosis. Limitations of this study are that patients enrolled had one or two target lesions not involving the central veins. Often times, patients will present with lesions not only within the cephalic or basilic vein component but also involving the subclavian and/or the brachiocephalic veins. The question is if the results would be impacted if both types of lesions were to be treated with DCB. Currently, there is limited to no data on central vein stenosis and use of DCB likely due to the limitation in balloon catheter diameter. Panagiotis et al. published a trial in Journal of Vascular Interventional Radiology in 2017 randomizing 40 patients to DCB or PTA for symptomatic central vein stenosis. Results were significantly favorable for DCB over PTA with freedom from intervention measured in days: DCB 179 days and PTA 129 days ($P = 0.02$). Again, these were single lesions treated in the central circulation. Nevertheless, these results provide for optimism in overcoming the myriad number of interventions often times required to prolong the viability of the HD access.

THE CHRISTIE CLINIC EXPERIENCE

DCB technology has definitely shown favorable results when treating lower extremity peripheral arterial disease. However, we were intrigued by the single center trials for AV access and the outcomes associated with those trials. This led us to study our own patient population. We looked at a snapshot small sample size to see what the outcomes may look like. We used the standard patency of ~30% at six months for the PTA arm in the literature to compare our outcomes. A prospective single arm nonrandomized study was performed utilizing the IN.PACT DCB in an outpatient Cath lab setting. A total of 22 patients were studied with 12 AVF and 10 AVG all of which had previous angioplasty procedures but no stent implantations and all involved the brachial artery as the conduit. Of the 12 AVFs, seven were brachio-cephalic and five were basilic vein transpositions. The 12 AVGs were all brachial-axillary vein heparin bonded polytetrafluoroethylene (PTFE) grafts. Primary endpoint was freedom from TLR at six months and dialysis circuit patency at six months. Follow-up was performed per protocol with a duplex ultrasound at six month intervals.

All types of lesions were included in the venous system including central veins. AV anastomotic lesions were excluded from the analysis. The 12 AVFs had 16 lesions that were as follows: (seven cephalic, five basilic, three subclavian, one brachiocephalic) and the 10 AVGs had 12 lesions that were as follows: (six graft-vein anastomosis, four mid-axillary vein, two subclavian vein). All of the lesions were predilated with a standard conventional balloon catheter prior to the use of DCB. The brachiocephalic vein was treated with a conventional balloon only since a DCB is not available in a size greater than 7 mm. The average diameter of the DCB was 6.4 mm. An average of 1.3 lesions were treated in each fistula/graft.

Freedom from TLR at six months for AVF was 56% (9/16 lesions) and 58% (7/12 lesions) for AVG. The dialysis circuit patency was 66% for AVF and 60% for AVG. Reinterventions were performed on four AVF within six months and two AVG. Two AVG thrombosed at six months and required declot therapy. No AVFs or AVGs were unsalvageable. Nevertheless, compared to standard PTA outcomes in the literature, these results were very encouraging. Clearly, this was a small sample size but definitely in line with other single center trials and the multicenter randomized Lutonix trial. Our practice has begun to adopt this as a first line therapy for all of our HD access stenoses. Since this analysis, we have implemented HPBA prior to DCB in all lesions. This was a limitation in our analysis as we did not have HPBA catheters available at the time in our outpatient Cath lab setting. Another limitation is the diameter of the currently available DCB catheters. The limited diameters render it difficult to treat some larger venous circuits. However, optimism hangs on as future trials will allow for these larger DCB catheters to be available commercially.

FUTURE DIRECTIONS

Multiple new trials are currently underway regarding HD access and the role of DCB in treating those lesions. Currently, Medtronic is starting the IN.PACT Admiral AV access trial which is set to begin enrollment second half of 2017. The purpose of the trial is to evaluate the safety and efficacy of the IN.PACT Admiral DCB catheter in de novo or nonstented restenotic lesions of the native AVF in the upper extremity.

It is a prospective, global, multicenter, randomized, single-blinded study involving 30 global sites with a 330 patient enrollment. There will be a 24-month follow-up with 1:1 randomization and lesions up to 10 cm in length. The primary safety endpoint is to look at 30 day serious adverse event rate and primary efficacy endpoint is to look at six month freedom from clinically driven TLR and six-month thrombosis rate postprocedure.

In addition, multiple other trials around the world are also looking at obtaining data on this matter: the Paclitaxel-coated balloon fistuloplasty versus plain balloon fistuloplasty only to preserve the patency of AVF used for hemodialysis (PAVE) trial, which is a randomized trial in the United Kingdom, a randomized trial evaluating cephalic arch stenosis in Israel, the APERTO trial in the Netherlands, which is a randomized controlled trial of paclitaxel drug eluting balloon compared to standard PTA in dialysis fistulas, and the FISBAL randomized trial in Spain which is looking at primary patency in postangioplasty dysfunctional AVF in renal dialysis: paclitaxel-releasing PTA balloon catheter versus PTA balloon.

These trials will help to amass enough randomized data to show if DCB technology will be a favorable player for treatment of HD access stenosis. With ongoing changes in health care and concerns for both cost and outcomes looming over every physician, minimizing the number of interventions will become paramount. DCB has shown early on to be a potential tool to help accomplish that end in this difficult patient population. With the encouraging results from the Lutonix AV study and many other randomized trials underway, the maintenance of HD access will become more palatable for the patients, physicians, and payors going forward.

REFERENCES

1. Saran R, Robinson B, Abbott KC, et al. US Renal Data System 2016 Annual Data Report: epidemiology of kidney disease in the United States. *Am J Kidney Dis.* 2017;69:S1–S688.
2. Al-Jaishi AA, Oliver MJ, Thomas SM, et al. Patency rates of the arteriovenous fistula for hemodialysis: a systematic review and meta-analysis. *Am J Kidney Dis.* 2014;63:464–478.
3. Lumsden AB, MacDonald MJ, Kikeri D, Cotsonis GA, Harker LA, Martin LG. Prophylactic balloon angioplasty fails to prolong the patency of expanded polytetrafluoroethylene arteriovenous grafts: results of a prospective randomized study. *J Vasc Surg.* 1997;26:382–390.
4. Munda R, First MR, Alexander JW, Linnemann CC Jr, Fidler JP, Kittur D. Polytetrafluoroethylene graft survival in hemodialysis. *J Am Med Assoc.* 1983;249:219–222.
5. United States Renal Data System. 2015 USRDS annual data report: epidemiology of kidney disease in the United States. Paper presented at: National Institute of Diabetes and Digestive and Kidney Diseases; 2015; Bethesda, MD: National Institutes of Health.
6. Kanterman RY, Vesely TM, Pilgram TK, Guy BW, Windus DW, Picus D. Dialysis access grafts: anatomic location of venous stenosis and results of angioplasty. *Radiology.* 1995;195:135–139.
7. National Kidney Foundation. NKF-KDOQI clinical practice guidelines for vascular access. *Am J Kidney Dis.* 2006;48:S176–S275.
8. Roy-Chaudhury P, Sukhatme V, Cheung A. Hemodialysis vascular access dysfunction: a cellular and molecular viewpoint. *J Am Soc Nephrol.* 2006;17:1112–1127.
9. Yamamoto Y, Nakamura J, Nakayama Y, Hino H, Kobayashi H, Sugiura T. Relationships between the outcomes of stent placement and the properties of arteriovenous graft outflow vein stenotic lesions. *J Vasc Access.* 2012;13:426–431.

10. Sivanathan G, Menashe L, Halin NJ. Cephalic arch stenosis in dialysis patients: review of relevance, anatomy, current theories on etiology and management. *J Vasc Access.* 2014;15:157–162.
11. Miller GA, Freidman A, Khariton A, Preddie DC, Savransky Y. Access flow reduction and recurrent symptomatic cephalic arch stenosis in brachiocephalic hemodialysis arteriovenous fistulas. *J Vasc Access.* 2010;11:281–287.
12. Steiner K. Pathophysiology of stenosis within AV fistulas and mechanisms of PTA. *Endovasc Today.* 2016;15(6):28–32.
13. Nobuyoshi M, Kimura T, Ohishi H, et al. Restenosis after coronary angioplasty: a proposal of new comparative approaches based on quantitative angiography. *J Am Coll Cardiol.* 1991;17:433–439.
14. Roy-Chaudhury P, Sukhatme V, Cheung A. Hemodialysis vascular access dysfunction: a cellular and molecular viewpoint. *J Am Soc Nephrol.* 2006;17:1112–1127.
15. Kim SJ, Masaki T, Leypoldt JK, Kamerath CD, Mohammad SF, Cheung AK. Arterial and venous smooth-muscle cells differ in their responses to antiproliferative drugs. *J Lab Clin Med.* 2004;144:156–162.
16. Kerlan RK, LaBerge JM. Fistula first, stent graft second. *N Engl J Med.* 2010;362:6.
17. Fu N, Joachim E, Yevzlin, Shin JI, Astor BC, Chan MR. A meta-analysis of stent placement vs. angioplasty for dialysis vascular access stenosis. *Semin Dial.* 2015;28(3):311–317.
18. Vesely T, DaVanzo W, Behrend T, Dwyer A, Aruny J. Balloon angioplasty versus Viabahn stent graft for treatment of failing or thrombosed prosthetic hemodialysis grafts. *J Vasc Surg.* 2016;64(5):1400–1410.
19. Krokidis M, Spiliopoulos S, Katsanos K, Sabharwal T. Peripheral applications of drug-coated balloons: past, present and future. *Cardiovasc Intervent Radiol.* 2013;36:281–291.
20. Portugaller RH, Kalmar PI, Deutschmann H. The eternal tale of dialysis access vessels and restenosis: are drug-eluting balloons the solution? *J Vasc Access.* 2014;15:439–447.
21. Diskin CJ. Novel insights into the pathobiology of the vascular access: do they translate into improved care? *Blood Purif.* 2010;29:216–229.
22. Lee JM, Park J, Kang J, et al. Comparison among drug-eluting balloon, drug-eluting stent, and plain balloon angioplasty for the treatment of in-stent restenosis: a network meta-analysis of 11 randomized, controlled trials. *JACC Cardiovasc Interv.* 2015;8(3):382–394.
23. Bittl JA. Catheter interventions for hemodialysis fistulas and grafts. *JACC Cardiovasc Interv.* 2010;3:1–11.
24. Aftab SA, Tay KH, Irani FG, et al. Randomized clinical trial of cutting balloon angioplasty versus high-pressure balloon angioplasty in hemodialysis arteriovenous fistula stenosis resistant to conventional balloon angioplasty. *J Vasc Interv Radiol.* 2014;25:190–198.
25. Haskal Z, Trerotola S, Dolmatch B, et al. Stent graft versus balloon angioplasty for failing dialysis-access grafts. *N Engl J Med.* 2010;362:494–503.
26. Katsanos K, Karnabatidis D, Kitrou P, et al. Paclitaxel-coated balloon angioplasty for symptomatic central vein restenosis in patients with hemodialysis fistulas. *J Endovasc Ther.* 2012;19:263–272.
27. Kitrou PM, Spiliopoulos S, Katsanos K. Paclitaxel-coated versus plain balloon angioplasty for dysfunctional arteriovenous fistulae: one-year results of a prospective randomized controlled trial. *J Vasc Interv Radiol.* 2015;15:348–354.
28. Patane D, Giuffrida S, Morale W, et al. Drug-eluting balloon for the treatment of failing hemodialytic radiocephalic arteriovenous fistkaulas: our experience in the treatment of juxta-anastomotic stenosis. *J Vasc Access.* 2014;15:338–343.
29. Kitrou P, Spiliopoulos S, Papadimatos P, et al. Paclitaxel-coated balloons for the treatment of dysfunctional dialysis access. Results from a single-center, retrospective analysis. *Cardiovasc Intervent Radiol.* 2017;40:50–54.
30. Swinnen JJ, Zahid A, Burgess DC. Paclitaxel drug-eluting balloons to recurrent in-stent stenoses in autogenous dialysis fistulas: a retrospective study. *J Vasc Access.* 2015;16:388–392.
31. Treretola SO. *Lutonix AV Clinical Trial.* Liepzig, Germany: LINC; January 2017.

13

HeRO Grafts in Patients with Central Vein Occlusions: When and How to Incorporate Them in Your Practice

Virginia L. Wong, MD

Central venous obstruction (CVO), whether due to high grade stenosis or occlusion, is a frequently encountered condition in end-stage renal disease (ESRD) patients who rely on hemodialysis (HD) as their form of renal replacement therapy. With over half a million prevalent ESRD patients in the United States, reported CVO rates of 11–40% affect a large number of patients in this population.[1] The HeRO graft is a technology devised to circumvent the problem that CVO presents for construction and maintenance of functioning HD access in ESRD patients. While data are available to describe the clinical use of HeRO and expected outcomes, these are mainly retrospective reviews and case series, which do not provide definitive answers as to where HeRO grafts belong in the HD access algorithm. Further, there are specific anatomic and physiologic considerations when considering HeRO implantation, and the monitoring and maintenance of these devices differs a bit from that of conventional arteriovenous fistula (AVF) or arteriovenous graft (AVG). An understanding of these particulars can help a dedicated access surgeon incorporate HeRO grafts into a practice where such challenging patients are frequently encountered.

CENTRAL VENOUS OBSTRUCTION

The principal risk factor for development of CVO appears to be the use of indwelling central venous catheters. While CVO is also reported to occur with smaller catheters such as implanted ports or peripherally inserted central catheters (PICC lines), for the ESRD population the tunneled hemodialysis catheter (TDC) is the chief culprit. Unfortunately, TDC use has increased in recent years, partly due to the large number of incident patients who begin HD with a catheter and a greater emphasis on construction of AVF, which have a higher primary failure rate and longer maturation period than AVG, thus prolonging the need for bridging TDC.

Patients with CVO often remain asymptomatic, as compensatory collateral venous drainage is usually sufficient to drain the limb. However patients with a patent AVF or AVG have a much greater volume of blood flow returning to the central veins and may experience severe manifestations when venous drainage becomes sufficiently impeded. Diminished access flow and dialysis clearance, cannulation difficulties, prolonged cannulation site bleeding, progressive access aneurysm enlargement, or access thrombosis may occur. Typical symptoms of upper extremity CVO include ipsilateral limb, face, neck or breast edema; development of large shoulder and cervical varicose veins; ipsilateral hearing loss.[2]

Traditional treatment for symptomatic CVO that also preserves the AVF or AVG includes percutaneous transluminal balloon angioplasty (PTA), with or without stenting, and often results in satisfactory initial results, with improved access function and symptom relief. However, recurrence is common. Repeat intervention to maintain sufficient venous drainage is the rule, rather than the exception, and will be required at varying intervals throughout the remainder of the life of the access. In some cases, where access patency cannot be maintained or adequate symptom relief cannot be achieved due to CVO, ligation or abandonment of the access becomes necessary and the limb cannot be used for subsequent conventional AVF or AVG. CVO that affects drainage from both upper extremities results in abandonment of the arms for further arteriovenous access, leaving femoral access as the only option before catheter dependence. However, CVO can also affect the lower extremities, where disease in the iliac veins or the inferior vena cava (IVC) causes similar problems for femoral AVF or AVG, such as lower limb edema, genital and lower extremity varicosities, poor access function or thrombosis.

HeRO GRAFT AND THE HD ACCESS ALGORITHM

In 2008, the Hemodialysis Reliable Outflow (HeRO) graft (Merit Medical, South Jordan, UT) was introduced and approved by the United States Food and Drug Administration (FDA) for use in patients with CVO. This unique device combines a standard expanded polytetrafluoroethylene (ePTFE) graft component with an entirely internalized central venous catheter component to direct venous return beyond any CVO that would preclude use of a conventional AVG configuration (Figure 13-1). The obvious benefit of such a device is the ability to use a limb for HD access that previously would have been abandoned because of inadequate venous drainage due to CVO. However the exact place that HeRO grafts should occupy in the access algorithm has not been well established, leaving the decision to proceed with HeRO up to provider experience and judgment.

ESRD patients who are considered for HeRO implantation typically have had numerous prior AVF and AVG and no further conventional upper extremity access options due to CVO. Such patients may still have a femoral option for AVF or conventional femoral AVG (fAVG), and as such may not yet have exhausted every option or be truly catheter-dependent for HD access. However, the available data have not established

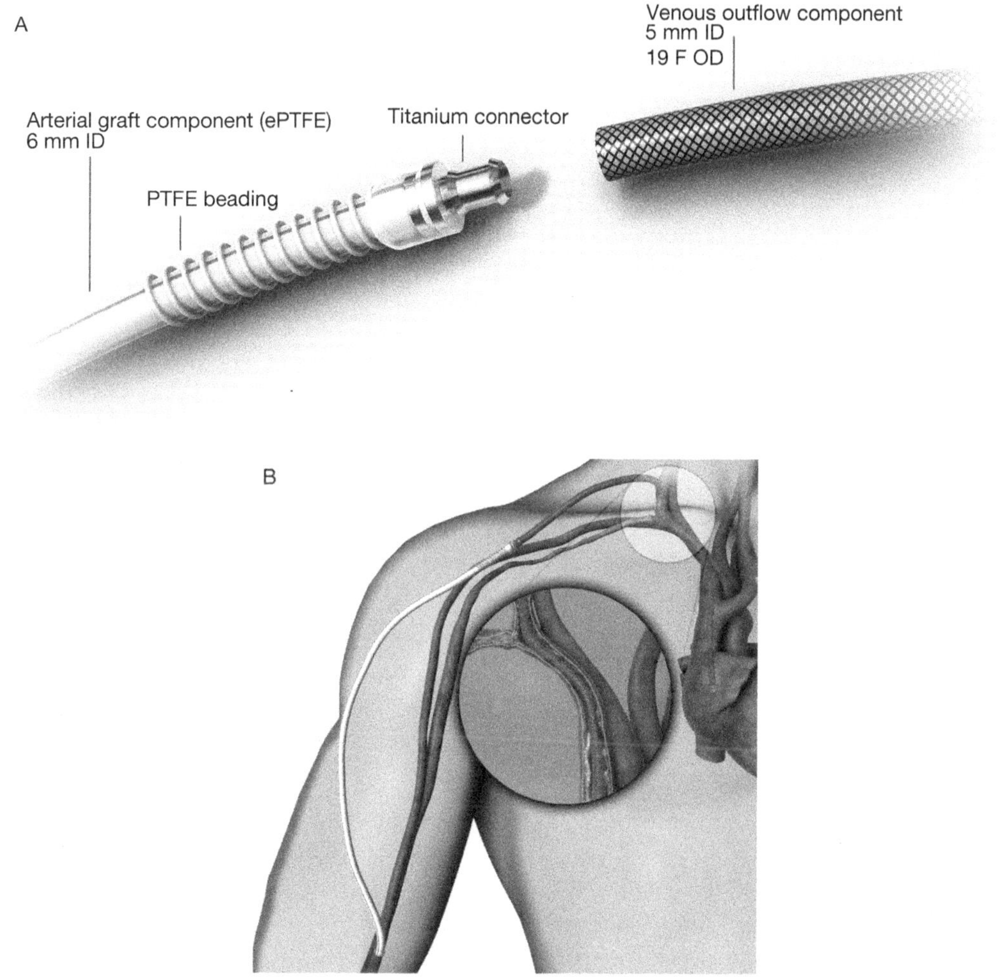

Figure 13-1. (**A**) Hemodialysis Reliable Outflow (HeRO) Graft components. *ePTFE*, Expanded polytetrafluroethylene; *ID*, internal diameter; *OD*, outer diameter. (Merit Medical; reprinted by permission.) (**B**) Depiction of HeRO graft implanted in a standard configuration. Arterial inflow is from the brachial artery and the venous outflow component is inserted via the right IJ vein. (Merit Medical; reprinted by permission.)

definitively the next best step for such patients: upper extremity HeRO or femoral access? Two retrospective studies directly comparing HeRO to fAVG showed similar 12-month secondary patency and similar rates of infection. Differences in re-intervention rates were noted between HeRO and fAVG in one study,[3] but not in the other.[4]

A recently published review of the literature regarding the use of HeRO in clinical practice sought to summarize outcomes across multiple relevant publications.[5] Pooled mean 1-year secondary patency was 59% for HeRO, which is fair, but lower than a literature reported secondary patency rate of 62–76% for conventional upper extremity AVG, and far lower than established patency rates for upper extremity AVF. HeRO-related bacteremia ranged from 0.13–0.7 per 1000 implant days, compared to a reported 2.3 infections per 1000 implant days for TDC.[8] Pooled re-intervention rate was 1.5–3.0 procedures per year for HeRO, compared to a TDC re-intervention rate of 5.8 per year (Table 13-1).

TABLE 13-1. SUMMARY OF HeRO OUTCOMES FROM EIGHT STUDIES[a]

Reference	Number of HeRO	Early failure rate (%)	Primary Patency rate (%)	Secondary Patency rate (%)	Dialysis access associated steal syndrome (%)	HeRO graft infection (%)	HeRO related bacteraemia per 1000 days	Rate of intervention per year	Mean time with HeRO (d/patient)
Katzman[5]	38	2.6	38.9[b]	72.2[b]	2.6	2.6	0.7	2.5	276
Gage[6]	164	NS	48.8	90.8	1.4	NS	0.14	1.5	NS
Steerman[7]	60	NS	15	57	1.7	22	0.61	2.2	NS
Kokkosis[8]	12	8.3	9.1	45.5	NS	25	NS	1.5	NS
Wallace[9]	21	14	11	32	22.2	NS	0.5	3	186
Nassar[10]	52	3.8	34.8	67.6	3.8	3.8	0.13	2.2	238
Kudlaty[11]	20	30	29	53.5	4.8	10	0.53	1.7	238
Torrent[12]	41	NS	8.4	53.7	NS	NS	NS	2.8	380
Weighed Pooled rate % (95% CI)		9.2 (1.9–19.9)	21.9[c] (9.6–37.2)	59.4[c] (39.4–78.0)	6.3(1–14.7)	10.1 (2.5–21)			

NS = not specified
[a] Studies reviewed by Al Shakarchi et al.[5] Reproduced with permission from the *European Journal of Vascular and Endovascular Surgery*.
[b] 8.6 months rates.
[c] Pooled rate excluding Katzman et al paper.

These data suggest that conventional upper extremity options should be exhausted before moving on to alternative access modalities, and that either HeRO or femoral access should be considered before deeming a patient catheter-dependent. The experience with HeRO so far also indicates that factors specific to patient anatomy and physiology should be taken into account when deciding if HeRO is an appropriate next step for that individual.

CENTRAL VENOUS ACCESS

Implantation of a HeRO graft requires large bore access to the central venous system. The venous outflow component (19 Fr OD) is intended to be sited with its exit at the superior vena cava (SVC)-right atrium junction. Passage of this component may require balloon venoplasty during insertion past a stenotic venous segment or may be achieved by exchanging out an existing large bore hemodialysis catheter. If no wire traversal can be achieved across complete central venous obstruction, however, or if the pathway cannot be dilated sufficiently to allow passage of the HeRO venous outflow component into a central vein with adequate outflow, then HeRO graft cannot be used. Investigation of central venous patency or ability to traverse the venous anatomy may require pre-operative venography and attempts at wire traversal.

INFLOW AND ARTERIAL CONSIDERATIONS

HeRO is a low resistance circuit, largely due to lack of a venous anastomosis. This accounts for a less prominent thrill over the HeRO AVG, resulting in the recommendation to listen for a bruit when determining if the access is patent. Often, a thrill remains strong over the arterial anastomosis, where energy loss remains high due to changes in resistance and flow direction. Early reports cautioned about the risk of steal syndrome with HeRO,[6] though the subsequently published pooled steal rate was a modest 6.3%.[5] As with any ESRD patient, the presence of severe or extensive arterial disease and other risk factors for steal must be taken into account when planning laterality, type, and position of access to minimize the risk of distal ischemia. HeRO grafts are long conduits and may total more than 50 cm from the inflow artery to the right atrium. Thus, they tend to thrombose if adequate flow volume is not maintained. Manufacturer instructions for use (IFU) recommend using an inflow artery > 3 mm diameter in patients with left ventricular ejection fraction (LVEF) > 20% and the ability to maintain systolic blood pressure (sBP) greater than 100 mmHg for HeRO graft patency.[7] Consideration could be given to maintaining even higher sBP for HeRO coming from the left upper extremity, which requires a longer circuit. This last criteria can be challenging for ESRD patients, many of whom experience significant hypotensive episodes during dialysis sessions, or who are relatively hypotensive for a period of time afterwards. Even patients who initially lost their renal function due to hypertension may experience refractory hypotension after a number of years on dialysis. Examining recent dialysis run sheets and anti-hypertensive medication regimens can help screen out patients who would be poor candidates for HeRO based on insufficient systolic blood pressure or help identify those in whom maintaining HeRO patency may be a challenge. The use of midodrine hydrochloride in appropriate patients can be helpful and requires consultation and communication with the patient's nephrologist.

AVOIDING BRIDGING CATHETERS

By the time patients come to consideration for HeRO, they have had multiple prior AVF or AVG and many are dialyzing through a catheter. While HeRO may be useful for delaying progression to long-term catheter-dependence, limiting the number of current catheter days should be part of any access plan. For many HeRO patients, the existing hemodialysis catheter also represents the best pathway into the vena cava. During the early HeRO experience, use of an existing catheter for HeRO central venous access required the insertion of a bridging hemodialysis catheter in a different location for use until the newly implanted HeRO arterial graft component could be cannulated, usually two to three weeks later. Given bilateral upper extremity CVO, many of these patients required femoral TDC with a high rate of infection associated with that bridging catheter.[8] For some patients, the existing hemodialysis catheter is the only access to the central venous system and no additional sites exist through which to place a bridging catheter. Immediate- or early-use PTFE grafts (e.g., Gore Acuseal Vascular Graft, W.L. Gore & Assoc, Inc, Flagstaff, AZ and Flixene Graft, Atrium Medical Corp, Hudson, NH) have been in use for conventional AVG configurations, and surgeons are using them to avoid or limit the need for bridging catheters after HeRO insertion.[9–11] The technique replaces the standard HeRO ePTFE arterial graft component with an early-use PTFE graft. However, as the titanium connector remains permanently affixed to the standard HeRO ePTFE arterial graft component, this graft is transected a few centimeters from the titanium connector, near the termination of the ridged, PTFE beading. A length of early-use PTFE is then anastomosed to the remaining stump of standard ePTFE graft, preserving the titanium connector for insertion into the venous outflow component. Tunneling of the early-use PTFE graft and construction of the arterial anastomosis is per routine.

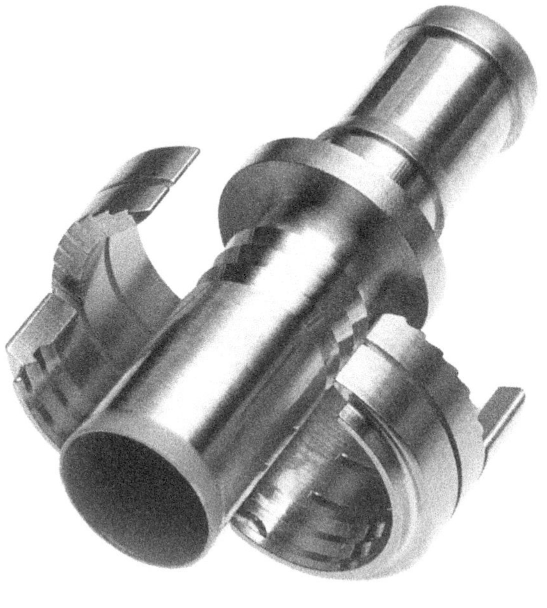

Figure 13-2. HeRO Adapter (due for release late 2016). This component is designed to allow mating of the HeRO venous outflow component with alternative ePTFE grafts, including early-use grafts intended for cannulation soon after implantation. (Merit Medical; reprinted by permission.)

The advantages of such a modification in HeRO insertion technique are clear. Disadvantages include the presence of an anastomotic graft-to-graft suture line and increased time for device implantation. Merit Medical intends US release (late 2016) of an adapter and support seal piece that will allow the HeRO venous outflow component to mate with alternative PTFE grafts, including an early-use variety, without the need for an additional suture line (Figure 13-2). This should further facilitate avoidance of bridging catheters in patients receiving or requiring revision of a HeRO graft.[12]

HeRO AND SALVAGE (RESCUE) OF EXISTING ACCESS

The HeRO graft can also be useful for salvage of HD access that remains functional, but which is failing or threatened by intractable CVO.[13] Insertion of the HeRO venous outflow component bypasses arteriovenous flow beyond the CVO, while the HeRO ePTFE arterial component with its titanium connector can be anastomosed to the existing AVF or AVG, thus preserving the previously incorporated access for continued cannulation (Figure 13-3). This technique not only reduces or eliminates symptoms of CVO, but it also preserves the limb and site for HD access and avoids the need for a bridging catheter. For the patient with no further upper extremity access options, preservation of the remaining upper extremity is a desirable goal. However, it is less clear whether HeRO should be used to salvage an existing access that is failing due to ipsilateral CVO if the contralateral upper extremity remains available for conventional access and is not affected by CVO. The available data regarding patency, infection, and re-intervention suggest that HeRO would not be superior to a functioning

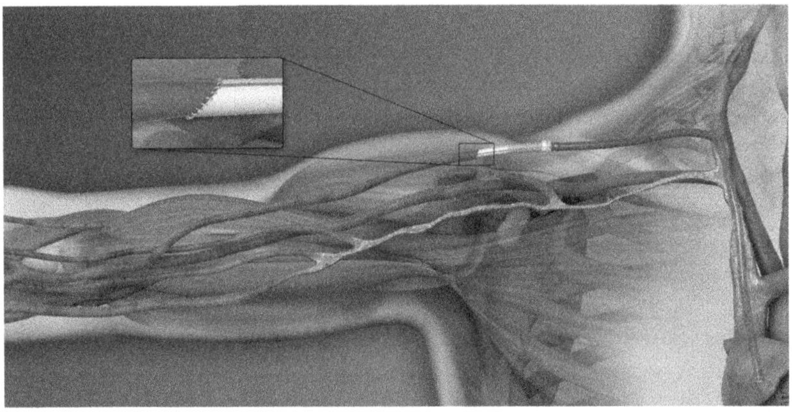

Figure 13-3. Depiction of HeRO used for salvage (rescue) of existing AV fistula. Truncated HeRO arterial graft component anastomosed to terminal AV fistula (inset) and venous outflow component inserted via right IJ vein. (Merit Medical; reprinted by permission.)

contralateral upper extremity AVF or AVG. Further, it is not known if the HeRO venous outflow component contributes to SVC stenosis that jeopardizes venous return from the opposite side, as can be the case with other types of central venous catheters. Therefore, until data are available to guide this decision process further, individual factors such as the desire to preserve a particular site for HD access, the estimated amount of time before complete failure of the current access, and how much time before a contralateral access could become functional must be taken into account.

UNUSUAL HeRO CONFIGURATIONS

In most patients, femoral access is avoided for a number of reasons including fewer fistula options, higher risk of surgical incisional complications, a higher associated infection rate than upper extremity access, risk of distal limb ischemia in patients with increased prevalence of peripheral artery disease (PAD), and the need to disrobe more fully at the dialysis unit. Femoral catheters are particularly undesirable in patients who still have a femoral AVF or AVG option or who are renal transplant candidates, due to the risk of iliac vein and inferior vena cava (IVC) thrombosis and stenosis (i.e., lower extremity CVO). In patients who have truly exhausted upper extremity access options, however, femoral AVF or AVG would be preferable to catheter dependence. If conventional femoral AVF or AVG are affected by CVO, use of a HeRO via the common femoral vein may be helpful to preserve the site. Femoral HeRO grafts have been included in most published series, though they constitute a minority of the patient cohort, and no particular outcomes appear attributable to their location when compared to upper extremity HeRO. The tip of the venous outflow component can be positioned so that it lies just beyond the CVO, shortening the HeRO circuit and potentially limiting the risk of caval thrombosis, which would impair venous drainage from both lower limbs and further limit access options. Another consideration is to preserve sufficient central veins for a future renal transplant, if that option remains available for the patient. In some cases, the IVC may be employed for renal allograft venous outflow, provided that sufficient renal venous conduit or extension can be achieved.

Another alternative HeRO configuration has been described for salvage of existing HD access using the contralateral central veins for outflow.[14] In these cases, preservation of the existing access was desired, however there was no opportunity for access to the SVC from the same side. Therefore, the HeRO venous outflow component was implanted from the contralateral IJ vein and tunneled subcutaneously across the upper chest, where the HeRO arterial graft component and titanium connector were sewn to the existing AVF or AVG for inflow. Such a configuration necessarily lengthens the circuit by a significant amount, potentially jeopardizing patency, however could still be useful for immediate access salvage and without any need for a bridging catheter. As outlined in the section above, it is not clear that this is preferable over contralateral upper extremity access if that option exists, but this could be a helpful technique in cases where the opposite arm is not available for reasons other than CVO.

MAINTENANCE, THROMBECTOMY, AND REVISION

Once implanted, a HeRO graft behaves much like any other implanted AVG. The patient, other providers, and dialysis unit staff should be made aware that the patient has a HeRO and be familiar with the patient's specific configuration. The venous outflow component is visible by various radiographic imaging modalities, and is MRI compatible within limits.[7] As described above, a thrill may be less prominent, but is usually detectable over the arterial anastomosis; a bruit should be audible as long as the HeRO graft remains patent. Any change in the strength or character of the thrill compared to a prior baseline may warrant further evaluation. Regular monitoring of HeRO graft performance and function, as with any other type of HD access, may reveal flow disturbances or signs of impending failure. As is the case with conventional AVG, HeRO grafts can develop inflow stricture at the arterial anastomosis or in the inflow artery, as well as strictures at the cannulation areas. However, as the HeRO has no venous anastomosis (the Achilles heel of conventional AVG), outflow stenosis generally does not occur in a HeRO graft, whose terminal outflow is in the vena cava. Routine endovascular techniques can be used for treatment of inflow and cannulation area strictures.

Published series have clearly established that HeRO grafts may undergo successful thrombectomy using routine techniques, thus achieving the reasonably acceptable secondary patency rates that have been reported. There are some specific considerations during thrombectomy of the HeRO venous outflow component, thus the interventionalist needs to be aware that the patient has a HeRO graft and should be comfortable with that prior to proceeding. The venous outflow component is not fixed within the vena cava and excessive manipulation or traction with balloon catheters and other devices can dislodge or alter the position of the tip. Larger volumes of thrombus can collect within the long length of a thrombosed HeRO graft, potentially exposing the patient to significant pulmonary embolism during thrombectomy procedures. In cases where prolonged hypotension was the suspected underlying cause of thrombosis, no culprit anatomic lesion will be identified. Future attention to baseline sBP and fluctuations, particularly toward the end of and immediately following a dialysis session, require investigation and follow up. If underlying lesions such as inflow or cannulation area stenosis cannot be sufficiently managed by standard endovascular techniques, surgical revision or replacement of the ePTFE component may become necessary. Finally, once patency has been restored, venography of outflow into the vena cava should be checked to confirm final position of the venous outflow component tip and to be sure that outflow remains sufficient to support ongoing HeRO graft patency. Extension or progression of caval stenosis or interval caval thrombosis could result in obstruction of outflow and immediate re-thrombosis of the HeRO graft.

When necessary, the various components of a HeRO graft can be revised or replaced surgically to maintain or restore patency and proper function. Cannulation area stricture that is resistant to standard endovascular technique may require replacement of the HeRO ePTFE arterial graft component. This can be accomplished by exposure of the terminal ePTFE graft. A new ePTFE graft can be implanted for inflow and cannulation. Until the HeRO Adapter becomes available, this requires graft to graft anastomosis to preserve the titanium connector to the venous outflow component. The venous outflow component can be replaced, its position altered, or length adjusted as necessary by gentle disconnection from the titanium connector and exchange over a guidewire, using fluoroscopic guidance.

Evaluation and management of distal limb hypoperfusion (steal syndrome) should proceed as for other types of arteriovenous access suspected of causing the same problem. For HeRO grafts, in addition to treatment of any significant inflow lesions, distal revascularization with interval ligation (DRIL) or proximalization of inflow (PAI) may be considered in appropriate patients for relief of symptoms while preserving the HeRO access. Abandonment has been reported as the most frequent treatment of steal induced by HeRO grafts.[4,6] Inflow restriction has been used and should be considered carefully, as this may result in HeRO graft thrombosis, given the length of the circuit and the flow volume needed to maintain patency.[3]

Management of infected HeRO grafts is as for other infected HD access, with appropriate antimicrobial therapy and removal of involved prosthetic material. As with many thrombectomy procedures, the original surgeon may not be the one providing urgent care when a patient presents with graft infection, and this provider must be aware that the patient has a HeRO graft.

HeRO GRAFT LONGEVITY AND FATE OF THE VENOUS OUTFLOW COMPONENT

As reported in the review of HeRO literature by Al Shakarchi, et al., the mean time patients had a HeRO graft in place ranged from 200 to nearly 400 days per patient.[5] Some reported that patients had a functioning HeRO up to the time of renal transplantation and that HeRO was a significant factor in being able to bridge that patient to definitive renal replacement therapy while avoiding catheter-dependence.[4] The fate and long-term effect of the HeRO venous outflow component are not known. Theoretically, a large bore central venous catheter could continue to cause venous injury, resulting in progression or worsening of CVO, with symptoms of increasing venous hypertension or development of SVC syndrome. Such a device might also remain a nidus for thrombus collection and source of emboli, particularly if continuous flow is no longer maintained through it. While a patient continues to require HD and is using the HeRO graft, benefit may outweigh risks, especially when access options are so limited. However, it is reasonable to conclude that if the HeRO graft has been abandoned for any reason, the venous outflow component should be removed at the earliest reasonable opportunity. Improvement in central venous collateral drainage and reduction in central venous wall trauma with cardiopulmonary and diaphragmatic excursion are theoretical advantages to removing the device after it is no longer needed. With venous outflow components inserted via the standard IFU approach, removal is a relatively simple procedure, requiring only local anesthesia. The titanium connector is exposed and the venous outflow component clamped. The ePTFE graft component is ligated and divided. It can be left *in situ*, as with any incorporated PTFE AVG, or removed if indicated. The venous outflow component generally slips out without much effort, though manual compression of the venous entry site and the subcutaneous tunnel must be maintained until hemostasis is achieved, as with the removal of any tunneled central venous catheter. Additionally, care must be taken to prevent embolization of air or thrombus through the large bore catheter during the removal procedure. If the patient requires a standard TDC, the HeRO venous outflow component can be exchanged out over a guidewire, thus providing access for an upper extremity TDC, which is preferable to a femoral TDC. Venous outflow components that have been placed via a non-standard approach (e.g. trans-axillary, subclavian, femoral) may require surgical closure of the venous entry site, as there is little to no subcutaneous tunnel tract associated with these approaches.

SUMMARY

Central venous obstruction affects a large segment of the ESRD population and presents a challenging problem for providers who construct and maintain functional HD access. HeRO grafts present an additional option for such patients, with reasonably acceptable outcomes, in terms of patency, infection, and re-intervention rates. The available data suggest that conventional upper extremity options should be exhausted before alternate HD access, including HeRO graft and femoral access, is considered. However, in anatomically and physiologically suitable patients, HeRO represents a way to avoid femoral access, or preserve femoral access if that is the sole remaining non-catheter option. HeRO is a superior choice to catheter-dependence and can buy more time for renal transplantation. More robust clinical trials and direct comparison with other types of dialysis access should help further define the role of HeRO grafts in the dialysis access algorithm. At the current time, there appears to be enough experience to conclude that HeRO grafts should be incorporated into the practice of a dedicated access surgeon, who is trained and experienced in open surgical and endovascular techniques for assessment, construction, monitoring, maintenance, and revision of dialysis access. While HeRO will not be the answer for every patient with CVO, its innovative design does provide one more tool for meeting the needs of a very challenging patient population.

REFERENCES

1. National Kidney Foundation. KDOQI Clinical Practice Guideline for Diabetes and CKD: 2012 Update. *Am J Kidney Dis*. 2012; 60: 850–86.
2. Ribeiro P, Patel S, et al. Case Report: Unilateral conduction hearing loss due to central venous occlusion. *J Vasc Access*. 2016; 17: e37–8.
3. Steerman SN, Wagner J, et al. Outcomes comparison of HeRO and lower extremity arterio-venous grafts in patients with long-standing renal failure. *J Vasc Surg*. 2015; 57: 776–83.
4. Kudlaty EA, Pan J, et al. The End Stage of Dialysis Access: Femoral Graft or HeRO Vascular Access Device. *Ann Vasc Surg*. 2015; 29: 90–97.
5. Al Shakarchi J, Houston JG, et al. A Review on the Hemodialysis Reliable Outflow (HeRO) Graft for Haemodialysis Vascular Access. *Eur J Vasc Endovasc Surg*. 2015; 50: 108–113.
6. Wallace JR, Chaer RA, et al. Report on the Hemodialysis Reliable Outflow (HeRO) experience in dialysis patients with central venous occlusions. *J Vasc Surg*. 2013;58:742–7.
7. HeRO Graft Instructions for use. https://www.merit.com/wp-content/uploads/2016/06/HeRO-IFU-Multilingual-2016_03_16.pdf. (Accessed 8/24/2016.)
8. Katzman HE, McLafferty RB, et al. Initial experience and outcome of a new hemodialysis access device for catheter-dependent patients. *J Vasc Surg*. 2009; 50: 600–7.
9. Vasquez JC, DeLaRosa J, et al. Conversion of Tunneled Hemodialysis Catheter into HeRO Device Can Provide Immediate Access for Hemodialysis. *Vasc Endovasc Surg*. 2010; 44: 687–690.
10. Schuman E, Ronfeld A. Early use conversion of the HeRO dialysis graft. *J Vasc Surg*. 2011; 53: 1742–4.
11. Hart D, Gooden C, et al. Modification of the HeRO Graft Allowing Earlier Cannulation and Reduction in Catheter Dependent Days in Patients with End Stage Renal Disease: A Single Center Retrospective Review. *TSWJ. l* 2014; 1–4.
12. Merit Medical, South Jordan, UT. Product Management and Support, personal communication. 2016.
13. Gage SM, Ahluwalia HS, et al. Salvaging Vascular Access and Treatment of Severe Limb Edema: Case Reports on the Novel Use of the Hemodialysis Reliable Outflow Vascular Access Device. *Ann Vasc Surg*. 2011; 25: 387.e1–387e5.
14. Allan BJ, Prescott AT, et al. Modified use of the Hemodialysis Reliable Outflow (HeRO) graft for salvage of threatened dialysis access. *J Vasc Surg*. 2012; 56: 1127–9.

14

Management of Infected AV Grafts

Samir K. Shah, MD and C. Keith Ozaki, MD

In 2010, there were approximately 384,000 patients with end-stage renal disease on hemodialysis in the United States.[1] The prevalence of renal failure and its attendant costs—$23.6 b in Medicare costs in 2010—has led to a focus on renal replacement strategies and outcomes generally in the renal failure population.[1] Hemodialysis stands as the most common renal replacement therapy. Despite the manifold advantages of autogenous reconstructions for hemodialysis access, including improved patency, decreased infection rates, and lower medical costs, arteriovenous grafts (AVGs) remain a common form of hemodialysis access.

INCIDENCE, RISK FACTORS, AND PREVENTION

Of the numerous complications that can affect AVGs perhaps the most important is infection. Indeed, infection affects 3.5 to 17% of prosthetic AVGs and is the second most common cause of access loss.[2-4]

AVG infection is most common in the first year after surgery: Minga[5] reported that 59% of infections occurred within one year of surgery while Ryan[2] reported that 86% were apparent within six months. In the latter report, 75% of infections occurring within a month were located at an incision while 78% of those presenting later than a month occurred in the body of graft, remote from any incisions. These observations prompted the authors to speculate that infections in the immediate postoperative period may reflect contamination at the time of surgery while later infections represent inoculation during graft access.

Factors associated with AVG infection include hypoalbuminemia,[5,6] number of surgical revisions,[7] lower extremity grafts,[3] diabetes,[6] limited ambulatory ability,[8] frequent hospitalization,[8] graft age,[8] patient age,[6] and poor hygiene.[7] Not all of these variables have been consistently associated with infection; for example, Minga has found that diabetes and lower extremity grafts are not associated with infection.[5]

Generic measures employed to prevent perioperative surgical site infections should also be applied to AVG surgery. Examples include maintenance of sterile technique, perioperative antibiotic use, avoiding contact between prosthetic material and skin surfaces, intraoperative normothermia, and optimization of diabetes to avoid hyperglycemia. Special mention should be made of vancomycin prophylaxis, which was shown by Zibari and colleagues in a randomized trial to reduce AVG graft infection compared to no antibiotics.[9] Aseptic technique at dialysis centers is also critical: 47% of AVG infections in one trial occurred in the body of the graft, suggesting infection during access.[2]

BACTERIOLOGY

Gram-positive pathogens are involved in an overwhelming majority of AVG infections. Specifically, *Staphylococcus aureus* is the most common cultured pathogen, accounting for 60% of infections, followed by *Staphylococcus epidermidis* (15%–22%). Gram-negative bacteria cause a minority of infections.[2,5] Intraoperative cultures are not uniformly positive, likely because of the effect of pre-culture antibiotic administration and the difficulty of culturing some organisms such as *Staphylococcus epidermidis.*

DIAGNOSIS

AVG infection most often presents with local signs. In a series of 57 PTFE infections from the Cleveland Clinic, all patients had at least one local sign, most commonly induration, while 28% had no systemic signs whatsoever.[10] In Ryan's series of 51 infected grafts, the most common presentation (occurring in 45%) was exposed graft or a sinus tract (Figure 14-1).[2] Alternative local presentations include purulent drainage, erythema, pseudoaneurysm, and hemorrhage (Figures 14-2 and 14-3). Hemorrhage can be controlled by direct pressure over the inflow and outflow of the conduit. If there is difficulty then a blood pressure cuff is temporarily placed on the affected limb proximal to the graft, and inflated to a pressure greater than the patient's systolic pressure. Patients may additionally present with remote manifestations (e.g. septic emboli, generalized sepsis) with or without local signs.

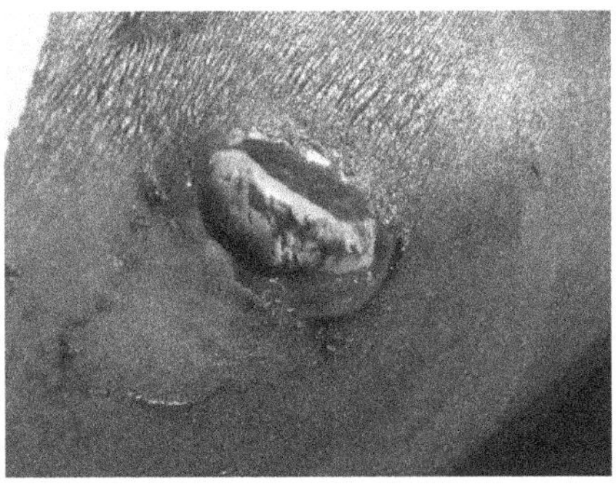

Figure 14-1. Exposed PTFE AVG with evidence of repeated cannulation. Image provided courtesy of Dirk Hentschel, MD.

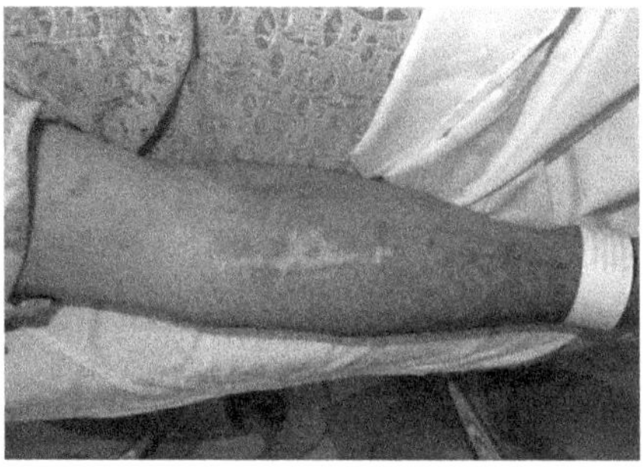

Figure 14-2. Erythema associated with a thrombosed AVG superinfected by repeated cannulation attempts. Extensive perigraft purulence was found during excision. Image provided courtesy of Dirk Hentschel, MD.

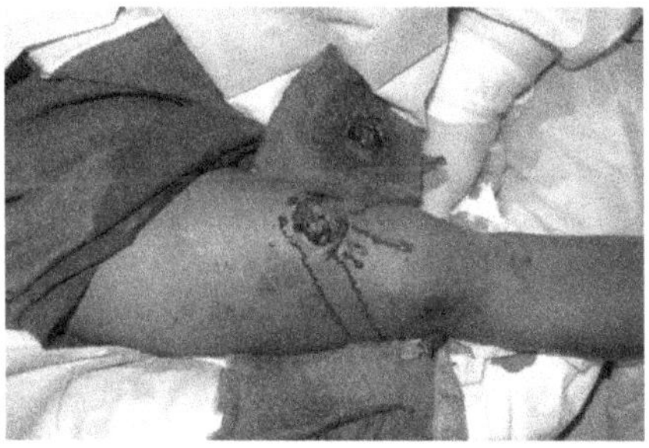

Figure 14-3. AVG infection presenting with focal hemorrhage. Image provided courtesy of Dirk Hentschel, MD.

Ultrasound is a useful adjunct to physical examination to gauge the extent of infection, particularly gross involvement of the anastomoses, which will impact management (see below). Ultrasound can also help identify vein for autogenous reconstruction or patching, and to clarify arterial anatomy.

In cases of suspected infection without clear localizing signs, groups have described the use of PET[11] and indium-111-labeled leukocyte scintigraphy[12] to clarify the status of the graft. Palestro reported a series of 30 indium scintigrams on patients with suspected PTFE AVG infections.[12] Of these 15 occurred in patients ultimately shown by intraoperative exam to have infection, all of who had scintigraphy consistent with infection. Only one patient with a thrombosed AVG had a false positive study. An added advantage of nuclear imaging was the ability to identify infections remote from the graft, which occurred in two patients in Palestro's report.

MANAGEMENT AND OUTCOMES

Prosthetic AVG infection generally mandates surgical excision. Strategies fall into three major categories: total, subtotal, and partial graft excision. Total excision consists of complete removal of prosthetic material and is indicated for extensive infection along the length of the graft, anastomotic involvement, or presentation with severe sepsis or shock. After debridement and irrigation of infected tissues, the wounds are left completely or partially open for drainage. Total graft excision has the advantage of removing all potentially infected prosthetic material and thereby theoretically minimizing recurrent infection. Disadvantages include the sacrifice of existing dialysis access and the corollary need for a temporary dialysis catheter and dissection through previously operated fields. Some arteriotomies may be amenable to primary closure while others will require vein patching. The venous outflow is closed primarily.

Subtotal graft excision implies removal of the entire graft save for a portion at the arterial anastomosis. Any open wounds are excluded by way of occlusive barriers from the field, and the clean arterial portion of the graft is exposed, divided, oversewn, then the outflow pushed into the soft tissue tunnel and sealed over. This clean wound is then closed, and again a barrier dressing applied. Finally, the infected portion of the conduit is explored and the inflow limb is pulled into the field through the now contaminated incisions. Subtotal graft excision has a profile of advantages and disadvantages similar to total graft excision except that the prosthetic cuff may be oversewn to close the arteriotomy. However, prosthetic cuff infection is a possible source of recurrent infection, and Schild reported that this was the cause in 17% of 132 procedures to address graft infection.[4] His group consequently argues against subtotal graft excision.

Partial graft excision involves segmental excision with bypass around the infected field to restore AVG continuity. As above, the infected field is initially excluded and dissection performed on uninfected, well-incorporated graft proximally and distally. Conduit is then tunneled around the infected field. Incisions are closed and covered before excising the infected graft segment. It is employed by some groups for focal AVG infection with no anastomotic involvement or systemic sepsis. This option preserves the AVG for hemodialysis and avoids extensive anastomotic re-operative dissection, but at the risk of incomplete removal of infected material.

Outcomes after partial graft excision have been mixed. Ryan reported a 74% success rate albeit at a short median follow up of 8 months.[2] Schutte and Schwab in series of 17 and 91 patients had salvage rates of 70% and 91%, respectively.[13,14] Nevertheless, relative to total excision, partial graft excision has been associated with more infectious complications and need for additional surgical procedures.[10,13] Thirty-day mortality is similar.[10] Schutte's report had a statistically insignificant trend toward more hemorrhage and systemic sepsis in patients undergoing partial graft excision compared to total excision[13]; Ryan reported no life-threatening hemorrhages or infections from attempts at graft salvage.[2]

Reconstruction of the arterial system (via autogenous patch or interposition vein graft) is the standard practice when grafts are removed from an artery. Brachial artery ligation is usually unnecessary but may be performed safely if there is concern about the integrity of the arteriotomy closure in an infected field. Schanzer reports on 21 patients with AVF graft infection with brachial anastomotic involvement where the brachial arteriotomy was oversewn followed by routine ligation distal to the profunda brachii artery.[15] Normal hand perfusion was assessed clinically preoperatively and again postoperatively at 6 months—there were no cases of hemorrhage or hand ischemia.

While creation of new access at an alternative site may be deferred until resolution of sepsis, some groups have reported success with immediate cryopreserved vein reconstruction. Matsuura and colleagues reported a series of 43 PTFE AVG infections treated with total graft excision and immediate cryopreserved femoral vein reconstruction.[16] Thirty-two of these preserved femoral veins were placed in tunnels parallel to the excision site while the remaining 11 patients had *in situ* reconstruction because of adjacent thrombosed AVGs and the lack of alternative tunneling sites. All were accessed within 14 days. Postoperative infection was rare: one patient with *Candida albicans* infection constitutes the sole case of the series, presenting with wound dehiscence and hemorrhage on postoperative day 94. Primary and secondary patencies at one year were 42% and 68%. However, this strategy can be expensive and care must be taken to avoid use in renal transplantation candidates because of the risk of allosensitization that may preclude transplantation.

Irrespective of the surgical strategy adjunctive antibiotic administration is an essential component of the treatment. Empiric antibiotics to cover methicillin-resistant *S. aureus* and Gram-negative bacilli are initially appropriate. Cultures should be used when available to tailor therapy. Antibiotic therapy durations in the literature range from two to six weeks after surgery.

In summary, with the rising incidence of the metabolic syndrome and aging population it is likely that prosthetic AVG infections will remain a morbid problem for patients and an expensive challenge for providers. Management strategies tailored to individual patient circumstances offer reasonable clinical outcomes in these patients.

REFERENCES

1. Malas MB, Canner JK, Hicks CW, et al. Trends in incident hemodialysis access and mortality. *JAMA Surg.* 2015;150(5):441–8. doi:10.1001/jamasurg.2014.3484.
2. Ryan SV, Calligaro KD, Scharff J, Dougherty MJ. Management of infected prosthetic dialysis arteriovenous grafts. *J Vasc Surg.* 2004;39(1):73–8. doi:10.1016/j.jvs.2003.07.002.
3. Akoh JA, Patel N. Infection of hemodialysis arteriovenous grafts. *J Vasc Access.* 2010;11(2):155–8.
4. Schild AF, Perez E, Gillaspie E, et al. Arteriovenous fistulae vs. arteriovenous grafts: A retrospective review of 1,700 consecutive vascular access cases. *J Vasc Access.* 2008;9(4):231–5.
5. Minga TE, Flanagan KH, Allon M. Clinical consequences of infected arteriovenous grafts in hemodialysis patients. *Am J Kidney Dis.* 2001;38(5):975–8. doi:10.1053/ajkd.2001.28583.
6. Powe NR, Jaar B, Furth SL, et al. Septicemia in dialysis patients: Incidence, risk factors, and prognosis. *Kidney Int.* 1999;55(3):1081–90. doi:10.1046/j.1523-1755.1999.0550031081.x.
7. Nassar GM, Ayus JC. Infectious complications of the hemodialysis access. *Kidney Int.* 2001;60(1):1–13. doi:10.1046/j.1523-1755.2001.00765.x.
8. Anderson JE, Chang AS, Anstadt MP. Polytetrafluoroethylene hemoaccess site infections. *ASAIO J Am Soc Artif Intern Organs. 1992.* 2000;46(6):S18–S21.
9. Zibari GB, Gadallah MF, Landreneau M, et al. Preoperative vancomycin prophylaxis decreases incidence of postoperative hemodialysis vascular access infections. *Am J Kidney Dis.* 1997;30(3):343–8.
10. Tabbara MR, O'Hara PJ, Hertzer NR, et al. Surgical management of infected PTFE hemodialysis grafts: Analysis of a 15-year experience. *Ann Vasc Surg.* 1995;9(4):378–84. doi:10.1007/BF02139410.
11. Carlos MG, Juliana R, Matilde N, et al. Hidden clotted vascular access infection diagnosed by fluorodeoxyglucose positron emission tomography. *Nephrol Carlton Vic.* 2008;13(3):264–5. doi:10.1111/j.1440-1797.2007.00837.x.
12. Palestro CJ, Vega A, Kim CK, et al. Indium-111-labeled leukocyte scintigraphy in hemodialysis access-site infection. *J Nucl Med Off.* 1990;31(3):319–24.
13. Schutte WP, Helmer SD, Salazar L, Smith JL. Surgical treatment of infected prosthetic dialysis arteriovenous grafts: Total versus partial graft excision. *Am J Surg.* 2007;193(3):385–8; discussion 388. doi:10.1016/j.amjsurg.2006.09.028.

14. Schwab DP, Taylor SM, Cull DL, et al. Isolated arteriovenous dialysis access graft segment infection: The results of segmental bypass and partial graft excision. *Ann Vasc Surg*. 2000;14(1):63–6.
15. Schanzer A, Ciaranello AL, Schanzer H. Brachial artery ligation with total graft excision is a safe and effective approach to prosthetic arteriovenous graft infections. *J Vasc Surg*. 2008;48(3):655–8. doi:10.1016/j.jvs.2008.04.030.
16. Matsuura JH, Rosenthal D, Wellons ED, et al. Hemodialysis graft infections treated with cryopreserved femoral vein. *Cardiovasc Surg*. 2002;10(6):561–5.

15

Arteriovenous Access-Associated Ischemia ("Steal")—A Hemodynamic Analysis and Evaluation of Treatment Options

Karl A. Illig, MD

As of 2015, approximately 468,000 persons in the United States are dependent on dialysis, and in 2013, an estimated 117,162 patients were placed on dialysis for the first time.[1] While more than 50% of patients with brachial artery-based arteriovenous (AV) access have retrograde flow in the artery immediately distal to the arterial anastomosis, 5%–8% develop AV access-associated hand ischemia, or steal, that is significant enough to need corrective surgery.[2,3] Even if only half of these patients eventually undergo any form of brachial-based AV access, the yearly incidence of significant steal in the United States is thus 2500 patients.

Technically, the concept of steal refers to the phenomenon whereby enough blood is supplied to the hand to preserve normal health, but the resistance is low enough at the AV anastomosis to allow retrograde flow back into the fistula—blood is "stolen" from the forearm. In practice, the term is used broadly to describe any situation when there is inadequate flow into the limb as a whole to provide both the flow through the fistula as mandated by its low resistance plus the flow needed to adequately perfuse the forearm and hand. If minor, this lowered flow can produce ischemic pain, but if significant (the 4% generally quoted), it can lead to rest pain and/or tissue death, both situations not generally felt to be compatible with a comfortable life.

Because this is such a common situation, multiple procedures have evolved over the years to address this problem. In addition to ligation of the fistula (which fixes the steal but obviously sacrifices the access), the fistula can be "banded," made globally smaller ("long-segment plication" [LSP]), or modified by means of proximalization of arterial inflow (PAI), revascularization using distal inflow (RUDI), or distal revascularization/interval ligation (DRIL). What is the issue? These are all dramatically different procedures, seemingly with nothing in common schematically or theoretically, yet data exist showing that all of them can be effective, albeit perhaps in different situations.[3,4] Our task is thus to determine what they all have in common, and/or why they all seem to work? A secondary issue, albeit one that is critical, is to see if we can identify under what circumstances each will work, and ideally to predict under what circumstances which is preferred.

A note regarding methods. For the following analysis, we will generally assume a fistula (one anastomosis) created at the antecubital fossa. Our analysis is obviously generalizable to an AV graft (two anastomoses), and the huge majority of steal occurs with anastomoses at this level. Further, we will discuss radius and diameter as the scenario dictates, and trust the reader to make the (very complex) transitions themselves. Finally, we will use the term "hand" to denote all tissues distal to the AV access.

WHY DO EACH OF THESE SEEM TO WORK?

First of all, we will accept as a given that they do. The literature as a whole seems to suggest the best results with DRIL,[3,4] and reasonable results with RUDI,[5,6] PAI,[7] and the minimally invasive limited ligation endoluminal-assisted revision (MILLER) procedure,[8,9] when done in the right circumstances, although multiple caveats exist, as described below (LSP, while very effective for fistula salvage,[10,11] has not been evaluated in terms of treatment of steal). Given this fact, how can we explain why they all work? Or, put in another way, how can we describe what they all have in common?

At least in the short term, let us assume a given amount of inflow to the arm. This is obviously low in the native situation, approximately 80–100 cc/min, but can increase massively if an AV fistula (AVF) is created. This flow includes both the axial inflow to the fistula via named vessels, but also the collateral flow to the forearm which includes enough blood to be "stolen" by the fistula without creating a cadaveric hand. Given this fixed inflow (in the short term), "steal" (functionally, hand ischemia) is determined by the ratio of blood supplying the fistula and the hand. How is blood flow determined? Flow (and, more conveniently resistance) is expressed in the ideal situation by Poiseuille's law:

$$\text{Flow} = \pi r^4/\eta L,$$

or

$$\text{Resistance} = \eta L/\pi r^4$$

where r is the radius of the vessel, L is the length of the conduit, and η is the viscosity of the fluid.

While this formula ignores many physiologic issues (and assumes a constant pressure gradient), the *relationships* it describes are critical. Because viscosity may be assumed to be a constant, the two factors that are most important are L and r, the length and radius of the conduit, respectively. Resistance in this situation according to L is determined by the (integrated) sum of planar resistances created by laminar flow, and is directly related to distance (1:1). As such, a change of a certain amount will be reflected in a change in resistance and flow, all other factors being equal, of exactly the same amount. By contrast, the radius affects resistance and flow according to its fourth

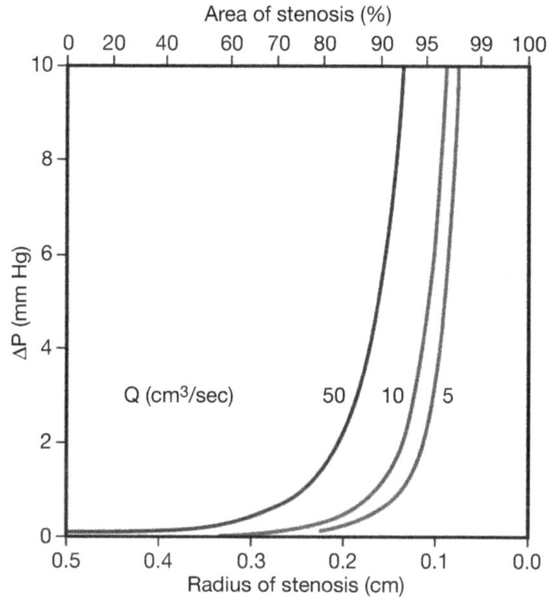

Figure 15-1. Relationship of pressure drop (ΔP) to inside radius of a cylindrical tube 10 cm in length at various rates of steady laminar flow (Q) otherwise under normal physiological conditions. Note the extreme changes in the shapes of the curves at radii between 1 and 3 mm, illustrating the fact that resistance is proportionate to the fourth power of the radius. From Zierler et al.[12]

power. But it is more complex than this. First, in the human body, there is a very large asymptote at large radii—at physiologic temperature and viscosity, a radius of 10 mm (e.g., the infrarenal aorta) brought to 5 mm does NOT produce a 16-fold increase in resistance (or, if it does, the absolute value is still too low to make a difference). However, dropping the radius from 6 to 3 mm DOES produce a highly measurable change. This change, moreover, is very steep, as it is related to the radius by the fourth power. As such, very small differences in radius will produce very large differences in resistance and flow (Figure 15-1).[12]

Given a fixed amount of inflow (in the short term), we can thus analyze steal and methods available to correct it in terms of the ratio of flow to the access versus flow to the hand.

Flow to the Fistula

Flow to the fistula is via a single conduit and is thus best analyzed according to Poiseuille's law. In simpler terms, access flow is most conveniently analyzed as being proportional to the fourth power of the radius (over a critical value), and inversely proportional to the length of the access:

$$\text{Flow}_{\text{Access}} \sim r^4/L$$

Both of these are subject to qualifications that must be kept in mind. The length of the fistula only matters when the radius is compressed to physiologically relevant levels—perhaps 3 or 4 mm (diameter 6–8 mm) or less—and a segment of radius interposed within an already dilated circuit can act as a critical or limiting resistance factor, independent of its length. We will consider then flow in the access in terms of length (linear) and radius (fourth power), but within these caveats above. Finally, this flow must be at least 600 cc/min or so, but can be anywhere above this for effective dialysis.

Flow to the Hand

Flow to the hand obviously follows the same hemodynamic principles, but because of collateral input and retrograde brachial flow (essentially by definition), Poiseuille's law is less helpful. Let us alternatively consider this as a relatively simple "continuity" equation:

$$\text{Flow}_{\text{Hand}} = \text{Collateral flow} + \text{axial flow}$$

The point here is that retrograde collateral flow is a negative number. In physiologic terms, what gets to the hand is the amount of collateral flow less retrograde flow (steal) at the brachial artery. In other words, collateral flow must supply both the hand as well as the amount of flow that is "stolen" retrograde by the access. This flow does not need to be very high, perhaps between 60 and 80 cc/min.

We submit that each of the methods to correct steal can be analyzed according to their effects on flow to the access and to the hand. Each technique, currently available, affects these flows in different ways. It likely follows that each will be effective in different circumstances, and thus that identifying when such circumstances exist will allow the most rational decision-making.

WHAT ARE THE GOALS WHEN WE NEED TO CORRECT STEAL?

The first step is to ensure adequate inflow to the arm. As above, normal flow is in the range of 80–100 cc/min, while a fistula can create flows of 4–6000 cc/min in extreme situations. Based on global empiric experience (with hundreds of thousands of fistulas), most of the time the inflow vessels (heart to anastomosis) can deliver enough blood to adequately perfuse hand as well as provide fistula flow. Exact evidence and predictive factors are, however, sparse. Again empirically, usually a visibly normal vessel will be able to supply this flow, and thus inflow is not usually the problem if all visible lesions have been corrected.

Given the assumption of normal inflow, our goal is again to change the *ratio* of flow between the hand and the fistula, taking into account both axial flow in named vessels and collateral flow to the forearm (some of which is "stolen" via retrograde flow). We do this by affecting the resistance of these two general circuits, using the principles discussed above. In turn, this ratio can be affected by either reducing the flow in the fistula (increasing its resistance), increasing the flow to the arm (reducing the resistance of the collaterals), or both. Each method to be discussed can be analyzed according to this philosophy.

Finally, flow to the hand does not need to be high at all and likely will not appreciably change very much over time. What changes is flow in the access, both at the time of creation (zero to several hundred cc/min) and as the vessels dilate (particularly in native fistulas). We (and many others) argue that the first factor to examine in patients with steal is thus the amount of flow in the access. This situation has been extensively analyzed both theoretically and in vivo,[13–16] and using these analyses and empiric experience, it seems that two general types of steal exist: High flow, very broadly defined as flow over 1500–2000 cc per minute, and low flow, flows that are below this. The two different situations may, in fact, represent two different "types" of steal (obviously with broad overlap), with high-flow steal being a situation where anatomy is fundamentally normal but compensatory mechanisms to perfuse the hand have failed, while "normal flow" steal representing a situation where anatomy and/or physiology is abnormal (i.e., collateral and/or forearm vessel disease).

Putting all of this together, treatment of steal will thus depend upon the flow in the fistula. The goal is always to increase flow to the hand, and this is always done by adjusting the ratio of flows in the fistula and to the hand (collaterals plus axial flow [which is negative in those with retrograde flow]). Patients with high-flow steal can simply be treated by methods to reduce the flow in the fistula, as dialysis will continue to be effective at much lower rates of flow than they currently have. However, there is not much room for error if flow is already normal—patients with normal-flow steal need methods to more subtly change the ratios of flow, perhaps by increasing flow to the hand as well as decreasing that to the fistula. Treatment of normal flow steal requires a lot more finesse!

STEAL IN PATIENTS WITH HIGH-FLOW ACCESS

There is no agreement, and certainly no empiric evidence, as to what constitutes "high flow." Most would classify flow less than 1000 cc/min as normal and flow greater than 2000 cc/min as high, but between obviously lies a gray zone, and treatment in this area will depend on local experience and resources.

As described above, most common physiology of the arm is relatively normal, and steal simply represents one in which all compensation has been exhausted. Supporting this is the fact that most of these patients develop late steal over time, as their (mostly) fistulas dilate over the years. In addition, as above, there is plenty of margin for error, as a flow of 2000 cc/min, for example, is three times higher than that needed for efficient dialysis. We thus submit that the goal in a high-flow fistula is thus simply to reduce the flow in the fistula, returning the situation to the point at which perfusion to the hand was not a problem. This can be done by decreasing the radius (assuming within an effective range, as shown in Figure 15-1) or by increasing the length. We also should reemphasize that this situation is almost always seen in patients with fistulas rather than grafts, for the reason discussed above.

Banding

Banding refers broadly to the technique of decreasing the radius of the fistula at one point, focally increasing resistance. In practice, most now refer to this as the MILLER procedure.[8] While this refers to one technical method of banding, the term is broadly descriptive of partial ligation of the fistula over an internal bougie, usually a 3-mm balloon (Figure 15-2). In their original report, all 16 patients so treated (using 4–5 mm balloons at this point) were improved and no fistulas were lost at a mean follow-up of three months.

Based on the premise of this discussion, banding increases resistance and decreases flow by solely affecting the radius of the access, but does not change flow to the hand directly—this flow is increased given the assumption that by increasing pressure at the access anastomosis, retrograde flow in the brachial artery will be decreased, hence making the relationship (collateral flow—retrograde brachial flow) more positive.

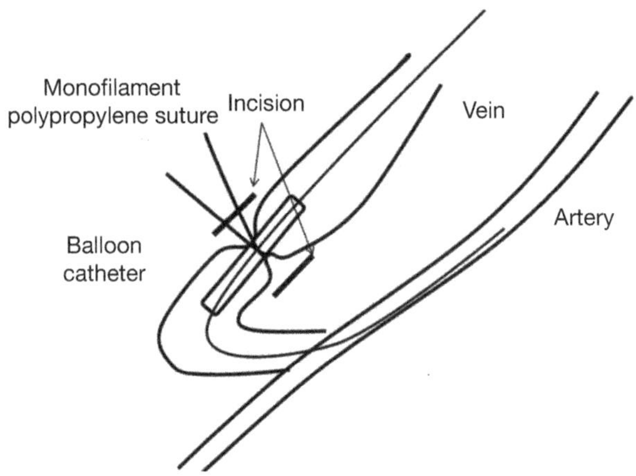

Figure 15-2. A schematic view of the MILLER procedure (minimally invasive limited ligation endoluminal-assisted revision) procedure. The salient point is that the fistula is partially ligated over an endoluminal bougie (here, a balloon) to provide an objective result. From Shintaku et al.[9]

The first criticism of this technique is that because radius affects resistance according to its fourth power, the inflection point is so severe and the curve is so steep (Figure 15-1) that there is little room for error. Further, while what may be perfect while on table may be too severe (or not severe enough) at other times—with higher or lower blood pressures, alterations in intravascular fluid volume, and so on. The second criticism is that this technique would seem to create a perfect model for intimal hyperplasia, as a very high volume of blood is forced through a pinhole opening, creating extreme local turbulence.

The former argument has been addressed in part by a premise loosely called "precision banding." The MILLER procedure, using an empirically derived but objective internal bougie to control the end diameter, is a good first step. Many now perform banding in general over a bougie of a defined size (MILLER procedure) plus using some objective measure of effect, such as measuring fistula flow,[9] forearm blood pressure, and/or differential angiographic flow to the forearm after banding. In addition, awareness has evolved that banding in general is most applicable in the setting of a high-flow fistula. Although results were not optimal in one recent preliminary series,[9] experience within our group has been encouraging and this is an area of active investigation.

Long-Segment Plication

An alternative technique to increase resistance and hence decrease flow in patients with high flow fistulas is LSP. This has been described by several groups using several different techniques,[10,11,17] but in general, this technique involves full exposure of a long segment of massively dilated fistula (Figure 15-3) with resection of redundant tissue and plication down around a 20 Fr red rubber catheter as a bougie (Figure 15-4). With one exception, however, these series have described this technique only for treatment of aneurysmal degeneration, not flow reduction per se.

LSP increases resistance and decreases flow by manipulating both L and r. The radius of the fistula is reduced, although not to the degree with banding (20 Fr bougie being approximately 6.3 mm), but the length of this area of reduced radius, the length plicated,

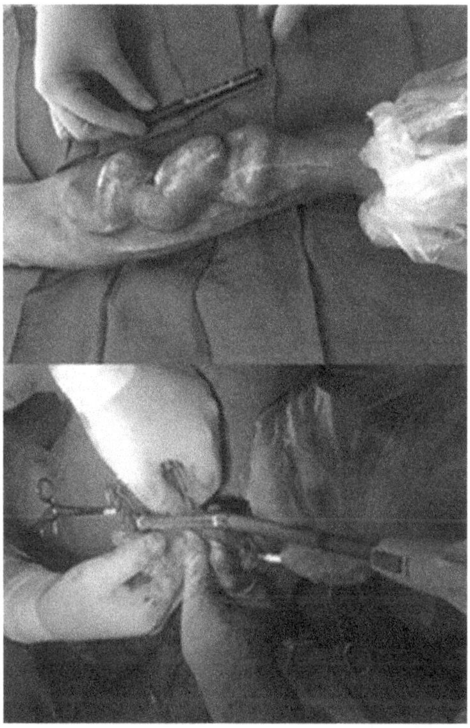

Figure 15-3. A patient with a hugely dilated fistula (top). After full exposure and excision of excess length, the fistula is plicated over a 20 Fr red rubber catheter internal bougie using a GIA stapler with vascular staples (bottom).

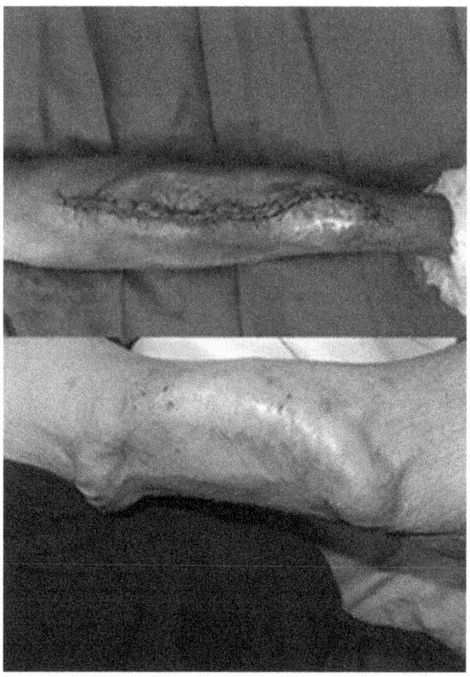

Figure 15-4. Patient in Figure 3, immediately postoperative (top) and 18 months later (bottom).

is much longer than the pinpoint focality of banding. Again, flow to the hand is thus increased by increasing the pressure at the anastomosis, again reducing retrograde brachial flow and making the relationship (collateral flow–brachial retrograde flow) more positive.

Published evidence that is helpful for high flow steal is entirely lacking, with one partial exception. Baker and Malgor recently reported a single patient with steal in the setting of a (minimally) aneurysmal fistula with flow measured at 2400 cc/min. They performed staple aneurysmorrhapy "by eye," but also then banded the fistula to 4 mm. At 12 months, flow was 717 cc/min and the patient was asymptomatic.[18] Unfortunately, because both precision banding and plication were performed at the same time, which actually made the difference is unknown. We have treated four patients using this technique for hemodynamic problems (two for congestive heart failure and two for steal). All four were essentially cured and flow reduced. We are planning on looking at these patients more carefully in the future with this concept in mind.

Other Techniques

DRIL, RUDI, and PAI are also theoretically applicable to high-flow fistulas, as each will add a segment of resistance and thus theoretically reduce flow. RUDI and PAI add the resistance of the new interposition conduit, and PAI and DRIL add the resistance of more artery proximal to the fistula anastomosis (PAI thus does both, although with the shortest length of both). These can be considered in patients with high-flow fistulas, but we believe they are more appropriate when flow is normal and will thus be discussed below.

STEAL IN PATIENTS WITH NORMAL-FLOW ACCESS

To reset the stage, for our purposes, a "normal flow access" in a patient with steal is defined at one with flow of 1000 cc/min or less (with anything up to 2000 cc/min residing in a gray zone). In this situation, we cannot just drop flow in the fistula by brute force; a more nuanced approach is needed. Such an approach can be thought of as trying to affect the overall ratio of flow in the fistula versus that to the hand.

Distal Revascularization/Interval Ligation

First described by Schanzer in 1988[19] and with results now approaching a thousand reported patients in the literature, this must be regarded as the standard of care (Figure 15-5). Results are excellent, with reported "cure" rates (significant improvement with maintenance of access) routinely 80%–90% or more.[3,4,20] DRIL accomplishes our objectives in several ways. First, the ligation of the brachial artery increases flow to the hand by eliminating the retrograde flow through the brachial artery, thus simplifying hand flow to (collateral flow) alone. Second, and probably most significantly, the bypass component provides a very low resistance artificial collateral to the forearm, increasing this term. Finally, the fact that by ligating the brachial artery the fistula is physiologically converted into a much longer length, now including the brachial artery, both increases the length of the fistula and adds a limiting segment with a smaller radius than the fistula itself.[20] By thinking of this in terms of the ratio between

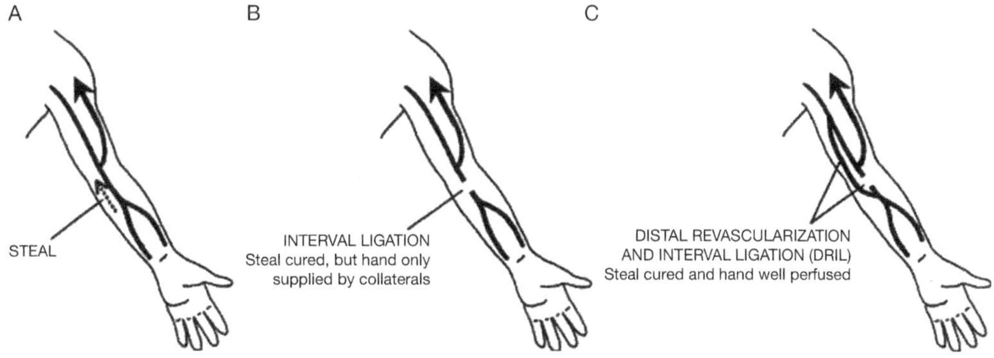

Figure 15-5. Schematic representation of DRIL (distal revascularization/interval ligation). From Illig et al.[21]

flow to the access and to the hand, support is also provided for the concept that the proximal anastomosis of the bypass should be as high as possible in the arm to add as much length of artery to the fistula.[21]

The major argument against DRIL is, of course, the fact that by ligating the brachial artery you are committing the patient to the bypass—if this fails, arm perfusion might be compromised. The one glaring error in this suggestion is, of course, that flow through the (now ligated) brachial artery was, and would remain, retrograde—even if the bypass failed with the brachial artery still open, the arm would not only be provided by blood from this route, but blood provided by the (undisturbed) collaterals would continue to be "stolen" from the arm! In other words, brachial artery ligation (IL) is of benefit whether or not the new collateral (DR) is provided and/or stays patent. This argument notwithstanding, to our knowledge, there has never been a reported case (or one discussed among those who perform this procedure) of a hand or arm being lost after failure of the bypass, powerful empiric support for the soundness of this procedure. Based on this, in fact, we have been more aggressive with the use of artificial conduit for the bypass component in an effort to decrease the morbidity related to vein harvest.

Following this sequence of thought, however, brings us to an interesting point. What, exactly, is the "active ingredient" in DRIL? Is ligation of the brachial artery even necessary, and is the bypass component itself needed? At least two groups have analyzed this situation by means of electrical circuit analogies[13,14] and two others by means of mechanical benchtop fluid dynamic simulators.[15,16] In a very broad summation of findings, this work taken as a whole suggests that the interval ligation component of DRIL may in fact add very little to the effect of the procedure. We have a clinical trial underway to assess this in patients undergoing DRIL, and extremely preliminary results ($N = 3$ as of July 2017) seem to support this.

Revascularization Using Distal Inflow

First described by Minion in 2005,[5] RUDI refers to the technique whereby a brachial artery based access is "moved" distally onto the radial artery, usually by means of a short jump graft with ligation of the original anastomosis (Figure 15-6). This does not dramatically affect one or the other of our two resistances and flows, but adjusts the ratio in a manner that seems to be somewhat beneficial. It increases the resistance of

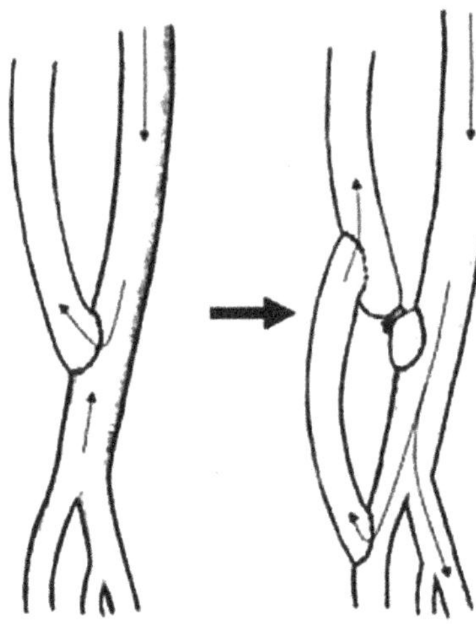

Figure 15-6. Schematic representation of RUDI (revascularization using distal inflow). From Minion et al.[5]

the fistula by adding a short additional length of brachial and radial artery, by adding a length of smaller radius radial artery, and by adding a short length of whatever conduit is used for the jump graft. Flow to the hand is perhaps increased by increasing the resistance to retrograde brachial flow (adding some radial artery), but this seems less significant than some of the other techniques.

The consequence of affecting resistances in a more subtle manner is, however, reduced effectiveness. Published experience is much less than with banding and DRIL, and in one large group's recently published experience, RUDI was associated with a lower rate of symptom improvement and a higher rate of access failure than DRIL.[3] A second paper with a slightly smaller *N* did not show a statistically significant difference between the two, but RUDI tended toward lower symptom resolution rate and higher access failure rate.[6]

Proximalization of Arterial Inflow

Described by Zanow in 2006, this technique is performed by providing a conduit from an inflow artery higher in the arm to the existing access, again with ligation of the original anastomosis (Figure 15-7).[7] At first glance, this appears to be exactly the opposite of RUDI—how can they both work? Again, we propose the benefit of PAI is the addition of resistance to the fistula by means of the new conduit, which adds length and perhaps a limiting radius. This explanation implies that the interposition conduit should be relatively small and high resistant (4 or 5 mm polytetrafluoroethylene, probably NOT vein), and as long as possible. Pursuing our argument above, in addition to this decrease in access flow, retrograde flow from the hand is perhaps lessened by the increase in resistance created by the length of brachial artery "added" by siting the access anastomosis higher. A theoretical drawback to this procedure is, of course, that the fistula may be brought far enough proximally to eliminate some collateral flow. While several series have reported some degree of improvement in all patients so treated,[3,7] currently published data are more sparse than with the other techniques.

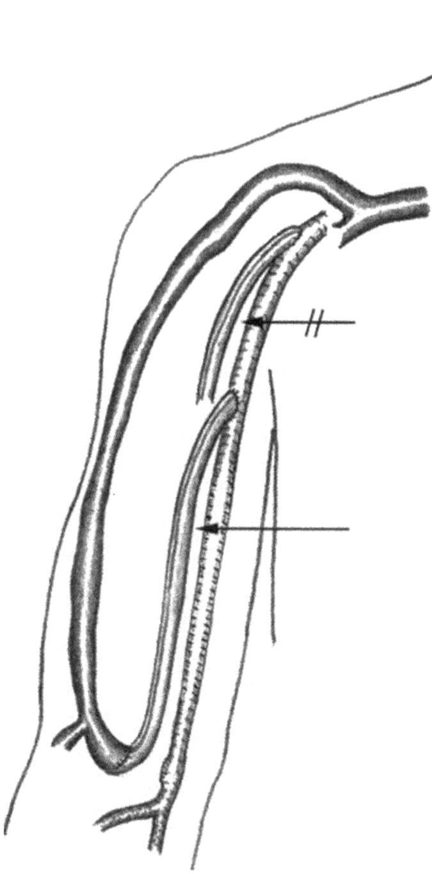

Figure 15-7. Illustration of PAI (proximalization of arterial inflow). Solid arrow illustrates proximalization to the level of the axillary artery, while broken arrow shows proximalization to a higher level. From Zanow et al.[7]

SO HOW DO WE TREAT STEAL?

First, it must be stressed that essentially no published report truly assesses outcomes according to the flow status of the access involved. Many investigators choose their procedures based on flow, but we could find no series expressly describing outcomes in those with different flow levels, or even discussing this issue explicitly, much less prospective trials using this as the independent variable. While this suggests a fruitful area for further research, treatment of steal and selection of procedures must be made with this caveat in mind.

Table 15-1 addresses the ratio of flow within the fistula as compared to flow to the hand, for each of the five procedures described above. It is obvious that the MILLER procedure (as a surrogate for banding, and with the assumption that this is based on physiologic rather than anatomic monitoring) is most effective in reducing the flow to the fistula, but DRIL seems to dominate otherwise. DRIL adds the same length to the fistula as does PAI (assuming the same philosophy of siting the new proximal anastomosis), but this length is brachial artery for DRIL, prosthetic for PAI. Does this make a difference? DRIL is then the only option that adds a collateral and is the only option that completely eliminates retrograde brachial flow.

TABLE 15-1. RELATIVE EFFECTIVENESS OF THE PROCEDURES DISCUSSED RELATING TO FLOW RATIOS

	Decrease Flow within Access		Increase Flow to Hand	
	Add Length to AVF	Decrease Radius of AVF	Addition of Collateral(s)	Elimination of Retrograde Flow
MILLER	No	+++ (focal)	No	No
LSP	No	++ (long segment)	No	No
DRIL	+++ (brachial artery)	++ (long segment)	+++	COMPLETE
RUDI	+	+ (limiting segment)	No	+
PAI	+++ (prosthetic)	+ (limiting segment)	No (or lose some)	+
BEST	DRIL, PAI	MILLER	DRIL	DRIL

Table 15-2 describes the general mechanism of action for the five procedures, along with the clinical outcome. Using these data, Table 15-3 summarizes what we propose as the critical clinical points to be kept in mind when planning and carrying out these procedures, as follows:

- Because the margin for error is so slight, banding must be carried out under objective size control and physiologic (flow or pressure) monitoring ("precision MILLER"). We suggest starting at a relatively large diameter (4 mm balloon or 11 Fr sheath) followed by assessment of outcome (e.g., angiographic flow from the axillary artery so as not to obturate the now-restricted lumen or forearm, duplex flow, or finger pressures) and reducing the size of the bougie if needed. We have found it useful to use a sheath rather than a balloon, as they provide a more gradual reduction in diameter (0.314 mm per French rather than 1 mm increments), and the sheath can also be used to "Dotter" a stenotic brachial outflow.
- Data regarding the effectiveness of **LSP** for steal are not available. It would seem to be prudent to perform the same physiologic assessment as with banding, and this can then be added if needed if the plication alone does not prove effective. For hemodynamic effect, it is likely that the longer the segment plicated the higher the resistance, with very little risk of fistula failure.
- The bypass component of **DRIL** should be a large, low-resistant conduit, either vein or 6–8-mm prosthetic. The proximal anastomosis should be sited as high in the axilla as possible, to add as much length of brachial artery to the access circuit (the added resistance of the additional bypass component would not seem to be very significant). There is some theoretical evidence that interval ligation may not be needed, but, in turn, the risks of bypass conduit failure are likely overstated.
- **RUDI** seemingly adds the least resistance to the fistula, and while perhaps reducing retrograde flow, seems to be the least powerful of the five options. Further data are needed.
- **PAI** adds resistance to the access in a manner exactly analogous to DRIL. Because this is a prosthetic, it should be as long and as narrow as possible. Vein should not be used as it defeats the whole purpose of the operation. PAI also seems to add reasonably significant resistance to retrograde flow, by the same mechanism as fistula resistance is increased after DRIL—the length of the brachial artery between anastomoses. Again, for both of these reasons, the new proximal anastomosis should be sited as high as possible in the axilla.

TABLE 15-2. PRESUMED MECHANISM OF ACTION AND RESULTANT OUTCOME

	General Mechanism of Action	Outcome
MILLER	Add focal stenosis to access	Flow reduction only
LSP	Add long segment of subtly higher resistance to access	Flow reduction only
DRIL	Add collateral to arm, eliminate retrograde flow Add length to fistula (brachial artery between anastomoses)	Large Increase flow to arm Moderate decrease flow to fistula via increasing its resistance
RUDI	Add length (resistance) to access via proximal radial artery and jump graft Small decrease in retrograde flow (longer pathway)	Small flow reduction Small decrease in retrograde flow
PAI	Add length (resistance) to access via jump graft Unknown influence on collateral by siting access more proximally	Flow reduction only

TABLE 15-3. CRITICAL CLINICAL POINTS RELATING TO PROSED MECHANISM OF ACTION TO TREAT STEAL

	General Mechanism of Action	Critical Clinical Implications
MILLER	Add focal stenosis to access	Must perform this under physiologic monitoring—"precision banding." Effectiveness depends on hemodynamic changes, not arbitrary size or distance.
LSP	Add long segment of subtly higher resistance to access	Empiric data lacking.
DRIL	Add collateral to arm, eliminate retrograde flow Add length to fistula (brachial artery between anastomoses)	Bypass should be low resistance—large conduit, and sited as proximally as possible. Role of interval ligation being reexamined, but implications of bypass failure likely overestimated.
RUDI	Add length (resistance) to access via proximal radial artery and jump graft Small decrease in retrograde flow (longer pathway)	Likely more effective if sited farther down the radial artery, with a concomitantly longer conduit, but unclear.
PAI	Add length (resistance) to access via jump graft Unknown influence on collateral by siting access more proximally	Diameter (small) and length (long) of the conduit likely very important.

Putting all of this together, we propose the following algorithm for the diagnosis and treatment of access-associated steal:

- First, steal is diagnosed clinically by documenting reduced flow in the forearm, improved by temporary occlusion of the access in a patient with appropriate symptoms.
- Next, flow should be measured, and the access categorized as "high" or "normal" flow. The cutoff between the two is not absolute, and choice of procedures in this situation will depend on local factors.
- Third, adequacy of inflow should be assessed, at least by duplex if not angiography. Even in a very high-flow fistula, if a problem is present proximally, fixing it may well treat the steal.

Once these three things have been done, treatment depends on flow:

- High flow access (usually fistulas) should be treated with a flow-reduction procedure.
    - If massively dilated: LSP over a 20 Fr bougie. This treats the dilation as well as the steal. We recommend real-time physiologic assessment.
    - If not massively dilated:
        - FIRST CHOICE: Precision banding (MILLER procedure over a defined bougie with real-time physiologic assessment).
        - ALTERNATIVES: PAI or possibly RUDI can be considered but only if flow is expected to be significantly reduced.
- Normal flow access:
    - FIRST CHOICE: DRIL. This provides the best overall correction of the problem and is supported by the most (and most favorable) evidence. The implications of bypass failure are probably overstated, and the morbidity of the procedure can be reduced by the use of prosthetic. Research is underway to determine whether interval ligation is needed.
    - ALTERNATIVES: PAI in theory produces the next strongest physiological improvement, while RUDI is theoretically the weakest option.

SUMMARY

In analyzing the problem in this regard, it is hard to escape several conclusions. First, banding may actually work after all, but ONLY in high-flow fistulas and ONLY when done using objective techniques and assessed using physiologic outcomes before leaving the operating room or angio suite ("precision MILLER"). Second, DRIL seems to address the problem in most cases when banding is not appropriate. Not only does it address every facet of the issue, but even in theory, the risks are likely overstated. A decade or more of outcomes, now approaching 1000 patients, have shown this to be safe and highly effective. PAI seems to have some benefit, but it is unclear what exactly the benefit of RUDI is over the others. Finally, LSP is attractive in that it fixes the functional and cosmetic issues in patients with massively dilated fistulas while in theory increasing resistance in a more gentle way. However, data in regard to steal are almost entirely lacking.

As all who work in this field will attest, there are numerous unanswered questions and areas where research is likely to be highly fruitful, including:

- What predicts adequacy of inflow short of invasive imaging?
- At what threshold fistula flow is inflow inadequate?
- Does interval ligation matter?
- Length and conduit for bypass in DRIL?
- Length and conduit relationships in PAI/RUDI?
- How to model collateral flow?
- Exact, empiric relationship between radius and flow/resistance at AVF measurements?
- Resistance and flow after LSP?
- Prospective randomized trials in patients with high- and low-flow fistulas—how does each procedure perform in each situation?

REFERENCES

1. US Renal Data System 2015 Annual Report. https://www.usrds.org/2015/view/Default.aspx. Accessed February 7, 2017.
2. Malik J, Tuka V, Kasalova Z, et al. Understanding the dialysis access steal syndrome. A review of the eitiologies, diagnosis, prevention, and treatment strategies. *J Vasc Access*. 2008;9:155–166.
3. Leake AE, Winger DG, Leers SA, Gupta N, Dillavou ED. Management and outcomes of dialysis associate steal syndrome. *J Vasc Surg*. 2015;61:754–761.
4. Russell. Treatment of steal syndrome. Kidney Health Australia CARI Guidelines. http://www.cari.org.au/Dialysis/dialysis%20vascular%20access/Treatment_of_steal_syndrome.pdf.2011. Accessed February 7, 2017.
5. Minion DJ, Moore E, Endean E. Revision using distal inflow: a novel approach to dialysis associated steal syndrome. *Ann Vasc Surg*. 2005;19(5):625–628.
6. Misskey J, Yang C, MacDonald S, Baxter K, Hsiang Y. A comparison of revision using distal inflow and distal revascularization-interval ligation for the management of severe access-related steal syndrome. *J Vasc Surg*. 2015;63(6):1574–1581.
7. Zanow J, Kruger U, Scholz H. Proximalization of the arterial inflow: a new technique to treat access-related ischemia. *J Vasc Surg*. 2006;43:1216–1221.
8. Goel N, Miller MC, Jotwani MC, Licht J, Schur L, Arnold WP. Minimally-Invasive Limited Ligation Endoluminal-assisted Revision (MILLER) for treatment of dialysis access-associated steal syndrome. *Kidney Int*. 2006;70:765–770.
9. Shintaku S, Kawanishi H, Moriishi M, Banshodani M, Ago R, Tsuchiya S. Modified MILLER banding procedure for managing high-flow access and dialysis-associated steal syndrome. *J Vasc Access*. 2015;16(3):227–232.
10. Powell A, Wooster M, Carroll M, et al. Long-segment plication technique for arteriovenous fistulae threatened by diffuse aneurysmal degeneration: short-term results. *Ann Vasc Surg*. 2015;29:1327–1331.
11. Vo T, Tumbaga G, Aka P, Behserescht J, Hsu J, Tayarrah M. Staple aneurysmorrhaphy to salvage autogenous arteriovenous fistulas with aneurysm-related complications. *J Vasc Surg*. 2015;61:457–462.
12. Zierler RE, Sumner DS. Arterial physiology. In: Cronenwett J, Johnston KW, eds. *Rutherford's Vascular Surgery*. 8th ed. Philadelphia, PA: Saunders/Elsevier; 2014.
13. van gemert MJC, Bruyninckx CMA. Simulated hemodynamic comparison of arteriovenous fistulas. *J Vasc Surg*. 1987;6:39–44.
14. Gradman WS, Pozrikidis C. Analysis of options for mitigating hemodialysis access-related steal. *Ann Vasc Surg*. 2004;18:59–65.
15. Zanow J, Krueger U, Reddemann P, Scholz H. Experimental study of hemodynamics in procedures to treat access-related ischemia. *J Vasc Surg*. 2008;48:1559–1565.
16. Varble N, Day S, Phillips D, et al. In vitro hemodynamic model of the arm arteriovenous circulation to study hemodynamics of native arteriovenous fistula and the distal revascularization and interval ligation procedure. *J Vasc Surg*. 2014;59:1410–1417.
17. Woo K, Cook PR, Garg J, Hye RJ, Canty TG. Midterm results of a novel technique to salvage autogenous dialysis access in aneurysmal arteriovenous fistulas. *J Vasc Surg*. 2010;51:921–925.
18. Baker J, Malgor RD. Concomitant staple aneurysmorrhaphy and flow-calibrated arteriovenous fistula banding over a coronary dilator to treat hand steal syndrome. *Vasc Endovascular Surg*. 2017;51(5):307–311.
19. Schanzer H, Schwartz M, Harrington E, et al. Treatment of ischemia due to "steal" by arteriovenous fistula with distal artery ligation and revascularization. *J Vasc Surg*. 1988;7:770–773.
20. Huber TS, Brown MP, Seeger JM, et al. Midterm outcome after the distal revascularization and interval ligation (DRIL) procedure. *J Vasc Surg*. 2008;48:926–932.
21. Illig KA, Surowiec S, Shortell SK, Davies MG, Rhodes JM, Green RM. Hemodynamics of distal revascularization-interval ligation. *Ann Vasc Surg*. 2005;19:199–207.

16

Utility of the Venous Window Needle Guide Device in Hemodialysis Access

Spencer W. Galt, MD

The arteriovenous fistula (AVF) is the gold standard for hemodialysis access. Unquestionably, the AVF is the safest and most effective method of hemodialysis access compared to arteriovenous grafts or dialysis catheters.[1,2] Accordingly, vascular access surgeons are striving to increase the proportion of patients being dialyzed utilizing an AVF. While the objective of increasing the number of AVFs has been successful, the unintended consequence is the simultaneous increase in the number of fistulas that are unusable without adjuvant intervention.[3] In particular, the widespread use of preoperative duplex ultrasound-guided venous mapping for planning of AVF placement has enabled creation of AVFs in obese patients whose superficial veins are not visible or palpable. Ironically, the veins in these obese patients are often of good quality, since their lack of palpability spares them percutaneous puncture. The National Kidney Foundation Kidney Disease Outcomes Quality Initiative Guidelines and Fistula First endorse the "Rule of 6s" for a functional AVF: the fistula is ≥6 mm in diameter (with tourniquet in place), ≤6 mm deep, and with a flow volume of ≥600 mL/min.[1] Additionally, a functional cannulation length of 6 in. is frequently recommended. Among the obese, a fistula may exhibit satisfactory diameter and flow volume, but may be too deep to reliably cannulate. This renders the AVF useless, and leaves the patient and dialysis team frustrated. The increasing prevalence of obesity in the United States[4] suggests that these uncannulatable fistulas will be created with increasing frequency.

Fistulas too deep to be cannulated require surgical revision. Most commonly these deep fistulas are superficialized, requiring a long skin incision with mobilization of the vein from its native position. Superficialization exposes the patient to operative morbidity, wound complications, and may adversely affect fistula patency.[5,6]

The Venous Window Needle Guide (VWING) was developed to address the challenge of the uncannulatable AVF. Specifically, the WVING was designed for AVFs that are uncannulatable because of excessive depth, fistula tortuosity, lack of

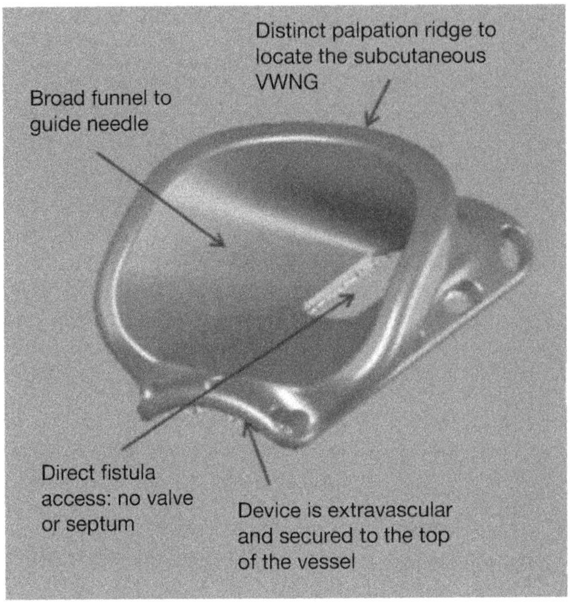

Figure 16-1. The Venous Window Needle Guide (VWING; Vital Access Corporation, Salt Lake City, UT). The device is comprised of a single piece of titanium that allows repeated access of an AVF though a single puncture site (buttonhole technique). Reproduced with permission from Elsevier, Inc.[8]

fistula palpability, or the presence of aneurysms(s), but are otherwise of sufficient diameter and flow volume to support effective hemodialysis. The VWING is a single-component titanium device designed to allow repeated access of an AVF though a constant-site (buttonhole) technique (Figure 16-1). It is surgically implanted on to the fistula wall. The upper surface of the device contains an arched ridge, designed to provide a palpable target for the dialysis needle. The broad funnel opening provides a wide target, and directs the needle tip into the channel. The needle exits the channel at the bottom surface of the device after it has become securely adherent to the fistula wall (Figure 16-2). The undersurface of the device, where it interfaces with the vessel, is composed of titanium beads that promote ingrowth of tissue, allowing the device to seal to the fistula. No septum is present at the base of the channel. Hemostasis is achieved after needle removal with gentle pressure, identical to conventional fistula puncture. The devices are 17.7 mm long, available in 7 and 9 mm widths, and 4, 6, 8, and 10 mm heights, accommodating a wide range of AVF widths and diameters (Figure 16-3).

CLINICAL EXPERIENCE WITH THE VWING

The VWING device was first implanted in nine dialysis-dependent patients in New Zealand,[7] whose fistulas were difficult to cannulate because of short length, lack of palpability, or excessive depth. Each patient had 1 VWING implanted on the venous limb of the fistula; the arterial limb was cannulated in the standard fashion, allowing each patient to act as his/her own control. Fistula cannulation through the VWING was successful in 94% attempts, compared to 77% at the arterial limb without the VWING.

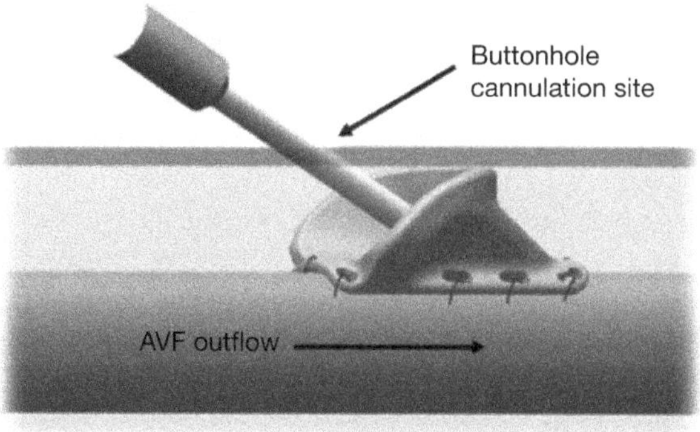

Figure 16-2. This schematic demonstrates the VWING sutured to the anterior AVF wall. Cannulation is accomplished using the buttonhole technique. Reproduce with permission, Elsevier, Inc.[8]

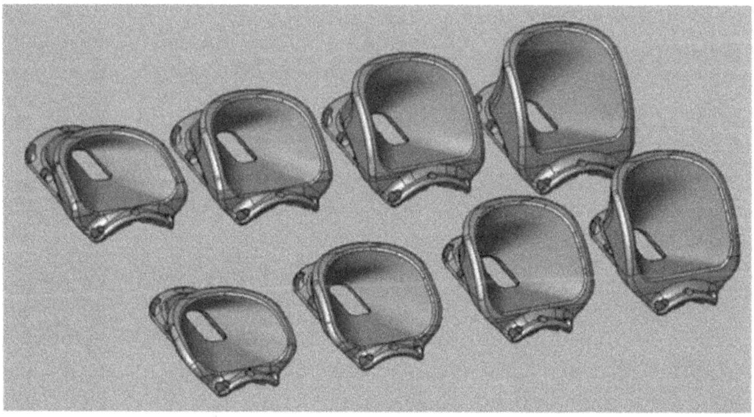

Figure 16-3. Each VWING device is 17.7 mm in length and available in 7 and 9 mm widths for variation in vessel diameter. AVF depth variation is accommodated by available 4-, 6-, 8-, and 10 mm heights. Reproduced with permission, Elsevier, Inc.[8]

No interventions were required at the VWING implant sites to maintain fistula functionality, and no device-related infections were identified over the course of 1367 subject days.

The favorable results in this small study lead to the launch of the VWING for the Salvage of AV Fistulae (SAVE) trial.[8] In this prospective, multicenter trial, subjects were eligible for enrollment only if an additional surgical procedure was required to establish reliable cannulation in an uncannulatable fistula. Confirmation that the fistula was suitable to support dialysis was obtained though ultrasonography. The prescribed depth of the fistulas, measured from the most superficial wall of the fistula to the skin surface, was 6–15 mm. One or two VWINGs were implanted on the fistula at the discretion of the surgeon. After three to five weeks of healing, the fistulas were cannulated though the VWING (s). Ninety-five percent of the implanted devices were cannulated within three months of implantation (median 36 days). Monitoring of the devices at three and six months demonstrated success in 92% and 86% of cannulations, respectively. Additionally, conversion to blunt needles was achieved in 91% of the successfully cannulated devices. The median number of sharp needle cannulations prior to blunt needle conversions was 14.

During the 6-month follow-up period of the SAVE trial, 39 interventions were performed on the fistulas to maintain functionality. Of those, 17 were considered to be device-related, and included: device explantation for pain, sepsis or device canting; percutaneous fistulaplasty, or seroma aspiration. One patient suffered sepsis from an infection of a VWING site, and three other patients were reported to suffer superficial access site cellulitis, treated with site rest and antibiotics. The overall cannulation site infection rate was 0.08/device-year, or 0.0007 per cannulation. The primary, assisted primary, and cumulative patency rates were 61%, 100%, and 100% respectively. Based upon the results of the SAVE trial, the Food and Drug Administration (FDA) approved the device in September 2013.

Implantation of the VWING is intended to provide continuous long-term access of the previously uncannulatable AVF. To confirm this, a follow-up study was conducted on the subjects enrolled in the SAVE trial,[9] examining the success of the device up to 18 months after implantation. At 18 months, the primary patency rate of the fistulas was 21%, and the assisted primary patency was 91%. While the primary patency was suboptimal, these patency rates demand comparison to either transposed brachiobasilic fistulas or superficialized cephalic-based fistulas. Two-year primary patency rates for transposed brachiobasilic fistulas broadly range from 10%–80%, with two-year secondary patency rates of 40%–90%.[10–13] The few data available for superficialized cephalic fistulas report one- and two-year primary patency rates of 60% and 50%, respectively and one- and two-year secondary patency rates of 70% and 61%, respectively.[5,6] The observed 91%, primary-assisted patency rate for the fistulas with the VWING implanted compares quite favorably to secondary patency rates of transposed brachiobasilic fistulas and superficialized cephalic fistulas, and therefore should encourage placement of the VWING. Moreover, wound complications when placing the VWINGs are rare.

Did VWING implantation adversely affect fistula primary patency? To investigate this possibility, interventions performed on the fistulas were segregated according to locus of intervention: at the VWING site, or remote from the VWING site. When accounting only for interventions at the VWING site, the primary patency was 78%; including only interventions remote from the VWING site, the primary patency was 38%. This demonstrates that implantation of the VWING has only a modest effect on fistula primary patency (Figure 16-4).

Implantation of a foreign body always raises concern regarding infection. During the entire 18-month postimplantation period, only one device was removed for infection, for an overall infection rate of 0.020 per patient-year, roughly 10% of the frequency of autogenous access site infections reported by the United States Renal Data System.[14] Possible reasons the infection risks was so low are: (1) the VWING is accessed after tissue ingrowth occurs, encapsulating the device. The first few cannulations may result in needle contact with the device, but as the cannulation site tract is developed and blunt needles are used, there is little contact between the needle and the device, probably reducing the chances of introducing bacteria onto the prosthetic device. (2) Wilson et al.[15] suggest that a well-functioning constant-site cannulation site has a cannulation tract that is >5 mm long. This distance between the skin puncture site and vessel puncture site provides adequate length to provide good hemostasis and infection protection. The patients with the VWINGs in place had fistulas that were 6 –15 mm deep. When approached at a 45° angle, the cannulation tract is 8–21 mm. (3) The dialysis units using the device were thoroughly trained to adhere to the "double preparation" technique, the best-demonstrated practice to minimize access site infection when constant-site cannulation is in use.[16]

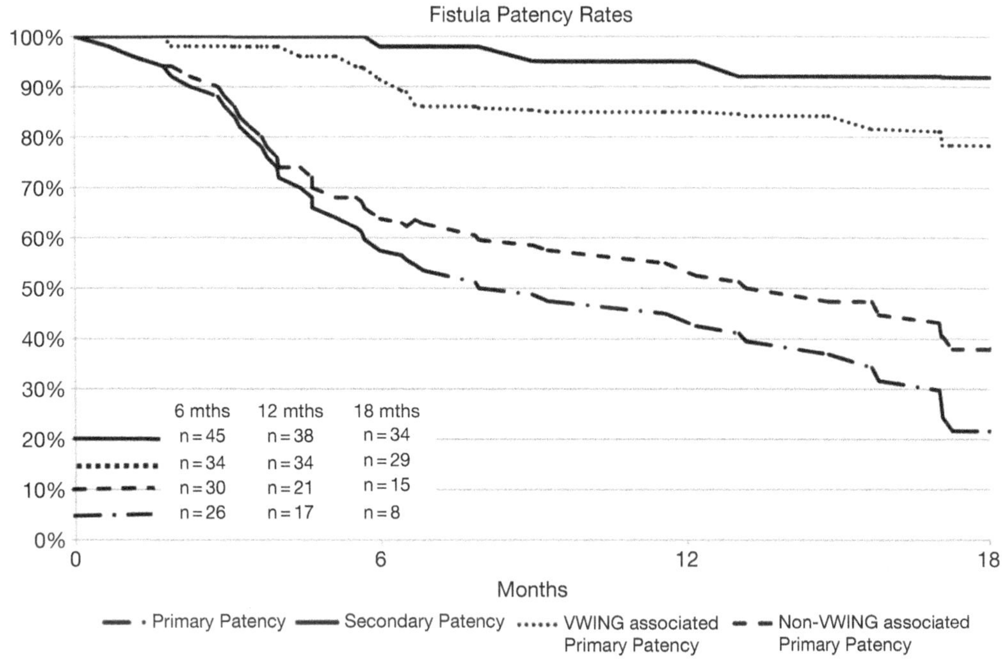

Figure 16-4. Kaplan-Meier survival curves demonstrating patency related to interventions at the VWING site compared to those remote from the VWING. Reproduced with permission, Elsevier, Inc.[9]

A potential alternative role for the VWING is enablement of access of brachiobasilic fistulas where transposition has been omitted, avoiding the morbidity of fistula mobilization. A recent review[17] of 94 VWINGs placed on 53 fistulas demonstrated that sharp needle cannulation was successful in 93% of attempted cannulations, and conversion to blunt needle cannulation was successful in 98%. The median time from VWING implantation to cannulation was 41 days. Ninety-one percent of fistulas that were cannulated through the VWINGs supported effective hemodialysis, and the fistula survival rate was 75% at 24 months. Complications related to the VWING were rare, and no infections were reported over 13,818 days of patient cannulation. In this limited series of patients, VWING implantation on nontransposed brachiobasilic fistulas appears to be a reasonable alternative to transposition.

TECHNIQUE

Implanting VWING(s) on an AVF is a simple outpatient procedure performed under local anesthesia. Nevertheless, careful attention must be paid to several details to ensure ultimate success: smooth, repetitive fistula cannulation in one that had previously been difficult of impossible to cannulate. First, complete ultrasound interrogation of the fistula is critical.[18] It is imperative to ensure that the fistula is of adequate size, and with sufficient flow volume to support hemodialysis. The "rule of 6s" guideline must be followed: the fistula should be at least 6 mm in diameter, and have a flow volume of at least 600 mL/min. If the diameter is smaller than 6 mm, the risk of back wall puncture with subsequent infiltration is increased. If the flow volume is below 600 mL/min, achieving satisfactory dialysis may not be possible. Placing a VWING on a fistula that cannot support hemodialysis is doomed to fail.

Measuring the depth of the fistula is also critical to successful fistula salvage with the VWING.[18] The optimal range of depths for the puncture site of the fistula is 4–13 mm below the skin surface; 15 mm is the maximum depth. Cannulation will fail in fistulas deeper than 15 mm despite VWING implantation. The tallest VWING is 10 mm, and hence will not be sufficiently palpable when implanted on a deep fistula. Furthermore, the dialysis needles will be too short to reach the fistula. Importantly, when measuring the depth of the fistula it is necessary to use the lightest touch possible with the ultrasound probe, with copious ultrasound gel. Pressure on the probe can distort the anatomy of the fistula, artefactually decreasing the distance between the skin and the puncture site.

Intraoperative ultrasonography must be employed at the time of implantation. Detailed B-mode mapping of the course of the fistula will facilitate successful placement. A 3 cm long straight segment of the fistula is required, and there should be no bends in the fistula within 1 cm of the VWING site. If one VWING is to be implanted (typically at the venous cannulation site), it should be at least 5 cm from the alternative cannulation site; if two VWINGS are implanted, they should be placed 5 cm apart to avoid recirculation. Implantation of the VWING on the arterial cannulation site of the fistula may suitably be done in a retrograde fashion, directing the needle toward the anastomosis. The venous cannulation site should always be place in the antegrade position, such that the dialysis needle is directed toward the central circulation. Placement of VWINGs near the axilla or antecubital fossa should be avoided, as cannulation at these sites is cumbersome.

After the appropriate site for implantation has been selected, local anesthesia is infiltrated. The skin is incised parallel to the fistula approximately 2 cm medial or lateral from the intended puncture site of the fistula. Typically, an incision of about 4 cm is required. The incision is deepened just through the dermis. A sub-dermal plane is developed to a point directly over the fistula, and the most superficial aspect of the fistula is exposed. Dissecting directly down to the fistula perpendicularly decreases the chances of tilting the VWING upon wound closure. The fistula is not fully mobilized;

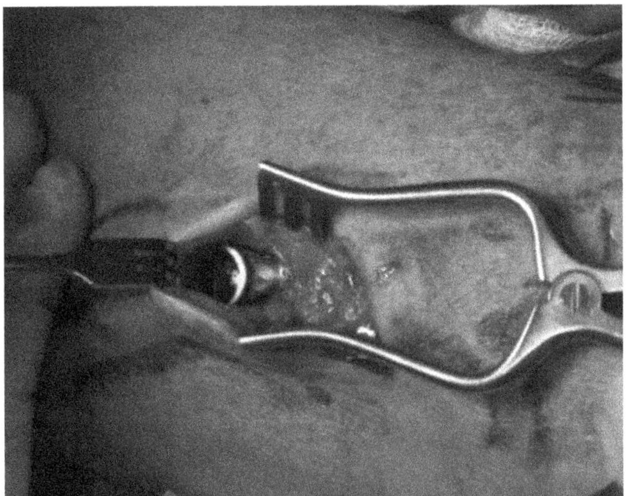

Figure 16-5. The VWING sutured to the anterior surface of the AVF just before closure of the incision. Surrounding adipose tissue is largely left in place to help stabilize the device. Reproduced with permission, Elsevier, Inc.[8]

only the anterior third is skeletonized, sufficient to suture the device in place. The correct device size is selected—typically, the height of the device approximates the fistula depth. The device is sutured to the fistula with a 6–0 monofilament permanent suture, using a BV-1 or RB-2 needle in a continuous or interrupted technique.

The skin is reapproximated over the device. Prior to closing the wound, easy palpation of the device is confirmed. This may require local excision of subdermal fat. Moreover, further lipectomy should be performed if the surrounding fat applies pressure to the VWING causing it to tilt as the skin is reapproximated, but extensive lipectomy should be avoided, since surrounding fat will help hold the device in place (Figure 16-5). The skin is then closed with a subcuticular suture.

The patient is seen in follow-up at three weeks. Ultrasonography should be repeated to ensure continued satisfactory diameter and flow volume in the fistula. If the swelling has subsided and the fistula is easily palpable, it is released for cannulation. Occasionally, local seroma may be present. Another two weeks of healing typically resolves this process, and cannulation can then be undertaken.

In summary, the VWING safely and effectively facilitates cannulation of AVFs that would otherwise require surgical revision for successful cannulation. The device is easily placed with minimal complications. It is a useful addition to the armamentarium of the dialysis access surgeon.

REFERENCES

1. NKF-K/DOQI clinical practice guidelines and clinical practice recommendations for vascular access. http://kidneyfoundation.cachefly.net. Updated 2006. Accessed May 20, 2017.
2. End Stage Renal Disease National Coordinating Center. Fistula first catheter last. http://fistulafirst.esrdncc.org/ffcl/. Accessed May 20, 2017.
3. Patel ST, Hughes J, Mills JL Sr. Failure of arteriovenous fistula maturation: an unintended consequence of exceeding dialysis outcome quality guidelines for hemodialysis access. *J Vasc Surg*. 2002;35:439–435.
4. Centers for Disease Control and Prevention. Adult obesity facts. https://www.cdc.gov/obesity/data/adult.html. Accessed June 2, 2017.
5. Bronder CM, Cull DL, Kuper SG, et al. Fistula elevation procedure: experience with 295 consecutive cases during a 7-year period. *J Am Coll Surg*. 2008;206:1069–1075.
6. Woo K, Farber A, Doros G, et al. Evaluation of the efficacy of the transposed upper arm arteriovenous fistula: a single institutional review of 190 basilic and cephalic vein transposition procedures. *J Vasc Surg*. 2007;46(1):94–99.
7. Hill AA, Vasudevan T, Young N, et al. Use of an implantable needle guide to access difficult of impossible to cannulate arteriovenous fistulae suing the buttonhole technique. *J Vasc Access*. 2013;14:164–169.
8. Jennings WC, Galt SW, Shenoy S, et al. The Venous Window Needle Guide, a hemodialysis cannulation device for salvage of uncannulatable arteriovenous fistulas. *J Vasc Surg*. 2014;60(4):1024–1032.
9. Galt S, Crawford M, Blebea J, et al. The efficacy and durability of the Venous Window Needle Guide implanted on uncannulatable arteriovenous fistulas. *J Vasc Surg*. 2016;64:708–714.
10. Vrakas G, Defigueiredo F, Turner S, et al. A comparison of the outcomes of one-stage and two-stage brachio-basilic arteriovenous fistulas. *J Vasc Surg*. 2013;58(5):1300–1304.
11. Korkut AK, Kosem M. Superficialization of the basilic vein technique in brachiobasilic arteriovenous fistula: surgical experience of 350 cases during 4 years period. *Ann Vasc Surg*. 2010;24(6):762–767.

12. Dix FP, Khan Y, Al-Khaffaf H. The brachial artery-basilic vein arterio-venous fistula in vascular access for haemodialysis-a review paper. *Eur J Vasc Endovasc Surg*. 2006;31(1):70–79.
13. Wolford HY, Hsu J, Rhodes JM, et al. Outcome after autogenous brachial-basilic upper arm transpositions in the post-National Kidney Foundation Dialysis Outcomes Quality Initiative era. *J Vasc Surg*. 2005;42(5):951–956.
14. United States Renal Data System. USRDS 2012 annual data report: atlas of chronic kidney disease and end-stage renal disease in the United States. Bethesda, MD: National Institute of Diabetes and Digestive and Kidney Diseases; 2012.
15. Wilson N, Shenoy S. Managing 'buttonhole' complications. *J Vasc Access*. 2014;15(suppl 7):S91–S95.
16. Ball L. The buttonhole technique: strategies to reduce infections. *Nephrol Nurs J*. 2010;37:473–477.
17. Galt S, Crawford M. The VWING vascular needle guide, a novel method to access non-transposed brachiobasilic arteriovenous fistulas. *J Vasc Surg*. 2016;63(6):192S.
18. Talukdar A, Wang S, Gupta, et al. Preoperative duplex characteristics predict successful use of the V-WING. *J Vasc Surg*. 2015;62(3):833.

17

What to Do with Patent Arteriovenous Fistulas after Successful Renal Transplantation?

Staci Canterino, MS, PA-C and David Fox, MD

After successful renal transplantation, patients with a patent vascular access will frequently approach their nephrologists or surgeons requesting removal or closure of their access. There are several factors that patients and physicians will state as reasons to ligate their access. For example, they will argue that they have no use for the access since there is no longer a need for dialysis. Cosmetic concerns are also a frequent motivator in patients' requests to remove their access (Figure 17-1).

The dilemma facing the surgeon is whether or not to ligate a patent access after successful renal transplantation. There are several questions that the surgeon should

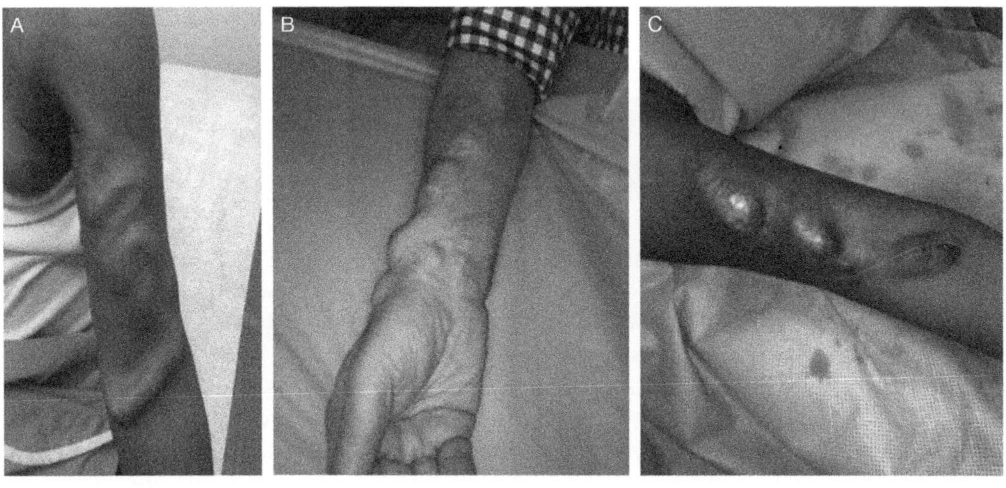

Figure 17-1. Representative cosmetic deformities associated with AV access. Tortuous mega-fistula (**A**). Aneurysmal radial cephalic fistula (**B**). AV fistula with diffuse hypopigmentation and puncture site aneurysms (**C**).

consider when contemplating ligation. The fundamental question of course, is will the transplanted patient need the access in the future? While patients are often under the impression that the transplanted kidney will last indefinitely, they are often unaware of the facts of kidney transplant graft survival. According to the 2010 OPTN data report, ten-year graft survival for deceased donors was 43%, whereas living donor graft survival was 61%.[1] Thus, a large number of transplanted patients will ultimately need either re-transplantation or resumption of dialysis. Another important consideration is the availability of donor kidneys. Many patients are under the impression that if their transplanted kidney fails, they can simply receive a new kidney. This is not often the case.

Despite an increasing number of candidates on the waiting list, the total number of kidney transplants in the US has not changed appreciably for a decade. In 2012, there were 92,000 patients on the waiting list for a donor kidney. During the same period, only 17,000 patients received a kidney transplant.[1] Thus, the demand for transplanted kidneys is five times greater than the supply. It is therefore unlikely, that the patient with a failing kidney transplant will be able to receive a new donor kidney in a timely fashion.

While one can cite the shortage of donor kidneys and the limited functional lifespan of kidney transplants as arguments in favor of maintaining the access, there are potential arguments for ligation of the access. These potential benefits include, improved cosmesis and correction of deformity, prevention of inflow artery aneurysmal degeneration with consequent mural thrombus formation and risk of embolization, improved cardiac function as well as increased patient survival.

There is limited literature to guide decision making on the management of AV access following successful transplantation. There have been no randomized trials on routine AV fistula closure following successful renal transplantation.[2] Remarkably, none of the current published vascular access or transplant guidelines such as the National Kidney Foundation Kidney Disease Outcomes Quality Initiative "DOQI Guidelines" provide recommendations for the management of vascular access following renal transplantation.[2] Indeed there are no established guidelines on this topic. Clinical practice varies widely and is a subject of controversy and debate. A number of recent review articles have supported the concept of access preservation following successful renal transplantation.[2,3,4,5] This chapter will review the available literature with the goal of developing and suggesting guidelines for the management of AV access following transplantation and point to future directions for research.

BRACHIAL ARTERY DILATATION

Dilation of the inflow artery after creation of a vascular access is a common phenomenon and a necessary response for fistula maturation. Less commonly, this process will go unchecked and patients will develop true aneurysmal dilatation of the brachial artery. This dilatation may be associated with mural thrombus formation, which can result in peripheral embolization, causing limb-threatening ischemia (Figures 17-2 and 17-3). The enlarged arteries may also cause pain as well as cosmetic deformity (Figure 17-4). Not much is known about the etiology, incidence and natural history of inflow artery aneurysms in AV access. Possible explanations for this phenomenon include increased flow in the inflow artery. High flow through this vessel may result in

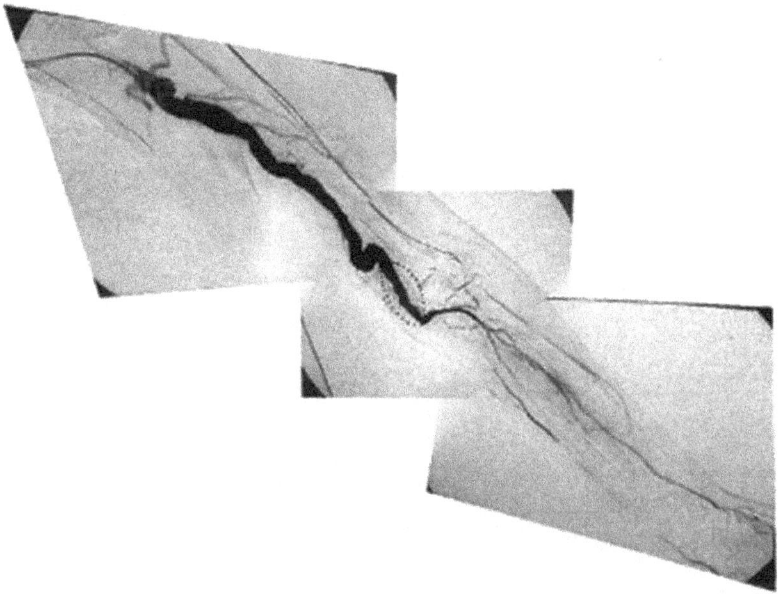

Figure 17-2. Angiogram of dilated left axillobrachial artery demonstrating distal embolic occlusions. *Dotted line* marks outer dimension of aneurysm. *Source: Eugster T, Wigger P, Bölter S, Bock A, Hodel K, Stierli P. Brachial artery dilatation after arteriovenous fistulae in patients after renal transplantation: a 10-year follow-up with ultrasound scan. J Vasc Surg. 2003; 37(3): 564–567; used with permission.*

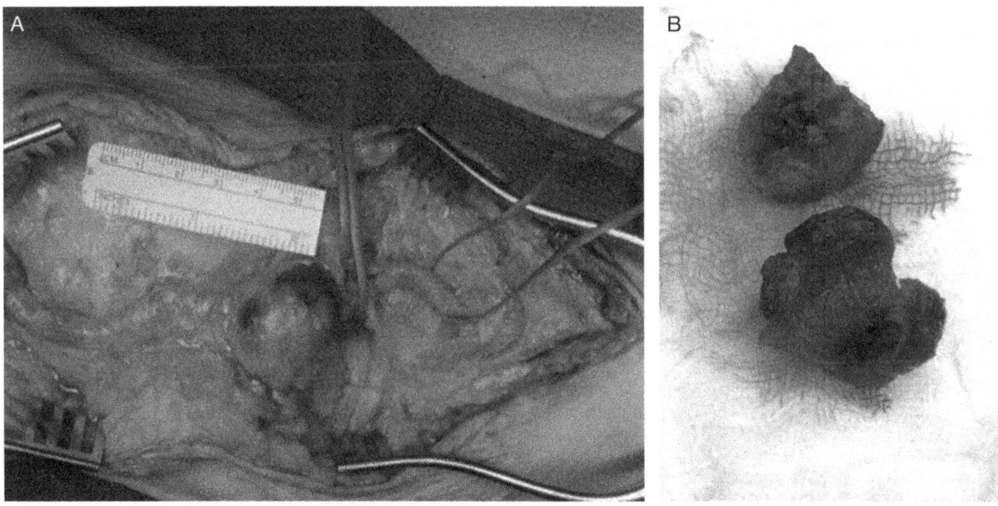

Figure 17-3. Dilated brachial artery with focal distal brachial artery aneurysm, intraoperative view (**A**). Laminated mural thrombus retrieved from brachial artery aneurysm (**B**).

abnormal shear stress, damaging the elastic fibers of the internal elastic lamina, often resulting in a progressive increase in diameter and tortuosity. Microscopic assessment of the arterial wall of operated aneurysms proximal to the arteriovenous fistula reveals characteristics similar to those of an arteriosclerotic aneurysm: fragmentation of the elastic tissue, increased fibrosis, muscle atrophy, intimal thickening and calcifications.[6]

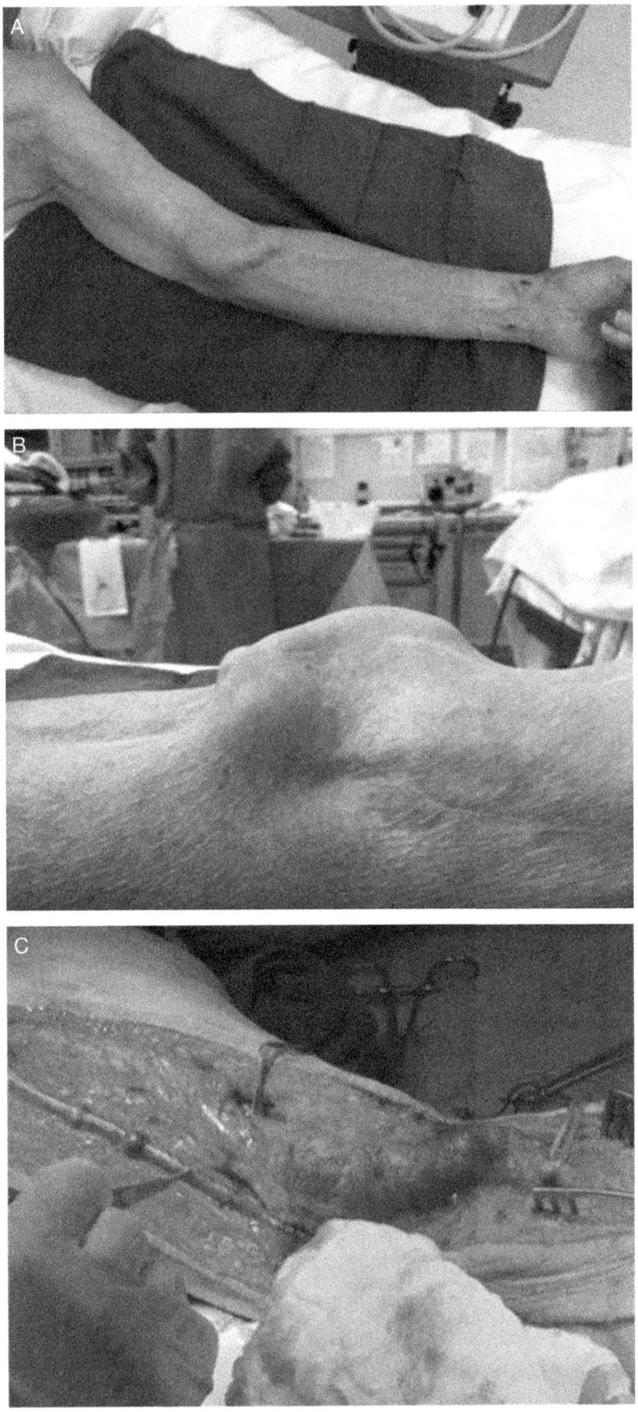

Figure 17-4. Fusiform brachial artery aneurysm, preoperative view AP (**A**), Closeup Lateral (**B**). Intraoperative view, note forceps holding basilic vein being used for bypass (**C**).

Development of brachial artery aneurysms after transplantation might additionally be explained by the duration of placement, use of corticosteroids or use of immunosuppressive medications especially sirolimus, which may adversely affect wound healing.[7] The influence of atherosclerotic risk factors, such as diabetes, tobacco use, and hypertension, on a previously diseased arterial wall has been implicated as well.[8]

There is a small body of literature that has attempted to document the incidence and natural history of inflow artery aneurysms status post AV access. Chemla et al. conducted a retrospective study describing a series of 13 patients with brachial artery aneurysms associated with AV access. They observed that the average time for aneurysmal formation was 40 ± 35.8 months. Ten of these patients presented with symptoms related to embolization. Chemla reported that all patients with patent brachial arteries following surgical repair experienced complete relief of the presenting symptoms (pain, ischemia, cold hands) at a median follow-up of 14 months.[7]

Eugster et al. performed a prospective study in order elucidate the natural history of brachial artery dilation in transplant patients.[6] They performed serial brachial artery diameter measurements over 10 years in 29 kidney transplant patients with AV fistulas using ultrasound. Nine patients with AV fistulas who had not received kidney transplants were studied as control.

They observed that the brachial artery diameters on the side with a fistula increased over time. This dilation occurred despite the fact that a third of the fistulas were occluded at baseline and half of all fistulas were occluded after ten years. Brachial artery diameters on the side contralateral to the fistula remained stable and were smaller than the brachial artery diameters on the fistula side at all time points (Table 17-1).

TABLE 17-1. DIAMETERS (MM) OF BRACHIAL ARTERIES ACCORDING TO SIDE AND TIME. EUGSTER ET AL.[(6)]

	Side with AF	*Contralateral side*	P *value*
1991 (n = 29)			
Patent (n = 20)	6.4 ± 1.8	4.3 ± 0.6	.001
Occluded (n = 9)	5.2 ± 1.5	4.0 ± 0.5	.02
P value	.066	.119	
1994 (n = 26)			
Patent (n = 14)	6.6 ± 1.7	4.2 ± 0.9	.001
Occluded (n = 12)	5.3 ± 2.0	4.0 ± 0.7	.008
P value	.029	.239	
2001 (n = 19)			
Patent (n = 10)	7.4 ± 1.3	5.1 ± 0.4	.005
Occluded (n = 9)	5.7 ± 2.8	4.5 ± 0.8	.173
P value	.022	.252	
Control (patent without transplantation; n = 9)			
	5.8 ± 0.6	4.4 ± 0.6	.001
Dilatation (mm) of brachial arteries with patent AF			
	Transplanted (n= = 14; 1994) 6.6 ± 1.7	Nontransplanted (n = 9) 5.8 ± 0.6	Not significant

Brachial artery diameters on the fistula side were greater in the transplanted patients versus the nontransplanted patients but these differences were not statistically significant. The magnitude of the brachial artery dilation was greater in arms with a patent fistula versus occluded fistula (16% versus 10%), however, the brachial arteries in arms with occluded fistulas continued to dilate over time despite the absence of flow in the fistula. Two patients required surgical treatment for embolic occlusions of peripheral arteries.

The finding that the brachial arteries in arms with occluded fistulas continued to dilate after the fistula was occluded provides a strong argument against surgical closure of the fistula in the transplanted patient for the purpose of preventing brachial artery dilation and its attendant potential morbidity.

True inflow artery aneurysmal dilatation in AV access patients seems to be a rare event. Marzelle et al. reported a retrospective study summarizing data from patients who presented with aneurysmal degeneration after access creation. They analyzed the characteristics, potential risks, and therapeutic options for donor artery aneurysms that developed in ten patients with AV fistulas. Patients with pseudoaneurysms were excluded from the study. Seven men and three women (mean age, 38.1 years) were identified with aneurysmal dilatation (mean diameter, 44.5; range, 24–80 mm). Mean duration of access was 83.6 ± 48.8 months. The diagnosis of aneurysmal degeneration was made at 117.5 ± 53.8 months after access creation. This is nearly three times later than that seen in Chemla's series.[7] The mean interval between AVF closure and diagnosis of the aneurysm was 11 years (range, 3–19 months). Presenting symptoms included pain, swelling as well as ischemia. They observed that the major risk of aneurysmal dilatation is related to the development of thrombus in the aneurysm. Like Eugster, they found that ligation of the access did not usually reverse or stop aneurysmal dilatation. They conclude that inflow artery aneurysmal dilatation is a rare but significant complication of vascular access. They recommend that surgical correction be advised in order to avoid the potential complication of thromboembolization. However, they did not provide definitive treatment recommendations.

In summary, aneurysmal dilatation of inflow arteries is a rare but potentially morbid process. The rare incidence and the failure of access ligation to prevent ongoing aneurysmal dilatation are not sufficiently compelling reasons to support access ligation in transplanted patients.

LEFT VENTRICULAR HYPERTROPHY (LVH)

LVH is the most common cardiac pathology seen in ESRD patients. It is found in almost 75% of the patients at the start of dialysis. LVH is associated with significant cardiac morbidity and mortality. Patients who develop LVH are at increased risk of heart failure, arrhythmias and sudden death.[9] The etiology of LVH in renal patients is multifactorial and includes factors such as hypertension, anemia, uremia, and the presence of an AV access. The results of studies evaluating the cardiac impact of functioning AV fistulas, however, has been discordant.[10]

There have been reports of negative hemodynamic effects of dialysis access resulting in what has been described by Amerling as fistula toxicity.[11] Cardiac and vascular complications have been described. Specifically, the AV access decreases systemic vascular resistance, resulting in increased stroke volume and increased cardiac output, possibly resulting in left ventricular overload, eccentric LVH and high output cardiac failure.[10] Fistula toxicity has been described as proportional to access flow rate, and inversely proportional to cardiac status.[11]

On the other hand there may be beneficial cardiovascular and other systemic effects associated with a patent AV fistula. The beneficial cardiovascular effects include lowered blood pressure, increased LVEF and reduced arterial stiffness. Increased arterial stiffness is associated with a higher risk of cardiovascular events. Another beneficial effect of a patent fistula is a reduction in the rate of decline of glomerular filtration rate (GFR) in patients with advanced CKD. Hypothetically one could extrapolate a salutary role in preserving late allograft function.[5] Another reason to maintain the access is so that it can be used as a conduit for phlebotomy and intravenous access for medications.[2] This would allow the superficial veins to be preserved for possible future AV access creation.

LVH may improve after renal transplantation, but complete regression is not usually achieved. It has been theorized that this may be attributable to the presence of a patent fistula.[3] The specific long-term contribution of a patent fistula on the development of LVH is not clearly defined. Studies have described high output cardiac failure resolving following ligation of high-flow AV fistulas; however, whether access ligation reverses the morphologic abnormalities is less clear. The literature reports disparate results regarding the effect of access ligation on LVH. We will now review the literature for and against access ligation.

LITERATURE ADVOCATING LIGATION

Several studies provide data supporting the practice of access ligation. Theses studies advocate ligation as a means of reducing LVH (Table 17-2).[10,12–14] Three of these are prospective studies, one is of matched-pair design. None were randomized trials. van Duijnhoven reported a prospective study of twenty patients with a well-functioning renal transplant.[12] Echocardiograms were performed at baseline and three to four months following fistula ligation. They observed that closure of the fistula following renal transplant resulted in decreased left ventricular mass index (LVMi) and decreased left ventricular end-diastolic diameter (LVEDD). The decrease in LVMi was significantly related to the magnitude of LVMi and LVEDD prior to the closure of the fistula. Of note, the reduction in LVMi did not correlate to fistula flow. It should be mentioned that the fistulas in this study were high flow fistulas with a mean fistula

TABLE 17-2. REPORTS ADVOCATING ACCESS LIGATION FOLLOWING RENAL TRANSPLANTATION

Authors	Design	Follow-up	Results[a]	Access Flow
Movilli, 2010[b]	Pro, $n = 25$	6 months	Reduced LVMI, etc.	–
Cridlig, 2008	Matched-pair $n = 38$	n/a	Reduced LVMI, etc.	1,040 ml/min
Unger, 2002	Pro, $n = 17$	3–10 week	Reduced LVMI, etc.	–
van Duijnhoven, 2001	Pro, $n = 20$	4–5 months	Reduced LVMI, etc.	1,790 ml/min

[a]No cardiac morbidity/mortality or survival data reported.
[b]Non-txp.

flow of 1,790 ml/min. It is conceivable that the higher flow in these accesses could have predisposed these patients to develop more significant cardiac effects.

Based on these observations, the authors hypothesize that patients with successful renal transplants and persistent LVH might benefit from closure of a fistula. This closure results in a decrease in eccentric LVH. It should also be mentioned that LV mass normalized in 33% of patients with LVH before fistula ligation. So not all patients may require or benefit from access ligation. While this study did show improvement of LVH, it did not report on cardiac morbidity and mortality.

Unger et al. conducted a prospective study of seventeen kidney transplant recipient patients referred for fistula closure.[13] The authors investigated whether surgical closure of the fistula is associated with reduction of abnormalities of left ventricular morphology in renal transplant patients. Echocardiograms, heart rate, and blood pressure were evaluated at baseline, during test fistula occlusion with pneumatic tourniquet, and following surgical fistula occlusion. They sought to determine which parameters would be the best predictors of post-operative improvements in cardiac morphology. The authors observed early and significant decreases in LVEDD and LVMi at three to ten weeks following fistula closure. These changes were not seen in the control renal transplant patients with patent fistulas. Unlike van Duijnhoven, they did not observe the relationship between the change in LVH after fistula closure and the LVMi and LVEDD prior to closure. They found that acute changes in total peripheral resistance and mean arterial blood pressure during pneumatic occlusions were the best predictors of post-ligation LVEDD and LVMi regressions. Like van Duijnhoven, these authors did not report on cardiac morbidity and mortality in the study population.

Other studies have reported the cardiac effects present in asymptomatic patients with high access flows. Cridlig et al. presented a case-controlled, match-paired study between renal transplant recipients with and without fistulas and evaluated the cardiac impact of a functioning fistula with echocardiography.[10] Seventy-six patients with a mean age of 49 years underwent echocardiography. These patients had no prior history of diabetes or cardiovascular disease Thirty-eight had a functioning fistula. Similarly to Unger and van Duijnhoven findings, Cridlig reported that LVMi was significantly higher in patients with a functioning fistula versus those without a fistula (135.1 $g/m^2 \pm 30.3$ g/m^2 vs. 112.4 $g/m^2 \pm 28$ g/m^2, $P = 0.001$). The presence of a fistula resulted in a fourfold increased risk of developing LVH.

They attempted to determine if a dose-effect of fistula flow was present. Their analysis revealed a trend towards increasing LVMi with higher fistula flows versus those without fistulas (142.6 $g/m^2 \pm 30$ g/m^2 vs.126.9 $g/m^2 \pm 23.9$ g/m^2, $P = 0.084$). Their results concerning the effect of access flow suggest that the fistula is a new circulation, characterized by low resistance and high flow back to the heart, leading to a higher cardiac flow rate, which becomes proportional to the fistula flow rate. This study suggests that, in stable asymptomatic renal transplantation patients, functioning fistulas have significant impact on cardiac mass, cardiac index and left ventricular dimensions. Like the previously cited studies, the effect on cardiac morbidity and mortality was not investigated.

Several studies have shown regression of LVH after fistula closure in kidney transplant recipients, yet whether this regression is a consequence of the restoration of normal fluid balance that follows transplantation or can be attributed to removal of the fistula is not clear. Movilli et al. conducted a prospective study of twenty-five consecutive hemodialysis patients with fistula malfunction who underwent closure and conversion to a tunneled dialysis catheter as well as thirty-six patients with a well-functioning fistula.[14] The authors evaluated the effect of fistula closure on functional and structural echocardiographic findings at baseline and six months after closure. The authors found that the presence of a fistula negatively influenced LV performance and cardiac geometry in dialysis patients, and its closure was associated with significant improvement in these parameters. Specifically, in the fistula-closure group, Left Ventricular Mass (LVM) decreased from 225 ± 55 to 206 ± 51 g (P <0.001) and LVMi decreased from 135 ± 40 to 123 ± 35 g/m^2 (P < 0.001). LV internal diastolic diameter, interventricular septum thickness, and diastolic posterior wall thickness decreased significantly, whereas left ventricular ejection fraction (LVEF) increased from 56% ± 7% to 59% ± 6% (P <0.001). Movilli concluded that fistula closure is associated with a significant improvement in LVEF, a significant decrease in LVM and LVMi, and a more favorable shift of cardiac geometry toward normality.

The findings of these studies favor the practice of access ligation, based primarily on the improvement of echocardiographic parameters such as LVMi and function. It must be emphasized, however, that none of these studies were designed to detect improvements in patient survival or reduced cardiac morbidity and mortality. Therefore a survival advantage cannot be attributed to access ligation and remains a matter of speculation.

LITERATURE ADVOCATING ACCESS PRESERVATION

Several studies support the practice of preserving AV fistulas in renal transplant patients (Table 17-3).[15–21] The majority of these studies are retrospective although two are of prospective design. Like the studies advocating access ligation none of these studies were randomized trials. Peteiro et al. conducted a prospective study of 30

TABLE 17-3. REPORTS ADVOCATING ACCESS PRESERVATION FOLLOWING RENAL TRANSPLANTATION

Author, Year	Design	Follow-up	Results of Ligation
Soleimani, 2012	Retro, n = 23[a]	6–18 months	No benefit (ECHO findings)
Manca, 2005	Retro, n = 542	–	Natural History Study
Sheashaa, 2004	Retro, n = 34[a]	10 years	No benefit (ECHO findings) Patient and TXP surviva
Patard, 2002	Retro, n = 160	69 months	Natural history study (Patent AVF = not morbid)
De Lima, 1999	Retro, n = 39 Pro, n = 10	62 months 7–0 days	No benefit (ECHO findings)
Peteiro, 1994	Pro, n = 30	10 months	"No fistula patency influence on LV mass and function"
Huting, 1992	Pro, n=24	41 months	"Fistula patency had no influence on LV mass or function"

[a] Spontaneous thromboses.

patients (19 men, 11 women, aged 37 ± 13 years) who underwent renal transplantation in order to examine changes in left ventricular mass and function at the time of transplantation and 10 +/− 1.8 months later.[16] Following renal transplantation there was a significant decrease in LVMi. The LVMi decreased from 201 ± 56 to 171 ± 41 g/m^2. Both LV diastolic diameter and the LV end–diastolic volume indices also decreased following transplantation.

Half of the patients in the study had a patent access, half had an occluded access. At follow up there were no significant differences in LV dimensions, mass, diastolic or systolic function between the groups with a patent or occluded access.

Following transplantation, 21 patients were observed to have significant reductions in blood pressure. Nine patients experienced an increase or no change in blood pressure following transplantation. In terms of cardiac mass and function the 21 patients who experienced a reduction in blood pressure were also found to have significant reductions in LV mass and volumes. No such reductions were seen in the patients whose blood pressure increased or remained stable. As the presence of a functional AV access was not associated with adverse cardiac morphology and function, the findings of this study favor access preservation.

Patard et al. performed a retrospective natural history study of one hundred and sixty renal transplant patients with fistulas.[17] The vascular access had been created at a median of 29 months prior to renal transplantation (Range: 0 to 312 months). The mean follow-up was 69 months from renal transplantation and 95 months from creation of the fistula. At follow up, the majority of accesses remained functional (61.9%). Spontaneous thrombosis had occurred in 30.6% of cases. All of the fistulas that thrombosed spontaneously were forearm fistulas. Access ligation was performed in 7.5% of cases. The indications for access ligation were high flow, painful thrombosis, aneurysm formation, steal syndrome, and other miscellaneous symptoms such as pain, paresthesia and cramping. The authors concluded that since most fistulas were still functional and seem to be well tolerated at long-term follow-up, systematic closure of fistulas after renal transplantation does not appear to be warranted and should be avoided as it would deprive patients of a useful access should dialysis be required in the future.

Soleimani et al. also conducted a retrospective study to evaluate the natural history of AV fistulas in kidney transplant recipients and also to study the effect of spontaneous AV fistula closure after kidney transplantation on cardiac status.[18] The records of 180 kidney transplant recipients were reviewed. 142 had AV fistulas prior to transplantation. At the time of study following kidney transplantation 99 (69.7%) had a functioning fistula.

Echocardiographic evaluation was performed in 23 of the patients with a functioning fistula and comparison was made to 17 patients whose fistulas had spontaneously closed. Both groups were found to have an improved left ventricular ejection fraction post-transplant. There was a trend towards lower left ventricular end-systolic and end-diastolic diameters in the group with patent fistulas, but this did not reach statistical significance. Of note, the mean fistula flow in these patients was relatively low at 560 ± 405 mL/min. So this was not a study of high flow fistulas.

Spontaneous AVF closure was not found to offer a significant beneficial cardiac effect. This is not surprising as lower flow fistulas are more likely to experience spontaneous thrombosis and are likely to induce cardiac morphologic and functional changes of lower magnitude than high flow fistulas. Based on these findings the authors conclude that there is insufficient data to promote systematic closure of AVF after successful kidney transplantation.

Sheashaa et al. also evaluated the effect of spontaneous fistula closure in the early period after renal transplantation on cardiac function and morphology.[19] The authors retrospectively studied seventeen transplant patients whose fistulas had thrombosed within the first month after transplantation and compared them to 34 transplant patients with patent fistulas. Echocardiographic assessment was done prior to transplantation and at one year after transplantation.

The echocardiograms performed at one year post transplantation showed no differences in LVM, LVMi and LV systolic and diastolic function between the patients with a patent fistula and those whose fistulas had thrombosed. They observed trends toward lower left ventricular end-systolic diameters (LVESD) and LVEDD in the group with thrombosed fistulas. The group with patent fistulas had higher cardiac output and cardiac index ($p < .05$). Information regarding access flow and forearm versus upper arm location of the access was not provided.

Unlike the other studies cited, this study did report outcomes data for the patient and allografts. No differences were found regarding actuarial 10 year patient and graft survival between groups with and without a patent AV access. They observed that spontaneous fistula thrombosis does not result in beneficial cardiac or survival effects and state that routine fistula closure is therefore not warranted. Unfortunately, as no information was provided regarding access flow the generalizability of their conclusions is limited. Again, it is worth mentioning that lower flow accesses are more likely to thrombose spontaneously and are less likely to be associated with adverse cardiac effects than high flow accesses. In addition, patients with a lower ejection fraction are more likely to experience access thrombosis and might therefore potentially be more likely to display abnormal cardiac morphology and dysfunction.

De Lima et al. reported a retrospective study that was designed to elucidate the relationship between echocardiographic outcomes and AV access flow. They compared echocardiographic findings in 39 patients with renal transplants and patent AV fistulas and 22 transplant patients whose fistulas had been ligated for esthetic reasons. These ligations had been performed within 2 months of renal transplantation. Echocardiograms were performed 14 months following transplantation. The mean access flow in the group with patent fistulas was 900 ± 350 mL/min (range: 500–1,600). They found that there were no significant differences between the groups in terms of LVM, cardiac index, ejection fraction and LVH. LVEDD was marginally higher in the group with patent fistulas (52.7 ± 4.8 vs. 49.2 ± 4.6, $p = 0.007$).

They also evaluated for changes in echocardiograpohic and hemodynamic parameters in the patients whose accesses were ligated. Measurements were obtained prior to and 7 to 10 days following ligation. No significant changes were seen in cardiac index, LV posterior wall thickness, LVEDD, ejection fraction and LVMi pre- and post-ligation. They conclude that their data does not support the practice of routine access closure in all patients following renal transplantation.

The disparate results of the studies for and against access ligation may have to do with bias induced by the emphasis of LVMi as a principal endpoint. Following transplantation body weight may decrease when fluid balance is restored and stabilized lowering body mass. On the other hand steroid use may increase fat and body mass. These changes in weight may influence the LVMi even if there has been no actual change in LVM.[2]

CONCLUSIONS AND FUTURE DIRECTIONS

Although several of the studies cited in this chapter suggest a benefit from access closure, the current evidence is inconclusive. As outcomes in transplantation improve it is possible that the balance may tip towards a benefit of routine access closure.

Systematic AV access closure in renal transplantation patients is not recommended. The literature has shown that AV fistula closure may reduce left ventricular volume and mass in renal transplant patients. In spite of that, whether fistula closure will reduce cardiac morbidity and mortality remains unknown.

Future research, particularly randomized prospective studies are needed in order to identify subsets of patients who would benefit from access ligation. Such subsets include patients with LVH and high-flow fistulas with outcomes predicting LVH reversibility and patients with an EF of <40% and/or significant pulmonary hypertension.[11] It would also be useful to better identify patients at increased risk for return to dialysis. Utilizing the estimated glomerular filtration rate (eGFR) at one year post-transplant has been suggested.[2] A randomized controlled trial evaluating the effect of access closure in asymptomatic patients with high-flow fistula has been proposed by a group in the Netherlands.[2]

GUIDELINES/RECOMMENDATIONS

Until the results of the proposed studies are available to guide decision making we suggest that clinicians refer to the following guidelines for managing AV access in the post-transplant patient.[5]

1. Do not ligate an asymptomatic access.
2. Do not ligate an access during the first year post transplant unless it is an emergency. The incidence of transplant failure and return to dialysis is highest in the first year following transplantion.[2]
3. After the first year assess the risk of transplant failure and only consider ligation after consultation with the nephrologist and/or transplant team.
4. Avoid ligating a forearm fistula, as these are associated with fewer local and systemic complications such as steal and high output failure.
5. Consider ligation of the fistula if the patients presents with significant symptoms such as severe venous hypertension, risk of rupture from aneurysms/pseudoaneurysms, significant high output failure or distal ischemia. Alternatively, consider managing these problems with appropriate interventions such as angioplasty, surgical revision or flow reduction procedures.

The philosophy of our practice is to preserve and maintain AV access in patients who have undergone renal transplantation. Our protocol for patients who are actively dialyzing is to perform a scheduled access evaluation by history and physical examination every three months. We recommend that patients who have received a transplant continue to return for quarterly access evaluations. If abnormalities are detected the access is evaluated with duplex ultrasound. If the viability of the access is threatened an intervention such as angioplasty is considered. When performing these interventions an effort is made to minimize the use of nephrotoxic contrast agents. We make liberal use of duplex ultrasound guidance to guide dialysis access interventions and also utilize alternative contrast agents such as carbon dioxide.[22] When iodinated contrast is used the dose is limited and hydration and *N*-acetylcysteine are administered.

REFERENCES

1. Matas AJ, Smith JM, Skeans MA, et al. OPTN/SRTR 2012 Annual Data Report: kidney. *Am J Transplant*. 2014;1:11–44.
2. Voorzaat BM, van Schaik J, Siebelink HM, et al. The pros and cons of preserving a functioning arteriovenous fistula after kidney transplantation. *J Vasc Access*. 2016;17 Suppl 1:16–22.
3. Yaffe HC, Greenstein SM. Should functioning AV fistulas be ligated after renal transplantation? *J Vasc Access*. 2012; 13(4):405–8.
4. Duque JC, Gomez C, Tabbara M, et al. The impact of arteriovenous fistulae on the myocardium: the impact of creation and ligation in the transplant era. *Semin Dial*. 2015; 28(3):305–10.
5. Wilmink T, Hollingworth L, Dasgupta I. Access ligation in transplant patients. *J Vasc Access*. 2016; 17 Suppl 1:64–8.
6. Eugster T, Wigger P, Bölter S, Bock A, Hodel K, Stierli P. Brachial artery dilatation after arteriovenous fistulae in patients after renal transplantation: a 10-year follow-up with ultrasound scan. *J Vasc Surg*. 2003; 37(3): 564–567.
7. Chemla E, Nortley M, Morsy M. Brachial artery aneurysms associated with arteriovenous access for hemodialysis. *Semin Dial*. 2010; 23(4): 440–4.
8. Marzelle J, Gashi V, Nguyen HD, et al. Aneurysmal degeneration of the donor artery after vascular access. *J Vasc Surg*. 2012; 55(4): 1052–7.
9. Silberberg JS, Barre PE, Prichard SS, Sniderman AD. Impact of left ventricular hypertrophy on survival in end-stage renal disease. *Kidney Int*. 1989; 36(2):286–90.
10. Cridlig J, Selton-Suty C, Alla F, et al. Cardiac impact of the arteriovenous fistula after kidney transplantation: a case-controlled, match-paired study. *Transpl Int*. 2008; 21(10): 948–54.
11. Amerling R, Ronco C, Kuhlman M, et al. Arteriovenous fistula toxicity. *Blood Purif*. 2011;31(1–3):113–20.
12. van Duijnhoven EC, Cheriex EC, Tordoir JH, et al. Effect of closure of the arteriovenous fistula on left ventricular dimensions in renal transplant patients. *Nephrol Dial Transplant*. 2001; 16(2):368–372.
13. Unger P, Wissing KM, de Pauw L, et al. Reduction of left ventricular diameter and mass after surgical arteriovenous fistula closure in renal transplant recipients. *Transplantation*. 2002; 74(1):73–79.
14. Movilli E, Viola BF, Brunori G, et al. Long-term effects of arteriovenous fistula closure on echocardiographic functional and structural findings in hemodialysis patients: a prospective study. *Am J Kidney Dis*. 2010; 55(4):682–9.
15. Hüting J. Course of left ventricular hypertrophy and function in end-stage renal disease after renal transplantation. *Am J Cardiol*. 1992; 70(18): 1481–4.
16. Peteiro J1, Alvarez N, Calviño R, et al. Changes in left ventricular mass and filling after renal transplantation are related to changes in blood pressure: an echocardiographic and pulsed Doppler study. *Cardiology*. 1994; 85(5):273–83.
17. Patard JJ, Bensalah K, Lucas A, et al. Management of vascular access for hemodialysis after successful kidney transplantation. *Scand J Urol Nephrol*. 2002; 36(5):373–376.
18. Soleimani MJ, Shahrokh H, Shadpour P, et al. Impact of dialysis access fistula on cardiac function after kidney transplantation. *Iran J Kidney Dis*. 2012; 6(3):198–202.
19. Sheashaa H, Hassan N, Osman Y, et al. Effect of spontaneous closure of arteriovenous fistula access on cardiac structure and function in renal transplant patients. *Am J Nephrol*. 2004; 24(4): 432–7.
20. De Lima JJ, Vieira ML, Molnar LJ, et al. Cardiac effects of persistent hemodialysis arteriovenous access in recipients of renal allograft. *Cardiology*. 1999; 92(4): 236–239.
21. Manca O, Pisano GL, Carta P, et al. The management of hemodialysis arteriovenous fistulas in well-functioning renal transplanted patients: many doubts, few certainties. *J Vasc Access*. 2005; 6(4):182–6.
22. Fox D, Amador F, Clarke D, Velez M, et al. Duplex guided dialysis access interventions can be performed safely in the office setting: techniques and early results. *Eur J Vasc Endovasc Surg*. 2011; 42(6): 833–41.

18

Incidence and Treatment of Central Venous Catheter-Associated Upper Extremity DVT

Timothy K. Liem, MD, MBA and Jeffrey D. Crawford, MD

Peripherally inserted central catheters (PICC) and central venous catheters (CVC) provide reliable access for the administration of parenteral nutrition, long-term antibiotics, chemotherapy, and numerous other medications. They also provide convenient access for patients who require dialysis or frequent laboratory testing. These multiple utilities have led to the placement of over 5 million CVCs every year.[1] Over the past decade, many hospitals have developed specialized nursing teams, whose primary function has been the placement and maintenance of intravenous catheters and PICC lines. The ease with which these PICC line may be ordered, and the added convenience for patients, have contributed to the rapid expansion of PICC line usage as well.

The use of CVCs and PICC lines may be complicated by arterial injury and hemorrhage, pneumothorax and lymphatic injury, deep or superficial vein thrombosis, central-line-associated blood stream infection (CLABSI), and central vein stenosis (potentially compromising options for future dialysis access). Some of these complications may be reduced with the use of a variety of best practices for insertion and maintenance. For example, ultrasound-guided CVC insertion reduces the rate of arterial injury and pneumothorax, and the use of "central line bundles" for insertion and maintenance may decrease the rate of CLABSI.[2,3] More recently, several professional societies also have made attempts to reduce the rate of catheter-associated upper extremity deep vein thrombosis (CA-UEDVT). This chapter will focus on the incidence, prevention, and treatment of CA-UEDVT.

INCIDENCE AND CLINICAL SIGNIFICANCE OF CATHETER-ASSOCIATED UPPER EXTREMITY DVT

The reported incidence of CA-UEDVT varies significantly (2% to 67%), and depends upon many factors, including the study methodology. Prospective evaluations are more likely to perform routine upper extremity venous duplex scans, which will identify symptomatic and asymptomatic CA-UEDVT. However, only a small percentage of patients develop clinical manifestations (0% to 12%).[4,5] In contrast, retrospective studies demonstrate a lower rate of CA-UEDVT, since in this setting, duplex scans are more likely to be performed after patients develop symptoms of pain and edema. We performed a recent review, identifying that retrospective studies had a PICC-associated UEDVT incidence ranging from 1.6% to 3.9%, while prospective studies had a higher rate, ranging from 3.0% to 19.4%.[6] In addition, the incidence of CA-UEDVT will depend on the presence or absence of certain co-morbidities. Malignancy and chemotherapy, increased age, and prior DVT are associated with an increased risk for CA-UEDVT.[5,6] The more common inherited hypercoagulable conditions (Factor V Leiden and prothrombin gene mutation) also may have an association, but studies remain inconsistent, suggesting that any association with CA-UEDVT is likely to be mild.[7–9]

Several technical factors, and the clinical setting in which the central line was inserted also affect the incidence of CA-UEDVT. Technical factors such as increased catheter size, increased lumen number, tip location (brachiocephalic versus caval-atrial), insertion site (left > right, femoral > subclavian), catheter material (polyethylene), and catheter duration all have been associated with an increased risk of CA-UEDVT.[5,10,11] PICC lines that are place in the ICU are associated with a significantly higher rate of CA-UEDVT, when compared with lines that are placed in the non-ICU setting (13.91% vs 3.44%).[12] In addition, when evaluating only studies that directly compared the incidence of PICC versus centrally-inserted CVCs, the CA-UEDVT was significantly higher with PICCs (Odds Ratio 2.55, 95% CI: 1.54 – 4.23).[12] Numerous other risk factors for CA-UEDVT are shown in Table 18-1.

In recent studies, we defined catheter-associated UEDVT as a deep vein thrombus in the same vein as, or immediately adjacent to, a recently placed CVC or PICC (≤ 30 days). Using this definition, we found that 35% of all UEDVTs during a 12-month period were associated with a recent PICC line, and 20% were associated with a CVC.[6] Figure 18-1. Conversely, since over 2,000 PICC lines were placed during that same 12-month period, the rate of symptomatic PICC-associated UEDVT averaged 2.6%. This rate falls well within the 1.6% to 3.9% incidence that was seen in numerous other retrospective clinical studies.

The natural history of treated and untreated lower extremity DVT is better known than that of upper extremity DVT. The limited available data suggests that after treatment with 3 months of anticoagulation, upper extremity DVT has a lower likelihood of causing pulmonary embolization and recurrent thromboembolism. However, the rate of developing UEDVT-associated post-thrombotic syndrome remained significant, ranging from 7% to 46%. There is some suggestion that catheter-associated UEDVT may be associated with a slightly decreased risk for post-thrombotic syndrome.[13–16]

TABLE 18-1. RISK FACTORS FOR CATHETER-ASSOCIATED UPPER EXTREMITY DEEP VEIN THROMBOSIS

High Risk	Low-Moderate Risk
Critically ill in ICU	Tip not at cavoatrial junction
Active malignancy	Small vein caliber accessed by PICC
Prior VTE	Surgery with catheter in place
Hypercoagulable disorders	Prior catheterization
PICCs	No pharmacoprophylaxis (PICCs)
Prior chest radiation therapy	CVCs (Hickman > port; femoral v. > subclavian > IJ)
PICC in paretic arm	Diabetes
Triple or double lumen catheter	Renal failure
Vancomycin/amphotericin B/chemotherapy	COPD
	Obesity (BMI >30)
	Recent trauma
	Catheter associated infection
	Catheter tip not at caval-atrial junction
	Inflammatory bowel disease
	Longer catheter dwell time

ICU, intensive care unit; PICC, peripherally inserted central catheter; VTE, venous thromboembolism; v, vein; IJ, internal jugular; CVCs, central venous catheters; COPD, chronic obstructive pulmonary disease.

Infusates with extremes of pH (<5 or >9) or caustic medications are higher risk for upper extremity deep vein thrombosis.

Source: Adapted from Crawford JD, Liem TK, and Moneta GL. Management of catheter-associated upper extremity deep venous thrombosis. JVS Ven Lym Dis 2015; August [ePub ahead of print].

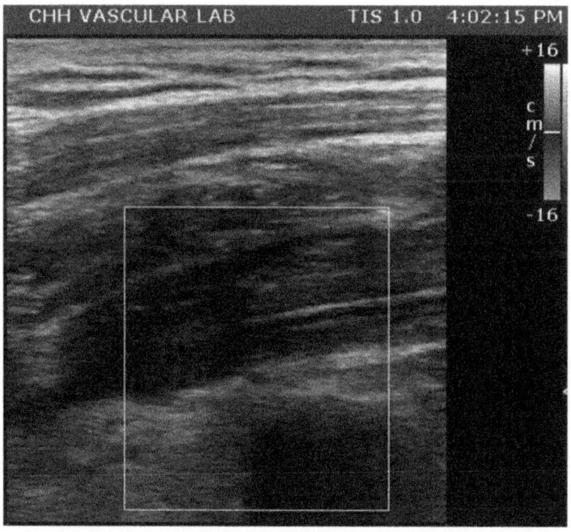

Figure 18-1. Duplex image of a subclavian vein with a PICC line and visible surrounding deep vein thrombosis.

PROPHYLAXIS AGAINST CATHETER-ASSOCIATED UEDVT

Prevention against CA-UEDVT begins with the judicious use of CVCs and PICC lines, and prompt removal when these catheters are no longer needed or functional. The Choosing Wisely® campaign, an initiative by the American Board of Internal Medicine in collaboration with various professional societies, has attempted to disseminate evidence-based recommendations for a variety of diagnoses and treatments.[17] The recommendations for the use of PICC lines are shown below:

1. Don't place, or leave in place, peripherally inserted central catheters for patient or provider convenience. (Society of General Internal Medicine).
2. Don't place peripherally inserted central catheters (PICC) in stage III-V CKD patients without consulting nephrology. (American Society of Nephrology).

Similarly, a position statement from the American Society of Diagnostic and Interventional Nephrology recommends to avoid PICC lines and subclavian-inserted CVCs in patients with chronic kidney disease stages III-V.[18] In these patients, the internal jugular (IJ) and external jugular veins are suggested for central access, and dorsal hand veins are suggested for phlebotomy and peripheral IVs. They also recommend that dialysis access should be coordinated with nephrology to minimize the need and duration of dialysis catheters.

If a PICC line is indicated, careful consideration should be given to the type of catheter to be used. The evidence is consistent that smaller catheter diameter and smaller lumen number are associated with lower rates of CA-UEDVT.[6,19–22] In addition, some preliminary data from our series of over 2000 PICC lines suggests that a cephalic PICC insertion site is associated with a higher rate of superficial vein thrombosis, but a lower rate of DVT.[6] However, the basilic and brachial veins still remain the most common sites for PICC insertion, probably related to several factors, including a greater ease of puncturing a larger target vein on ultrasound imaging, and a more direct route for passage of the catheter tip to the caval–atrial junction.

Some prospective trials demonstrate a mild benefit of thromboprophylaxis [fixed low-dose warfarin, prophylactic unfractionated heparin (UH) or low-molecular-weight heparin (LMWH)] compared to no prophylaxis, for prevention of *all* CVC-related UEDVT (symptomatic and asymptomatic). These same authors did not identify any benefit for prevention of *symptomatic* CVC-related UEDVT.[23] However, a Cochrane review of 12 randomized controlled trials (RCTs) failed to show a reduction in CVC-related UEDVT with prophylactic UH or low-dose warfarin, and thromboprophylaxis, therefore, is not recommended for CVCs.[24] The Jupiter trial in non-cancer patients and other studies in cancer patients have demonstrated decreased LEDVT with the use of statins by as much as 50%.[25,26] Statins reduce LEDVT by suppressing inflammatory mediators, but there is currently insufficient evidence to recommend statins for CA-UEDVT prevention.

TREATMENT OF CATHETER-ASSOCIATED UEDVT

The treatment of catheter-associated UEDVT is not well studied, and recommendations are largely based on extrapolation from data regarding lower extremity DVT (LEDVT). To date, there are no randomized clinical trials that have evaluated anticoagulation for initial and long-term therapy of CA-UEDVT. Because patients with UEDVT also may be at high risk for LEDVT, screening for LEDVT in patients with UEDVT may identify a clinically proven indication for short-term and intermediate-term anticoagulation. Based on the best available data, the 2012 American College of Chest Physicians (ACCP) Evidence-Based Clinical Practice Guidelines provide recommendations for the management of *acute* CA-UEDVT (Table 18-2).[27]

Of particular note, the Guidelines recommend *against* removal of the offending catheter unless it is no longer needed or nonfunctional (Grade 2C). This recommendation is in agreement with our experience, regarding the common reflex to remove the catheter and replacement it at a new access site. Although catheter removal is associated with improved thrombus resolution, the placement of a catheter at a different site is associated with an 86% incidence of developing CA-UEDVT at that new site.[28] This is a strong argument in favor of leaving the catheter in place, if it is functional and if there is ongoing need. A second caveat from the ACCP Guidelines also recommends continued anticoagulation, as long as the catheter remains in place, as opposed to a fixed-duration of therapy.[27]

New oral anticoagulants are FDA approved for VTE prophylaxis and treatment, but have not been studied for CA-UEDVT. Bleeding risk in CA-UEDVT specifically is not well-studied. However, small retrospective and prospective cohort studies suggest that major bleeding risk is slightly lower in the treatment of UEDVT compared to LEDVT with a rate of 2.0%–4.1% with either dalteparin or warfarin, compared to 4.9% for LEDVT.[29–31] Catheter-directed thrombolysis (CDT) for acute UEDVT has been evaluated only in retrospective and small prospective studies, and is not generally recommended except for patients with severe, acute (<14 days) symptoms and low bleeding risk (Grade 1C).[27] We rarely offer CDT to patients with catheter-associated UEDVT, since most patients usually have some relative or absolute contraindication to thrombolysis (e.g. recent surgery, active or recent malignancy, active infection). In addition, the rate of post-thrombotic syndrome seems to be lower with CA-UEDVT, when compared with non-catheter-associated thrombosis. There is no role for SVC filters in the management of CA-UEDVT as the risk of death from PE is believed to be extremely low and SVC filters carry significant risk of complications.[32]

TABLE 18-2. SUMMARY OF AMERICAN COLLEGE OF CHEST PHYSICIANS RECOMMENDATIONS REGARDING THE MANAGEMENT OF *ACUTE CATHETER-ASSOCIATED UPPER EXTREMITY DEEP VEIN THROMBOSIS*. LMWH, LOW-MOLECULAR-WEIGHT HEPARIN; IV, INTRAVENOUS; SC, SUBCUTANEOUS

1. **Acute UEDVT that involves the axillary or more proximal veins:** we recommend acute treatment with parenteral anticoagulation (LMWH, fondaparinux, IV unfractionated heparin, or SC unfractionated heparin) over no such treatment (Grade 1B).
2. **Most patients with UEDVT that is associated with a central venous catheter:** we suggest that the catheter NOT be removed if it is functional and there is an ongoing need for the catheter (Grade 2C).
3. **UEDVT that is associated with a central venous catheter that is removed:** we recommend 3 months of anticoagulation over a longer duration of therapy in patient with no cancer (Grade 1B), and we suggest this in patient with cancer (Grade 2C).
4. **UEDVT that is associated with a central venous catheter that is NOT removed:** we recommend that anticoagulation is continued as long as the central venous catheter remains in patients with cancer (Grade 1C), and we suggest this in patients with no cancer (Grade 2C).

Source: Adapted from Kearon C, et al. Antithrombotic Therapy for VTE Disease: Antithrombotic Therapy and Prevention of Thrombosis, 9th ed: American College of Chest Physicians Evidence-Based Clinical Practice Guidelines. Chest 2012; 141: e419S–e494S.

CONCLUSIONS

Upper extremity DVT is a common complication in patients who receive CVCs and PICC lines, with PICC lines having a slightly greater association with thrombosis. These catheters must be used judiciously, and not just for patient or provider convenience. Physicians and surgeons should be well versed with the various sizes and types of catheters which are being placed in their patients, and they should be familiar with clinical and technical factors that are associated with the development of UEDVT. Treatment consists of anticoagulation for at least 3 months, longer if the CVC or PICC line is left in place. If central venous access still is needed, and the catheter is functional, the access should NOT be removed, since a policy of remove and replace at another site is associated with a very high rate of thrombosis at the new access site.

REFERENCES

1. Radd I. Intravascular-catheter-related infections. *The Lancet*. 1998;351(9106):893–8.
2. Hind D, Calvert N, McWilliams R, et al. Ultrasonic locating devices for central venous cannulation: Meta-analysis. *BMJ*. 2003;327:361.
3. Guidelines for the prevention of intravascular catheter-related infections, 2011. http://www.cdc.gov/hicpac/pdf/guidelines/bsi-guidelines-2011.pdf. Updated 2011. Accessed June 2015.
4. Periard D, Monney P, Waeber G, et al. Randomized controlled trial of peripherally inserted central catheters vs. peripheral catheters for middle duration in-hospital intravenous therapy. *J Thromb Haemost*. 2008;6:1281–8.
5. Van Rooden CJ, Tesselaar MET, Osanto S, Rosendaal FR, Huisman MV. Deep vein thrombosis associated with central venous catheters – a review. *J Thromb Haemost*. 2005;3:2409–19.
6. Liem TK, Yanit KE, Moseley SE, et al. Peripherally inserted central catheter usage pattersn and associated symptomatic upper extremity venous thrombosis. *J Vasc Surg*. 2012;55(3):761–7.
7. Van Rooden CJ, Rosendaal RF, Barge RM, et al. Central venous catheter related thrombosis in haematology patietns and prediction of risk by screening with Doppler-ultrasound. *Br J Haematol*. 2003;123:507–12.
8. Fijnheer R, Paijmans B, Verdonck LF, et al. Factor V Leiden in central venous catehter-associated thrombosis. *Br J Haematol*. 2002;118:267–70.
9. Riordan M, Weiden P. Factor V Leiden mutation does not account for central venous catheter-related thrombosis. *Am J Hematol*. 1998;58:150–2.
10. De Cicco M, Matovic M, Balestreri L, et al. Central venous thrombosis: an early and frequent complication in cancer patients bearing long-term silastic catheter. A prospective study. *Thromb Res*. 1997;86:101–13.
11. Gould JR, Carloss HW, Skinner WL. Groshong cathteter-associated subclavian venous thrombosis. *Am J Med*. 1993;95:419–23.
12. Chopra V, Anand S, Hickner A, et al. Risk of venous thromboembolism associated with peripherally inserted central catheters" a systematic review and meta-analysis. *Lancet*. 2013;382:311–25.
13. Prandoni P, Polistena P, Bernardi E, et al. Upper-extremity deep vein thrombosis. Risk factors, diagnosis, and complications. *Arch Intern Med*. 1997;157(1):57–62.
14. Prandoni P, Bernardi E, Marchiori A, et al. The long term clinical course of acute deep vein thrombosis of the arm: prospective cohort study. *BMJ*. 2004;329(7464):484–5.
15. Kahn SR, Elman EA, Bornais C, et al. Post-thrombotic syndrome, functional disability and quality of life after upper extremity deep venous thrombosis in adults. *Thromb Haemost*. 2005;93(3):499–502.

16. Elman EE, Kahn SR. The post-thrombotic syndrome after upper extremity deep venous thrombosis in adults: A systematic review. *Thromb Res*. 2006;117:609–14.
17. American Board of Internal Medicine. Choosing Wisely®. http://www.choosingwisely.org. Updated June 2015. Accessed June 15, 2015.
18. Hoggard J, Saad T, Schon D, et al. Guidelines for venous access in patients with chronic kidney disease. A Position Statement from the American Society of Diagnostic and Interventional Nephrology, Clinical Practice Committee and the Association for Vascular Access. *Sem Dialysis*. 2008;21(2):186–91.
19. Grove JR, Pevec WC. Venous thrombosis related to peripherally inserted central catheters. *J Vasc Interv Radiol*. 2000;11(7):837–40.
20. Evans RS, Sharp JH, Linford LH, et al. Risk of symptomatic DVT associated with peripherally inserted central catheters. *Chest*. 2010;138(4):803–10.
21. Evans RS, Sharp JH, Linford LH, et al. Reduction of peripherally inserted central catheter-associated DVT. *Chest*. 2013;143(3):627–33.
22. O'Brien J, Paquet F, Lindsay R, Valenti D. Insertion of PICCs with minimum number of lumens reduces complications and costs. *JACR*. 2013;10(11):864–8.
23. Kirkpatrick A, Rathbun S, Whitsett T, Raskob G. Prevention of central venous catheter-associated thrombosis: a meta-analysis. *Am J Med*. 2007;120(10):901.e1–13.
24. Akl EA, Karmath G, Yosuico V, et al. Anticoagulation for thrombosis prophylaxis in cancer patients with central venous catheters. *The Cochrane database of systematic reviews*. 2007(3):CD006468.
25. Glynn RJ, Danielson E, Fonseca FA, et al. A randomized trial of rosuvastatin in the prevention of venous thromboembolism. *N Eng J Med*. 2009;360(18):1851–61.
26. Lotsch F, Konigsbrugge O, Posch F, et al. Statins are associated with low risk of venous thromboembolism in patients with cancer: a prospective and observational cohort study. *Thromb Res*. 2014;134(5):1008–13.
27. Kearon C, Akl EA, Comerota AJ, et al. Antithrombotic therapy for VTE disease: Antithrombotic therapy and prevention of thrombosis, 9th ed: American college of chest physicians evidence-based clinical practice guidelines. *Chest*. 2012;141(2 Suppl): e419S–94S.
28. Jones MA, Lee DY, Segall JA, et al. Characterizing resolution of catheter-associated upper extremity deep venous thrombosis. *J Vasc Surg*. 2010;51(1);108–13.
29. Rathbun SW, Stoner JA, Whitsett TL. Treatment of upper-extremity deep vein thrombosis. *J Thromb Haemost*. 2011;9(10):1924–30.
30. Savage KJ, Wells PS, Schulz V, et al. Outpatient use of low molecular weight heparin (Dalteparin) for the treatment of deep vein thrombosis of the upper extremity. *Thromb Haemost*. 1999;82(3):1008–10.
31. Munoz FJ, Mismetti P, Poggio R, et al. Clinical outcome of patients with upper-extremity deep vein thrombosis: results from the RIETE Registry. *Chest*. 2008;133(1):143–8.
32. Owens CA, Bui JT, Knuttinen MG, Gaba RC, Carrillo TC. Pulmonary embolism from upper extremity deep vein thrombosis and the role of superior vena cava filters: a review of the literature. *JVIR*. 2010;21(6):779–87.

19

Catheter-Directed Thrombolysis for Acute Finger Ischemia

Matthew A. Corriere MD, MS

Acute finger ischemia (AFI) is a relatively uncommon clinical presentation with specific considerations for diagnosis and management. In contrast to acute upper extremity ischemia, which presents with signs and symptoms (such as pain, pallor, paralysis, paresthesias, pulselessness, and poikilothermia) that involve and potentially threaten the limb,[1] AFI is distinguished by more focal symptoms involving one or more fingers but not the entire arm or hand. In fact, patients with AFI frequently (but not always) present palpable radial and/or ulnar pulses. The designation *acute* refers to symptoms and signs that are new-onset and have been present ≤ 30 days; although this time interval is somewhat arbitrary, it is meant to distinguish AFI from more chronic presentations where the time frame for diagnosis and treatment may be less urgent. AFI therefore does not include ischemic finger symptoms that are intermittent in nature or chronically wax and wane (as commonly seen with many rheumatologic disorders such as Raynaud's disease).

Within the limits of this relatively precise definition, diagnosis and treatment of AFI differs in several ways from more proximal upper extremity arterial occlusive disease. This chapter will review the epidemiology, diagnosis, and management of AFI with a focus on the role of catheter-directed thrombolysis. Because AFI resulting from penetrating trauma or known iatrogenic causes (such as an ipsilateral arterial catheter or arteriovenous hemodialysis access) involves distinct diagnostic and treatment considerations reviewed elsewhere, these presentations are more appropriately considered separately from *de novo* AFI and therefore will not be discussed.

EPIDEMIOLOGY

Although the epidemiology of AFI is poorly understood, limited data suggests several characteristics that distinguish these patients from those with lower extremity peripheral arterial disease (PAD): patients presenting with AFI are relatively younger and have a higher prevalence of both connective tissue disease. In a single center review of 35 patients treated with catheter-directed thrombolysis for AFI, Islam et al. noted a mean age of 48 years with a 31% prevalence of connective tissue disease.[2] Current or previous history of smoking was present in 65% of patients in this cohort, while 29% had a history of ipsilateral repetitive motion or minor blunt trauma, and 14% had a hypercoagulable disorder.

ANATOMIC CONSIDERATIONS

The upper extremity arteries are superficial, small in diameter (relative to the lower extremity arteries), and sensitive to temperature and mechanical stimuli.[3] The arterial circulation of the hand and fingers is highly variable, and the clinical manifestations of AFI usually depend on the amount of collateral flow between the radial, ulnar, and proper digital arteries. The normal arterial anatomy of the hand involves duplicated systems between the radial and ulnar arteries which communicate through the superficial and deep palmar arches. This rich collateral network makes it possible for acute occlusion of either the radial or ulnar arteries to occur without clinically apparent signs, symptoms, or severe alterations of either nutritional blood flow or thermoregulatory function.[4] An incomplete palmar arterial arch, however, has been reported in up to 65% of patients with AFI and may predispose patients to develop relatively severe ischemia from disease that otherwise might be tolerated in the setting of intact collateral flow.[2] AFI presenting with severe signs and symptoms therefore should prompt suspicion of atypical arterial anatomy as a potential predisposing factor.

Anatomic assessment and classification of AFI requires consideration of the level of the occlusive lesion(s) and the adequacy of collateral flow (Figure 19-1).[4] AFI is characterized by a high prevalence of both distal lesions and multi-level disease. Lesions distal to the level of the wrist have been reported based on angiography in over 90% of patients presenting with AFI,[2] while approximately 75% of patients with upper extremity ischemia have lesions of the forearm or hand.[4, 5] Ruch et al. reported multi-level occlusive disease in 76% of patients with upper extremity ischemia based on angiography, with lesions the distal forearm or Guyon's canal in combination with a second distal occlusion of one or more proper digital arteries as the most common combinations of occlusive disease levels.[4] Islam et al. reported disease involving the contralateral upper extremity among 32% of patients with AFI who were studied with bilateral upper extremity arteriography, although only 6% of patients presented with bilateral symptoms.[2] Other anatomic findings of interest reported from this study included a 23% prevalence of radial and/or ulnar artery aneurysms and a 20% prevalence of a proximally located (upper arm) brachial artery bifurcation.

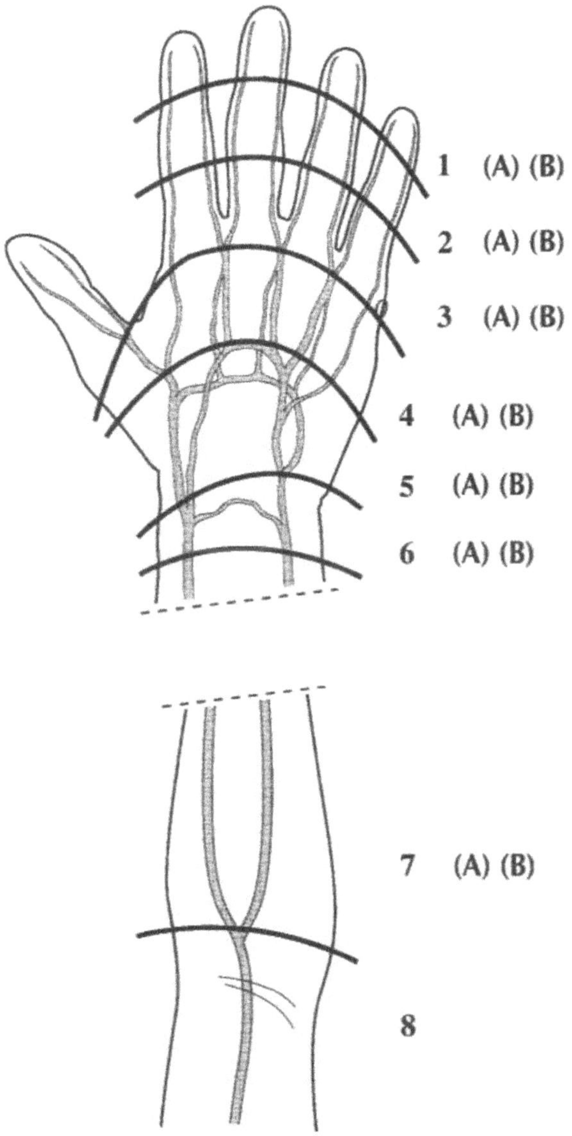

Figure 19-1. Classification system for describing arterial occlusive disease associated with acute finger ischemia. Numbers 1-8 indicate level of occlusion, while letters refer to whether occlusion of either the radial or ulnar (A) versus both the radial and ulnar sources of inflow (B) at the given level. (Figure originally published but Ruch et al, and used with permission from the publisher.[4])

CLINICAL PRESENTATION OF ACUTE FINGER ISCHEMIA

AFI usually presents with finger pain, numbness, and/or paresthesias; motor deficits are much less common. In more severe cases, patients may also present with digital ulcers or focal gangrene. Skin discoloration (including mottling or pallor) may also be seen with AFI but is more consistently associated with diseases characterized by intermittent vasospasm (such as Raynaud's), although AFI may also occur without visible skin changes. Patients with AFI often delay seeking medical evaluation for several days or weeks after onset, sometimes mistakenly attributing their initial symptoms to minor blunt trauma or other causes.[2] Symptoms may be vague and have multiple similarities to other conditions such as compressive neuropathy (Table 19-1).[4] AFI is seldom associated with significant finger or hand edema, so these symptoms should prompt consideration of alternative etiologies such as venous or lymphatic disease, local traumatic injury (including insect bites or stings), or focal allergic reactions (such as contact dermatitis).

DIAGNOSTIC EVALUATION AND TESTING

History and physical examination

When AFI is suspected, the history and physical examination can provide valuable information that helps to narrow the differential diagnosis and to focus subsequent diagnostic testing. The history of present illness interview should include focused questions exploring precipitating factors (such as cold exposure, positional changes,

TABLE 19-1. DIFFERENTIAL DIAGNOSIS FOR ACUTE FINGER ISCHEMIA

Embolism from proximal source	Aortic aneurysm
	Cardiac mural thrombus
	Patent foramen ovale
	Valvular heart disease/endocarditis
Embolism from ipsilateral arm	Subclavian artery aneurysm/psuedoaneursm
	Radial or ulnar artery aneurysm
Atherosclerotic disease	Subclavian steal syndrome
Non-atherosclerotic vascular disease	Buerger's disease
	Takayasu arteritis
	Giant cell arteritis
	Kawasaki disease
	Arterial dissection (aortic, subclavian)
	Collagen vascular disease
Vasospasm	Temperature-induced (e.g., Raynaud's syndrome)
	Drug-induced (e.g., cocaine, methamphetamine)
	Systemic shock
Neurologic	Compressive neuropathy (e.g., carpal tunnel syndrome)
	Cerebrovascular accident
	Complex regional pain syndrome
Steal syndrome	Proximal arteriovenous fistula
	Subclavian stenosis
	Hypothenar hand syndrome
Traumatic	Pectoralis minor syndrome
	Iatrogenic (arterial catheterization)
	Brachial artery injection
Other	Hypocalcemia
	Hypersensitivity

repetitive motion or blunt force, or other physical activities) or associated symptoms (including palpitations, transient ischemic attacks or other cerebrovascular manifestations, or hyperventilation) that might establish suspicion of a likely cause or alternative diagnosis. Physical examination should include a thorough pulse examination of all extremities, chest auscultation, and visual inspection of the symptomatic extremity with direct comparison to the contralateral arm and hand. Finger inspection should include examination of the nail beds for evidence of micro-embolization.[6] Ulcers or focal gangrene should be documented if present and may be identified in up to 20% of patients at the time of initial evaluation.[2] Visual inspection of the ipsilateral arm should also be performed to screen for ecchymosis, skin lesions, needle tracks, or other signs that may indicate a likely etiology. Photographs of both hands are useful to obtain at the time of presentation, particularly if these images can be added to the electronic medical record for longitudinal comparisons to assess wound healing and/or response to revascularization. The Allen test can assess the relative contributions from the radial and ulnar arteries to hand blood flow, but is less useful for AFI than for chronic disease.[6] Continuous wave Doppler evaluation of the palmar arch, proper digital arteries, and both the radial and ulnar arteries allows bedside assessment of these vessels but is inadequate for confirming the diagnosis or developing a treatment plan.[6] Nonetheless, abnormal continuous wave Doppler findings may establish increased suspicion for AFI, while normal signals may help lower AFI on the differential diagnosis and direct the subsequent workup toward other diagnoses if plausible alternative explanations exist.

Laboratory Testing

Laboratory testing for patients with AFI can inform both short-term and long-term management. Screening for thrombophilia should be considered at the time of presentation before initiating therapeutic anticoagulation, which can affect the results of several of these tests (including proteins C and S), making it difficult to interpret the results and sometimes necessary to obtain repeat testing. Assessment of coagulation parameters is also important for evaluating patients as candidates for thrombolysis; patients with severe coagulopathy (such as a profoundly elevated INR or low fibrinogen) may not be appropriate candidates due to increased risk of hemorrhagic complications. Longer-term considerations include testing for vasculitis, rheumatologic, or other inflammatory conditions that may not be critical to management during the acute presentation but may identify opportunities to decrease risk for disease progression or relapses through pharmacotherapy for systemic disease. From a practical perspective, it is also worth obtaining a serum creatinine for glomerular filtration rate estimation to determine risk of contrast-induced nephropathy. When contrast imaging is necessary in a patient with kidney disease, it is prudent to consider catheter arteriography as the primary modality to minimize the volume of iodinated contrast. Prophylactic hydration and medications should also be considered in patients with severe kidney disease. Although evidence supporting pharmacotherapy for prevention of contrast-induced nephrotoxicity is not robust, these medications are safe and inexpensive. We routinely administer prophylactic intravenous hydration for patients with an estimated glomerular filtration rate (eGFR) <60 ml/min/m^2 and add pharmacologic prophylaxis with oral N-acetylcysteine and vitamin C for those with an eGFR <30 ml/min/m.[2] Obtaining a serum pregnancy test in women at risk will maximize safety while avoiding subsequent delays if imaging requiring radiation exposure and/or thrombolysis are pursued. Table 19-2 summarizes laboratory tests worthy of consideration during initial evaluation of AFI; this list is not all-inclusive, and the tests ordered should be individualized based on the history, patient gender, and clinical suspicion.

Physiologic Testing

Digital brachial index assessment, digital plethysmography, and laser Doppler may be useful for confirming the symptom etiology and quantifying the severity of ischemia; these tests can also provide an assessment of the microcirculation (and related likelihood of wound healing with conservative management) that cannot be obtained through routine anatomic imaging tests.[4] A digital pressure <30 mm Hg or digital brachial index <0.5 indicates likely finger ischemia, while a digital brachial index <0.3 has been suggested as consistent with imminent digital gangrene.[6,7] Laser Doppler may

TABLE 19-2. USEFUL LABORATORY TESTS DURING INITIAL EVALUATION OF ACUTE FINGER ISCHEMIA

Category	Test(s)
Renal function and acid-base status	Electrolytes
	Serum creatinine (with estimated glomerular filtration rate)
	Serum creatine phosphokinase
Bleeding risk	Complete blood count (with platelet count)
	Prothrombin time with International Normalized Ratio
	Partial thromboplastin time
	D-dimer
	Type and screen
Thrombophilia	Protein C
	Protein S
	Plasminogen
	Antithrombin III
	Antiphospholipid antibodies (lupus anticoagulant, anti-cardiolipin, anti-beta-2 glycoprotein)
	Factor V Leiden
	Prothrombiin (Factor II) 20210 mutation
Connective tissue disorders, vasculitis	Antinuclear antibody
	Anti-neutrophil cytoplasmic antibody
	Erythrocyte sedimentation rate
	Serum complement
Miscellaneous	Ionized calcium
	Serum/urine pregnancy
	Drug screen

Note: Testing should be individualized based on the history, patient gender, and clinical suspicion, and list is not all-inclusive.

provide additional information related to cutaneous finger perfusion, although poor correlation has been reported between laser Doppler and arteriogram findings in the setting of finger ischemia.[4] Non-invasive physiologic testing can also sometimes provide useful information when attempting to rule out a non-vascular etiology, but may be less useful in the setting of bilateral disease, poorly tolerated in patients with severe finger pain, or inadequate if gangrene and/or ulcers warrant proceeding directly to a more definitive anatomic assessment. In contrast to evaluation of chronic symptoms, cold/warm stress testing and digital temperature evaluation are less useful for AFI.

Anatomic Imaging

Diagnostic imaging selection or AFI should be guided by the clinical presentation, pulse examination, and suspected anatomic location of the causative pathology. When a proximal brachial artery occlusion is suspected based on the clinical presentation, it may be most efficient to forego extensive imaging and proceed with immediate surgical exploration; one example of such a situation would be a patient who has chronic history of atrial fibrillation, is not therapeutically anticoagulated, and presents with numbness and weakness involving the arm and hand ipsilateral to an absent brachial pulse. When the clinical presentation does not clearly point to a likely etiology, however, anatomic imaging can provide useful information for both making the diagnosis and developing an appropriate treatment plan based on the findings.

Duplex ultrasound (DUS) is often helpful for assessing flow in the brachial and axillary arteries and can provide confirmation of suspected proximal disease (such as a brachial artery thrombus) sufficient for proceeding with exploration without need for contrast imaging. DUS may also serve as a non-invasive screening test that informs subsequent imaging selection; Barbiero et al. described using DUS confirmation of distal arterial ischemia as a criterion for proceeding with catheter angiography, while patients with non-diagnostic or equivocal DUS findings were instead studied with cross-sectional imaging.[3]

Cross-sectional contrast imaging (including both computed tomography angiography [CTA] and magnetic resonance angiography [MRA]) can provide useful information related to proximal sources of embolism (such as aneurysmal disease) or non-vascular anatomic findings relevant to both etiology and treatment (such as a cervical rib). Cross sectional imaging can also be used for imaging more distal arterial pathology involving the small vessels of the hand and fingers, although issues such as motion artifact, vascular calcification, and timing of image acquisition relative to contrast infusion (particularly for patients with multilevel occlusive disease) can sometimes result in an inadequate study. Cross sectional imaging systems may require patients to assume non-anatomic positions such as abducting the symptomatic extremity above their head while lying supine or extending their hand while prone in the "Superman" position so that the hand enters the imaging field first.[6,8] Because these maneuvers can sometimes reduce blood flow in asymptomatic patients without known arterial pathology, catheter angiography may be necessary when studies performed in this position suggest abnormal distal flow without a clear proximal lesion. MRA may also be limited by length of coverage or overlap between arteries and veins in the hand, and is contraindicated for patients with implanted devices that are not magnetic resonance compatible.[6] Given these considerations, cross-sectional imaging may be most useful for evaluating the aortic arch and subclavian vessels, particularly when clinical suspicion for AFI is low or there is reason to suspect proximal disease.

Catheter angiography is considered the gold standard for anatomic imaging of upper extremity arterial occlusive disease,[6, 9] and plays an even more prominent role in the diagnosis and treatment of AFI. Because AFI often results from occlusive disease affecting the more distal arterial circulation (including the radial, ulnar, palmar arch, and/or proper digital vessels), angiography can often provide the most definitive evaluation of the distal vasculature by avoiding issues related to motion artifact and timing of image acquisition relative to contrast infusion. This advantage is especially important in the setting of multi-level disease (as may be seen in the setting of an embolizing proximal lesion) (Figure 19-2). Catheter angiography also allows immediate initiation of endovascular treatment if anatomically suitable pathology is identified, resulting in greater efficiency while avoiding the additional time, contrast volume, and/or radiation exposure from an initial cross-sectional study if endovascular treatment is selected based on the findings. Catheter angiography also provides real-time evaluation of flow (including both direction and rate) that is not available with cross sectional imaging.[8] When distal vasospasm is suspected, intra-arterial

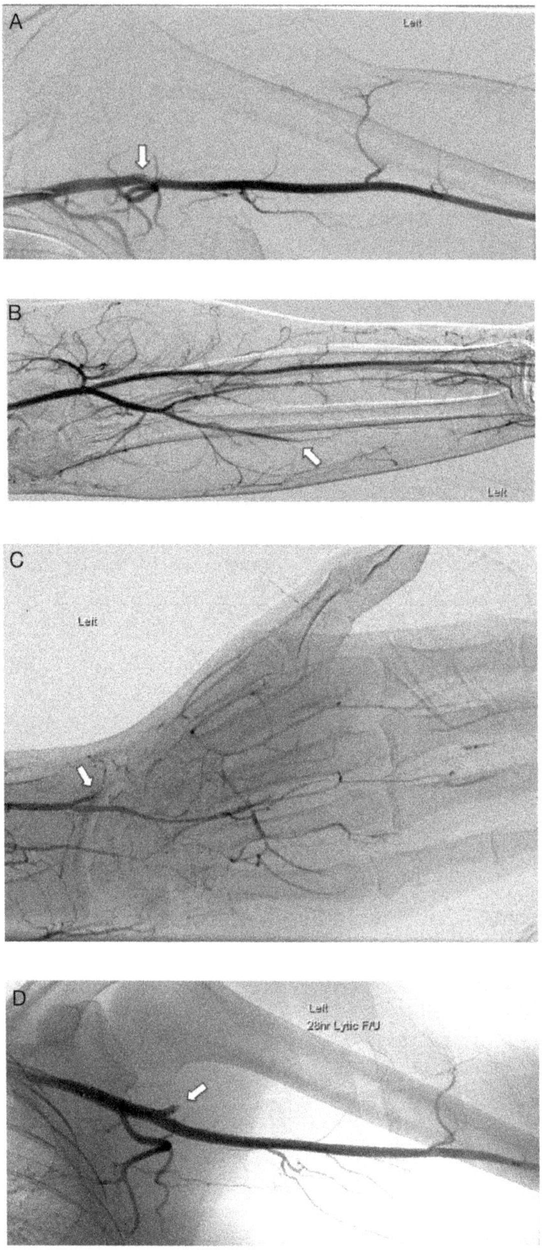

Figure 19-2. Proximal upper extremity arterial lesion with distal embolization to radial and ulnar arteries. The patient was a baseball pitcher who presented with acute finger ischemia. (**A**) Catheter angiogram demonstrates focal filling defect with intraluminal thrombus at junction between third portion of the left axillary artery and the brachial artery (arrow). (**B**) Forearm arteriogram performed using axillary artery injection demonstrates occlusion of the ulnar artery (arrow), with patent radial and interosseus arteries. (**C**) Distal catheter arteriogram performed using same injection indicates occlusion of the princeps pollicis artery (arrow) with absent deep and superficial palmar arches and pruning of the proper digital vessels. (**D**) Repeat catheter angiography after 28 hours if catheter-directed thrombolysis with alteplase (infused through an end-hole catheter positioned with its tip in the axillary artery) demonstrates thrombosed, aneurysmal subscapular artery as source of embolizing lesion. Patient was treated with ligation of the aneurysmal branch, axillary artery repair, and pectoralis minor tendon lengthening after a two week period of temporary anticoagulation.

administration of vasodilator medications (400 μg boluses of nitroglycerine can be administered every 3–5 minutes with minimal effects on systemic blood pressure) will sometimes reduce vasoconstriction adequately to allow angiographic characterization of distal small vessels (such as the metacarpal and proper digital arteries) that were not previously visible.

An additional advantage of contrast arteriography for diagnostic imaging of AFI is the ability to immediately initiate catheter-directed thrombolysis if anatomically suitable findings are identified. In contrast to arteriography for lower extremity ischemia, where it is common to identify lesions that are treatable with other endovascular techniques such as angioplasty, stenting, and/or atherectomy, these treatments are utilized less often for AFI for several reasons. Non-atherosclerotic pathology that is less often amenable to endovascular treatment (such as radial or ulnar artery aneurysm) is commonly identified during arteriography for AFI, and longer working lengths between the lesion and femoral artery access can create issues with reaching the lesion or delivering a device to its intended location.

Other Diagnostic Testing

An electrocardiogram should be obtained at the time of initial evaluation for AFI to rule out arrhythmia, particularly if the patient is tachycardic (as is often the case in the setting of significant pain or anxiety due to symptoms) and the ability to distinguish an irregular heart rhythm therefore may be limited based on physical examination alone. Additional evaluation with echocardiography and/or three-dimensional cardiac imaging should also be obtained when an arrhythmia is identified or physical exam findings (such as a murmur) suggest valvular or structural heart disease. Echocardiography with saline injection may also be useful for excluding paradoxical embolism associated with a septal defect (such as a patent foramen ovale) if the presentation is consistent with embolism and a proximal arterial source is not identified.

CATHETER ANGIOGRAPHY FOR ACUTE FINGER ISCHEMIA

Careful pre-procedure planning with anticipation of the necessary wires, catheters, and other equipment is therefore important for successful angiography. Anticipating challenges, carefully planning the approach, and minimizing potential for adverse circumstances related to equipment or technique can optimize imaging success. With the possible exception of trans-radial access for lower extremity angiography, catheter access of the brachial artery or more distal arm vessels from a femoral approach generally involves one of the longest distances between the access and target vessels routinely encountered, particularly for patients who are tall or lanky. Accordingly, it is wise to confirm availability of adequate length catheters and wires to avoid technical limitations during angiography. Providers who routinely perform carotid stenting will find many of the catheters used for this purpose (including vertebral, headhunter, and VTK catheters) also useful for selective innominate and/or subclavian artery access during upper extremity angiography. Although long (90 cm) sheaths and/or guide catheters are useful for treating disease of the proximal innominate or subclavian arteries, these devices are often impractical for dealing with more distal upper extremity pathology due to flow limitations, tendency to induce vasospasm, and (for right upper extremity disease) the disadvantage of leaving a larger diameter device positioned across the remaining arch vessels if catheter-directed thrombolysis is utilized. It is also helpful to anticipate what medications will likely be needed on the field for trans-arterial administration so that they can be prepared and immediately available during the procedure.

The patient is positioned supine on a radiolucent imaging table with one or both arms abducted depending on whether unilateral versus bilateral imaging is planned. To minimize potential for vasospasm, the room should be warmed and local warming of the affected hand should be arranged using forced heated air and/or a warmed intravenous fluid bag placed over the patient's hand. The hand should be taped to a radiolucent arm board to minimize motion artifact during angiography. At the time of positioning, it is useful to ensure that external devices with potential to obscure important anatomy or create imaging artifacts (such as ECG leads) are positioned outside the anticipated fields of view. If thrombolysis is being considered, it is wise to establish all invasive access and monitoring devices that will likely be needed prior to angiography to avoid bleeding complications resulting from invasive procedures performed during thrombolytic medication infusion. Relatively minor procedures (such as insertion of nasogastric tubes, urethral catheters, or intravenous lines) during catheter-directed thrombolysis can provoke significant bleeding during thrombolytic infusion, so it is better to perform these procedures beforehand to minimize risk of major complications or need to discontinue the infusion prematurely.

Although the additional diagnostic yield or therapeutic benefit gained from bilateral upper extremity imaging in the setting of unilateral AFI has not been definitively evaluated or proven, some providers advocate routine bilateral imaging to avoid the need for subsequent evaluation of the contralateral extremity with a separate procedure. This approach may be particularly wise when a systemic disease process is suspected as the most likely etiology for AFI, as information related to the contralateral upper extremity may be useful in confirming the diagnosis or potentially provide useful anatomic information if contralateral symptoms occur in the future. Contralateral imaging may also identify pathology warranting pre-emptive intervention under elective circumstances in the future (such as asymptomatic aneurysms of the radial or ulnar arteries). Conversely, bilateral imaging may have less benefit when the history or presenting signs and symptoms suggest a cause that is more likely to be unilateral (such as AFI involving the dominant hand in a throwing athlete or a history of repetitive hand trauma affecting one hand but not the other).

A large proportion of procedure-related adverse events related to upper extremity arteriography and thrombolysis are access-related,[2] and use of ultrasound guidance can minimize risk of iatrogenic complications resulting from repeated access attempts in multiple locations. If femoral access is utilized, the femoral head should be localized with fluoroscopy, and percutaneous access of the common femoral artery at this location should then be attempted after confirming that this site is free of dense plaque or calcification and proximal to the origin of the deep femoral artery. Antegrade brachial access has also been described for upper extremity arteriography and/o thrombolysis, but this approach does not permit imaging or treatment of more proximal disease and has a higher rate of access-related complications.[3,5,7,10] After infiltrating the overlying skin with local anesthetic and establishing access with a 4 French micro-catheter over an 0.014 "wire, an 0.035" wire can then be advanced and used to insert a short sheath. A 6 French sheath may be preferred due to easier infusion and blood sampling through the side port during thrombolysis, which is associated with greater resistance when performed around an infusion catheter through a smaller 5 French sheath. After establishing percutaneous access, the patient should be anticoagulated (unless anticoagulation was initiated preoperatively) with a bolus of unfractionated heparin prior to advancing a guide wire retrograde into the aortic arch. An activated clotting time (ACT) obtained 3–5 minutes following heparin administration allows confirmation of adequate anticoagulation before proceeding with selective catheterization. To minimize risk of cerebrovascular embolization during angiography and catheter manipulation, an ACT can be assessed every 30–45 minutes during the procedure with a target of >280 seconds as the criterion for repeat heparin administration.

Arch aortography is useful for identifying the location of the targeted access vessels and evaluating them for ostial disease, but is not always necessary. Aortography may be omitted if preoperative cross sectional imaging has been obtained and provides adequate information for procedure planning (including catheter selection), particularly if there is no proximal arch vessel disease. Arch angiography should be performed if cross-sectional contrast imaging has not been obtained, however, and may be preferred for patients with impaired renal function in order to minimize contrast volume. A reasonable arch aortogram can be obtained with a single dose of half-strength contrast while still managing to keep the total contrast volume for the procedure well below the volume needed for a routine CTA. Arch angiography should utilize a left anterior oblique (LAO) projection of 25°–30°, and the ideal projection can be identified by rotating the C-arm during live fluoroscopy until the maximum AP distance between the guidewire in the ascending versus descending thoracic aorta. Selective access to the targeted arch vessel is then established using a configured catheter in combination with an angled hydrophilic guide wire. Difficulty of arch access and catheterization may be anticipated using one of several scoring systems, such as that described by Schneider et al.[11] Left subclavian access is usually the least difficult and can often be accomplished using a catheter with a single angle such as a vertebral artery, Berenstein, or MP catheter. More difficult access in the setting of a severely angulated or diseased aortic arch may require more advanced catheter configurations such as a Simmons, Headhunter, or VTK catheter. Once selective access is established, the more distal subclavian artery can then be imaged using serial hand injections of dilute contrast with digital subtraction.

If proximal arch vessel disease suitable for endovascular treatment is identified, it is usually prudent to proceed with intervention prior to obtaining more distal imaging. Proximal disease is identified in only a minority of patients presenting with AFI, however, and is seldom the sole cause for symptoms other than arm claudication in the absence of distal embolization. If no proximal arch disease is identified, a 5 French angled diagnostic catheter is then advanced into the proximal axillary artery and used to image the distal axillary and brachial vessels. If appears satisfactory arteriograms of the brachial, radial, and ulnar arteries are obtained with the catheter tip positioned in the distal axillary artery, it may be worthwhile to also perform arteriography of the distal forearm and hand injecting from this same location. Alternatively, a catheter can advanced more distally into the brachial artery for more selective contrast injection but this approach risks provoking vasospasm which can be severe enough to result in arterial occlusion, may jeopardize both imaging and catheter-based therapy, and may be resistant to intra-arterial vasodilators.[3] For this reason, selective catheterization of the brachial, radial or ulnar arteries should be performed with an 0.018 "or 0.014" guide wire and a smaller diameter catheter (such as a 4 French catheter or microcatheter), although rapid injection may be more challenging due to increased resistance with the latter.

CATHETER-DIRECTED THROMBOLYSIS FOR ACUTE FINGER ISCHEMIA

Patient selection

Arteriography should guide selection of the most appropriate treatment strategy based on the anatomic findings and suspected disease etiology. A management algorithm proposed for imaging and use of thrombectomy versus catheter-directed thrombolysis for AFI is shown in Figure 19-3.[2] Catheter-directed thrombolysis should be considered for one or more of the following findings: pruning of the distal small

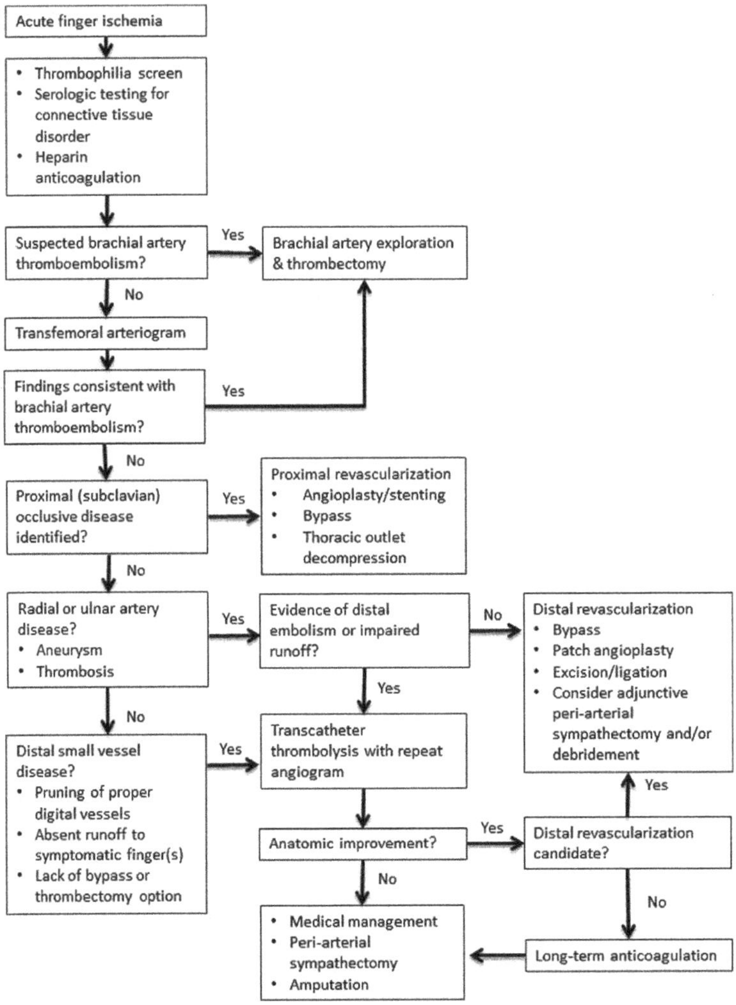

Figure 19-3. Proposed management algorithm for patients with acute finger ischemia. (Figure originally published by Islam et al. and used with permission from publisher.[2])

vessels consistent with proper digital vessel thrombosis and/or embolism, radial or ulnar artery aneurysm with thrombosis or distal embolization, or absent distal outflow to the fingers with lack of alternative revascularization options.[2] Digital emboli are present in the most patients with AFI resulting from radial or ulnar artery aneurysms[9]; because these small diameter vessels are poorly suited to thrombectomy, there are limited alternatives apart from catheter-directed thrombolysis for re-establishing their patency. Alternatively, when arteriography demonstrates more proximal large vessel thrombosis involving the brachial, radial, and/or ulnar arteries with patent palmar and digital vessels, exploration with thrombectomy should be considered as primary therapy rather than thrombolysis, as this treatment will allow more rapid and definitive restoration of arterial perfusion.[3,12] Thrombectomy and/or bypass should also be considered for patients who present with severe acute neurologic deficits, as the interval of time required for catheter-directed thrombolysis to achieve a clinically apparent effect may not be rapid enough to salvage function or prevent permanent neurologic symptoms. Patients with small diameter brachial arteries or those who develop significant arterial spasm during angiography are also suboptimal candidates for catheter directed thrombolysis. Patients with these symptoms who have limited alternatives for treatment may require intra-arterial vasodilator medications and/or withdrawal of the catheter tip to a more proximal location for contrast injection and/or thrombolytic infusion.

Prior to proceeding with angiography, it is critical to review the patient's history and ask specific questions to confirm that there are no contraindications to thrombolytic administration. Because many contraindications to thrombolysis cannot be identified based on physical examination alone (Table 19-3),[5,13–18] a detailed and accurate history is critical for minimizing risk of bleeding complications and may require confirmatory imaging (such as brain imaging) to ensure safety when details are unclear.

TABLE 19-3. CONTRAINDICATIONS TO CATHETER-DIRECTED THROMBOLYSIS

Contraindications to catheter-directed thrombolysis
Intracranial tumor
History of intracranial bleeding
Known peptic ulcer or history of gastrointestinal bleeding
Recent major surgery or trauma
Stroke within past 2 months
Thrombocytopenia
Coagulation disorder
Severe uncontrolled hypertension
Irreversible ischemia (i.e., severe motor deficit or rigor)
Sensory/motor deficit (inability to tolerate ≤24 additional hours of ischemia)
Infected bypass graft
Infective endocarditis
Pregnancy
Cardiopulmonary resuscitation

Approach and technical considerations

Tissue plasminogen activator (t-PA) (alteplase) is a naturally occurring serine protease that activates fibrin-bound plasminogen several hundred times more rapidly than circulating plasminogen.[18] t-PA is secreted naturally by vascular endothelial cells, plays an important role in normal endogenous fibrinolysis, and is primarily cleared by hepatic metabolism with a half-life of approximately 5 minutes.[13] Other recombinant variants of t-PA (sometimes alternatively abbreviated as rt-PA to specifically designate them as such, including reteplase and tenecteplase) have longer half-lives than native t-PA but are similar in terms of both efficacy and toxicity.[13,18] Catheter-directed thrombolysis using streptokinase and urokinase for upper extremity ischemia has also been described.[3,19,20] Limited evidence suggests that intra-arterial t-PA is more effective than either intra-arterial streptokinase or intravenous t-PA for improving vessel patency in people with peripheral arterial occlusion.[21] Recombinant t-PA is packaged in vials as a lyophilized powder that requires reconstitution prior to infusion.[13] When using alteplase for catheter-directed thrombolysis, a bolus dose of 6–10 mg is often administered prior to initiating an infusion at 1–2 mg/hr. When preparing the infusion, the alteplase should be reconstituted and diluted in an adequate volume. A practically useful concentration can be obtained by reconstituting 10 mg alteplase in 250 mL of saline, which yields a concentration of 0.04 mg/mL; this concentration permits easy dose adjustment for infusion at 1 mg (25 mL) or 2 mg (50 mL) per hour, allows easy bedside dose identification based on the infusion rate during rounds, and minimizes potential for accidental administration of large doses of atleplase as the result of line flushes (which may happen with more concentrated doses, although line flushes through the infusion catheter should be avoided if at all possible).

Once catheter angiography is complete and the decision has been made to proceed with catheter-directed thrombolysis, a bolus of thrombolytic agent can be administered through the catheter while the infusion is being prepared. An end-hole catheter positioned in the distal axillary or proximal brachial artery is well suited for both infusion and repeat arteriography to assess the treatment response. A proximally positioned catheter may also result in wider thrombolytic distribution through the radial, ulnar, and interosseus arteries.[7] Alternatively, infusion through a multiple side-hole catheter placed within the thrombus (as commonly performed for lower extremity arterial or venous thrombosis) has been described for upper extremity arterial thrombolysis,[3,7] but may be impractical due to relatively smaller arterial diameters, access length, and tendency to induce vasospasm. If arterial spasm is a problem but thrombolysis is necessary, a smaller diameter microcatheter or infusion wire can be used for thrombolytic infusion but usually requires exchange for a larger catheter to obtain adequate images during follow-up arteriography.

Once the thrombolytic infusion has been initiated, the catheter and sheath should be secured to one another and to the patient to avoid inadvertent withdrawal or repositioning during port manipulation or transportation. The infusion catheter can be secured to the sheath using adhesive strips wound in a spiral fashion, and the sheath then sutured to the skin before covering the entire apparatus with an adhesive barrier drape. When attached in this fashion, traction on the infusion catheter will transfer tension to the patient's skin without resulting in catheter withdrawal. Peri-catheter thrombosis has been reported as a complication of catheter-directed thrombolysis,[19,22] and a low-dose heparin infusion (500 units/hr) should therefore be administered through the side port of the sheath to minimize risk of local thrombus accumulation. The heparin dose should not be adjusted or titrated based on the pTT. To maximize safety and reduce risk of errors, it is wise to clearly label both the catheter and sheath in a manner consistent with the infusion orders (such as "catheter-TPA" and "sheath-heparin"), particularly if the patient will be cared for or observed (even temporarily) in a unit where experience with catheter-directed thrombolysis is limited. For this reason, it is worthwhile to routinely transport patients receiving thrombolytic infusions directly to the intensive care unit and personally review the orders, labeling, and intended infusion doses directly with the receiving nurse and other team members.

PATIENT CARE AND MONITORING

Patients treated with catheter-directed thrombolysis should be monitored in a unit staffed appropriately for high-acuity patients, preferably by a nursing and pharmacy team experienced with their specific care and monitoring needs. If circumstances require the patient to temporarily reside in a location other than the definitive care unit (such as a postoperative anesthesia care unit or imaging department), it is important that all personnel involved with medication administration, phlebotomy, and management of intravenous fluids are aware that the patient is receiving a thrombolytic infusion so that appropriate safety precautions can be followed. Patients should be closely monitored with a heightened sense of awareness for potential bleeding complications related to thrombolysis. Accordingly, any new symptoms that are potentially attributable to bleeding (including acute headache or back pain) must be pursued immediately with appropriate diagnostic imaging while the thrombolytic infusion is temporarily held until bleeding has been ruled out. As previously mentioned, any invasive procedures (including arterial or intravenous lines, Foley catheters, nasogastric tubes, or even suppositories) should be avoided during infusion if at all possible. In order to avoid needle phlebotomy during thrombolytic infusion (and associated bleeding risk), blood samples can be obtained from the side port of the access sheath provided that it is flushed with non-heparinized saline and an adequate amount of blood is temporarily aspirated to clear the sheath before obtaining the sample. Radial artery catheters and other upper extremity arterial lines, which are sometimes used for blood sampling in intensive care unit settings, should be avoided in patients with AFI (including in the contralateral arm).

During catheter-directed thrombolysis, patients should be re-evaluated after 8–24 hours of infusion with repeat angiography to determine whether treatment has resulted in anatomic improvement (i.e., partial or complete resolution of previously identified occlusive disease) and decide whether the infusion should be resumed or discontinued (Figure 19-4). Angiography can be performed through the infusion catheter without need for removal of the securing adhesive attachments if adequate rates of injection are possible. When anatomic improvement is observed but is incomplete (such as re-established radial artery patency with persistent proper digital artery occlusion), continued thrombolysis has potential to yield further improvement and should be considered. Conversely, catheter-directed thrombolysis should be discontinued in the absence of anatomic improvement, particularly if the total duration of the

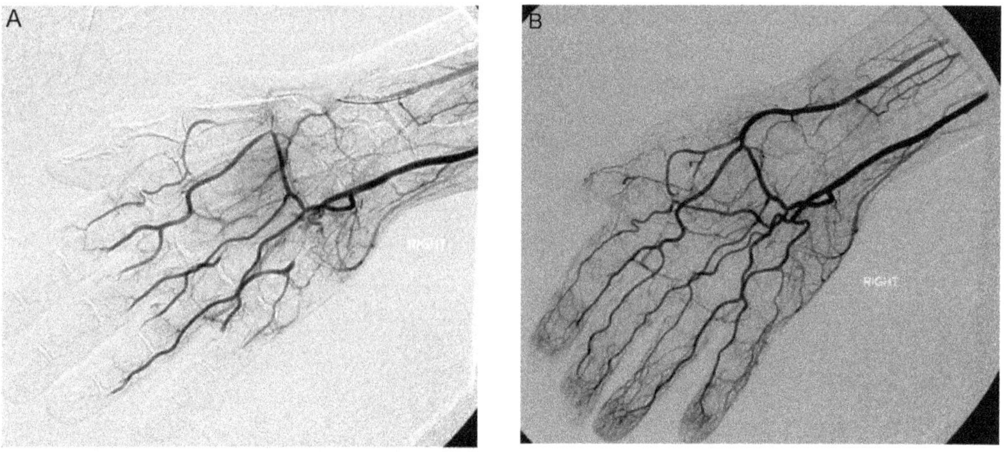

Figure 19-4. Interval anatomic improvement based on angiography following catheter-directed thrombolysis. (**A**) Catheter angiogram demonstrates occluded right radial artery, occluded superficial palmar arch, incomplete deep palmar arch with occlusion of multiple metacarpal arteries and pruning of the proper digital arteries. (**B**) Repeat angiogram following catheter-directed thrombolysis for 24 hours demonstrates re-established patency of previously occluded superficial palmar arch, metacarpal, and proper digital arteries.

infusion is approaching 48 hours, the total dose of alteplase has exceeded 20–25 mg, or severe and persistent vasospasm is observed.

Risk of bleeding during catheter-directed thrombolysis is related to both the dose and duration of infusion.[13,15] Use of weight-based dosing or a maximum total dose (such as 20 mg of alteplase) has been described by some and may limit the risk of bleeding complications.[1,20] During catheter-directed thrombolysis, patients should be monitored regularly (i.e., every 4–8 hours) with surveillance laboratory testing that includes fibrinogen, pTT, platelet count, and hemoglobin. A significant decrease in the hemoglobin, platelet count, or fibrinogen, or a fibrinogen level <100 mg/dL, should prompt an immediate patient assessment and consideration of either decreasing or discontinuing the infusion to avoid bleeding. Other reasons to discontinue the thrombolytic infusion include lack of improvement during the previous infusion interval (which may be assessed based on symptoms, physical examination, or arteriogram findings), restoration of flow without an identifiable need for continuation of thrombolysis, or infusion for a period >48 hours. When the infusion is discontinued, the catheter should be removed to avoid adjacent thrombus accumulation and associated risk of arterial thrombosis or embolization (unless repeat arteriography to assess the anatomy at the conclusion of thrombolysis is immediately pending). Sheath removal should be deferred for 2–4 hours following cessation of both the thrombolytic and heparin infusions to allow these medications to dissipate, and a repeat ACT should be obtained if the previous value was >200 seconds.

ADJUNCTIVE TREATMENTS

Several adjunctive treatments have been described in combination (either simultaneously or in a staged fashion) with catheter-directed thrombolysis for AFI.

Thromboaspiration in combination with thrombolysis has been described for endovascular management of organized thrombus embolizing from a proximal anatomic location.[20] Because aspiration catheters are seldom long enough to reach the distal arm from the femoral artery, this technique requires retrograde access from a patent distal arterial segment and often requires multiple aspiration sessions with a 6 French catheter. Use of pulse-spray thrombolytic infusion for acute upper extremity ischemia has also been described.[20]

Although use of ultrasound-accelerated thrombolysis has been associated with reduced thrombolysis time for acute lower extremity ischemia, this adjunctive treatment was not associated with a patency advantage has not been described extensively for upper extremity ischemia.[14] Proposed mechanisms of action for ultrasound-accelerated thrombolysis include increased thrombus permeability resulting from loosening of fibrin strands, increased exposure of plasminogen receptors, and acoustic cavitation.

OUTCOMES

Adverse procedure-related events occur in in 11%–12% of patients treated with catheter-directed thrombolysis for upper extremity disease, with access-related bleeding complications being the most common.[2] Rates of major bleeding reported from larger series of patients undergoing catheter-directed thrombolysis for lower extremity arterial disease range from 6%–13% with a 2%–3% rate of intracranial bleeding,[23–26] while a meta-analysis identifying a 9% rate of major bleeding within 30 days.[17] Bleeding risk is related to both the duration of the infusion and the total dose of the thrombolytic agent.[13] Other reported procedure-related adverse events include access site pseudoaneurysm, guide wire perforation of branch arteries, stroke or transient ischemic attack, and upper extremity compartment syndrome.[2,7,19,20,27] Compartment syndrome of the hand during catheter-directed thrombolysis is associated with instrumentation of the affected extremity;[27] avoiding ipsilateral antegrade brachial access may therefore be wise, particularly among patients with neurologic symptoms at the time of presentation (which may make clinical diagnosis of compartment syndrome challenging).

Rates of angiography-based anatomic improvement reported with catheter-directed thrombolysis for upper extremity arterial disease are between 33%–50%.[2,5] Finger amputation is necessary 5%–6% of patients and is usually performed within 60 days of initial evaluation; the majority of these patients present with ulcers or gangrene.[2] Surgical revascularization (including aneurysm resection, ligation, or bypass) was performed in approximately 12% of patients following angiography with or without catheter directed thrombolysis for AFI,[2] with a bypass patency of 77% reported at 2 years.[28]

Although one year amputation-free survival following presentation with AFI is 70%–80% overall, nearly half of patient report continued long-term symptoms.[2] Amputation-free survival appears similar between patients treated with versus without catheter-directed thrombolysis, limited data suggests a possible benefit associated with thrombolysis among those patients without ulcers or gangrene at the time of initial presentation (Figure 19-5).[2]

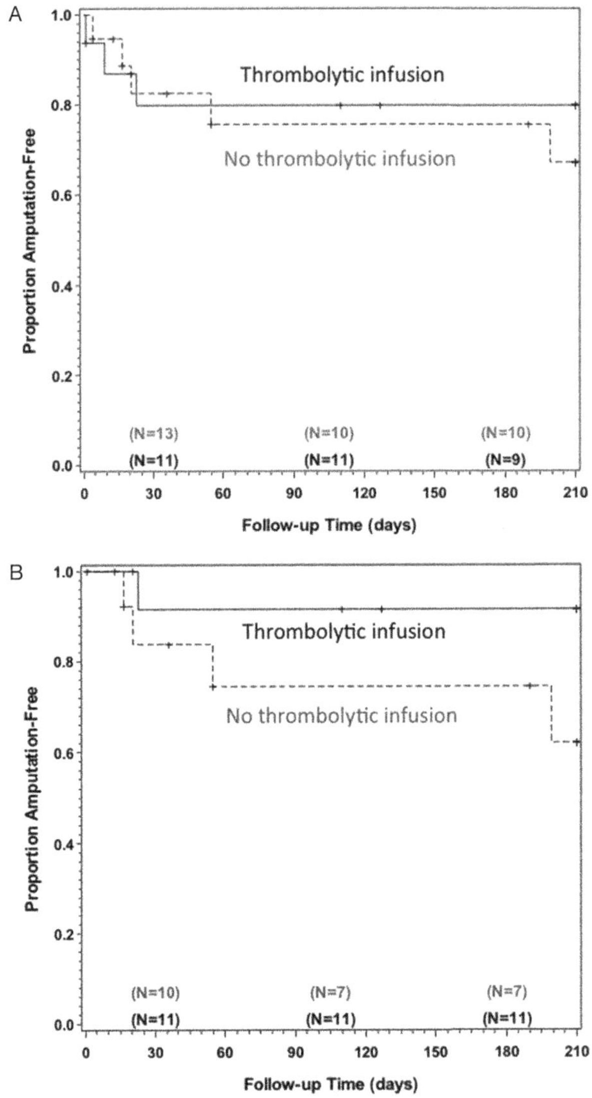

Figure 19-5. Estimated amputation-free survival following presentation with acute finger ischemia stratified by use of catheter directed thrombolysis. Figures represent overall cohort of 35 patients (**A**) versus subgroup without tissue loss or gangrene at time of initial evaluation (**B**). Solid line indicates group treated with catheter-directed thrombolysis, while interrupted line indicates those treated without catheter-directed thrombolysis.

REFERENCES

1. Schernthaner MB, Samuels S, Biegler P, et al. Ultrasound-accelerated versus standard catheter-directed thrombolysis in 102 patients with acute and subacute limb ischemia. *J Vasc Interv Radiol.* 2014;25(8):1149–56; quiz 1157.
2. Islam A, Edgerton C, Stafford JM, et al. Anatomic findings and outcomes associated with upper extremity arteriography and selective thrombolysis for acute finger ischemia. *J Vasc Surg.* 2014;60(2):410–7.

3. Barbiero G, Cognolato D, Casarin A, et al. Intra-arterial thrombolysis of acute hand ischaemia with or without microcatheter: preliminary experience and comparison with the literature. *Radiol Med.* 2011;116(6):919–31.
4. Ruch DS, Smith TL, Smith B,P et al. Anatomic and physiologic evaluation of upper extremity ischemia. *Microsurgery.* 1999;19(4):181–8.
5. Cejna M, Salomonowitz E, Wohlschlager H, et al. rt-PA thrombolysis in acute thromboembolic upper-extremity arterial occlusion. *Cardiovasc Intervent Radiol.* 2001;24(4):218–23.
6. Grasu BL, Jones CM, Murphy MS. Use of diagnostic modalities for assessing upper extremity vascular pathology. *Hand Clin.* 2015;31(1):1–12.
7. Breguet R, Terraz S, Righini M, et al. Acute hand ischemia after unintentional intraarterial injection of drugs: is catheter-directed thrombolysis useful. *J Vasc Interv Radiol.* 2014;25(6):963–8.
8. Friedrich KM, Frühwald-Pallamar J, Stadlbauer A, et al. Hypothenar hammer syndrome: long-term follow-up of selective thrombolysis by 3.0-T MR angiography. *Eur J Radiol.* 2010;75(2):e27–e31.
9. Vayssairat M, Debure C, Cormier JM, et al. Hypothenar hammer syndrome: seventeen cases with long-term follow-up. *J Vasc Surg.* 1987;5(6):838–43.
10. De Martino RR, Moran SL. The role of thrombolytics in acute and chronic occlusion of the hand. *Hand Clin.* 2015;31(1):13–21.
11. Schneider PA, Bohannon WT, Silva MB. *Carotid interventions.* Boca Raton, FL: Marcel Dekker; 2005.
12. Andersen LV, Mortensen LS, Lindholt JS, et al. Upper-limb thrombo-embolectomy: national cohort study in Denmark. *Eur J Vasc Endovasc Surg.* 2010;40(5):628–34.
13. Semba CP, Sugimoto K, Razavi MK, et al. Alteplase and tenecteplase: applications in the peripheral circulation. *Tech Vasc Interv Radiol.* 2001;4(2):99–106.
14. Schrijver AM, van Leersum M, Fioole B, et al. Dutch randomized trial comparing standard catheter-directed thrombolysis and ultrasound-accelerated thrombolysis for arterial thromboembolic infrainguinal disease (DUET). *J Endovasc Ther.* 2015;22(1):87–95.
15. Ebben HP, Nederhoed JH, Lely RJ, et al. Low-dose thrombolysis for thromboembolic lower extremity arterial occlusions is effective without major hemorrhagic complications. *Eur J Vasc Endovasc Surg.* 2014;48(5):551–8.
16. Yusuf SW, Whitaker SC, Gregson RH, et al. Prospective randomised comparative study of pulse spray and conventional local thrombolysis. *Eur J Vasc Endovasc Surg.* 1995;10(2):136–41.
17. Berridge DC, Kessel DO, Robertson I. Surgery versus thrombolysis for initial management of acute limb ischaemia. *Cochrane Database Syst Rev.* 2013;6 CD002784.
18. Weitz JI. Chapter 30. Blood Coagulation and Anticoagulant, Fibrinolytic, and Antiplatelet Drugs. In: Goodman LS, Brunton LL, Chabner B, et al. *Goodman & Gilman's Pharmacological Basis of Therapeutics.* 12th ed. ed. New York: McGraw-Hill; 2011.
19. Coulon M, Goffette P, Dondelinger RF. Local thrombolytic infusion in arterial ischemia of the upper limb: mid-term results. *Cardiovasc Intervent Radiol.* 1994;17(2):81–6.
20. Miyayama S, Yamashiro M, Shibata Y, et al. Thrombolysis and thromboaspiration for acute thromboembolic occlusion in the upper extremity. *Jpn J Radiol.* 2012;30(2):180–4.
21. Robertson I, Kessel DO, Berridge DC. Fibrinolytic agents for peripheral arterial occlusion. *Cochrane Database Syst Rev.* 2013;12 CD001099.
22. Wheatley MJ, Marx MV. The use of intra-arterial urokinase in the management of hand ischemia secondary to palmar and digital arterial occlusion. *Ann Plast Surg.* 1996;37(4):356–62; discussion 362.
23. Results of a prospective randomized trial evaluating surgery versus thrombolysis for ischemia of the lower extremity. The STILE trial. *Ann Surg.* 1994;220(3):251–66; discussion 266.
24. Cragg AH, Smith TP, Corson JD, et al. Two urokinase dose regimens in native arterial and graft occlusions: initial results of a prospective, randomized clinical trial. *Radiology.* 1991;178(3):681–6.

25. Duda SH, Tepe G, Luz O, et al. Peripheral artery occlusion: treatment with abciximab plus urokinase versus with urokinase alone—a randomized pilot trial (the PROMPT Study). Platelet Receptor Antibodies in Order to Manage Peripheral Artery Thrombosis. *Radiology.* 2001;221(3):689–96.
26. Ouriel K, Veith FJ, Sasahara AA. A comparison of recombinant urokinase with vascular surgery as initial treatment for acute arterial occlusion of the legs. Thrombolysis or Peripheral Arterial Surgery (TOPAS) Investigators. *N Engl J Med.* 1998;338(16):1105–11.
27. Freyer M, Vachalova I, Zirngibl B, et al. Compartment syndrome following thrombolysis: clinical features and associated conditions. *J Thromb Thrombolysis.* 2014;38(2):201–7.
28. Chloros GD, Lucas RM, Li Z, et al. Post-traumatic ulnar artery thrombosis: outcome of arterial reconstruction using reverse interpositional vein grafting at 2 years minimum follow-up. *J Hand Surg Am.* 2008;33(6):932–40.

20

Brachial Access for Peripheral Arterial Interventions

Matthew Mell, MD, MS

Newer strategies for percutaneous endovascular interventions have expanded the need for alternative access approaches. Although retrograde femoral access remains the most frequently used one, other important access techniques include antegrade femoral access, popliteal or pedal access, and brachial or radial artery access. An upper extremity approach may be beneficial with unfavorable aortoiliac anatomy. Examples may include previous open or endovascular aneurysm repair, open aortoiliac reconstruction for occlusive disease with a steeply angled and fixed aortic bifurcation, previous "kissing" iliac stents, or contralateral iliac artery occlusion. Additionally, arm access may be preferred when treating downward-pointing visceral or renal arterial lesions.

When considering brachial access, location of the disease and the type of treatment must be considered. Shaft lengths must be long enough to reach the vessel to be treated from the proposed access site. The artery must have a large enough diameter to accommodate the appropriate sheath size, and there should not be proximal subclavian artery, aortic arch, or significant descending aortic thoracic aortic disease.

TECHNICAL CONSIDERATIONS

Access

The brachial artery can be accessed by a percutaneous approach with fluoroscopic or ultrasound guidance, or with an open cutdown approach. Percutaneous access is most safely obtained by accessing the brachial artery with a 21-gauge micropuncture needle under ultrasound guidance. Fluoroscopy should confirm appropriate placement just proximal to the olecranon fossa to allow for compression against a bony structure after sheath removal. Once accurate placement is confirmed, the access is changed over a 0.035 wire to an appropriately sized sheath based on procedural goals. For larger sheaths, an open approach should be considered, as it may be associated with a lower complication rate.[1]

The axillary artery can be approached in a similar fashion to the brachial artery. Access may be facilitated by placing the patient's hands behind the head. (Figure 20-1) This position will elevate the artery closer to the surface and will allow for pressure over the humeral head when the sheath is removed.

Radial artery access is being used more commonly for coronary procedures due to fewer local complications. Even in centers with experience with radial artery cannulation, its use for peripheral arterial revascularization has been more limited due to the added shaft length needed to treat the affected vessel.[2] Sheath sizes larger than 6F and radial artery diameter <2 mm are generally contraindicated for a radial approach.

Because radial artery access may be complicated by radial artery thrombosis in up to 19% of patient,[3,4] it is important to document the presence of a complete palmar arch prior to attempting access with this approach. A complete palmar arch can be confirmed with a modified Allen's test or with pulse oximetry on the thumb with radial artery compression.[5,6] An incomplete palmar arch is a contraindication to radial artery access as radial artery thrombosis may result in significant hand ischemia and its sequelae.

More so than other arteries, the radial artery has a tendency to experience vasospasm once instrumented. To prevent this, it is our preferred technique to obtain radial artery access with ultrasound guidance and a hydrophilic 6F sheath over a 0.021 wire. Once access has been confirmed, the dilator assembly and wire are removed followed by administration of heparin (50 units/kg), verapamil (2.5 mg), and nitroglycerine (100 μg) diluted into 30 mL of blood. A second dose of heparin is given prior to treatment of the arterial lesion.

Closure

Traditional management of the access site at sheath removal is to apply manual compression for 20 minutes, followed by immobilization of the limb for four to six hours depending on the size of the sheath. Heparin if given should be reversed when feasible. It is our practice to reverse heparin with protamine to an activated clotting time (ACT) goal of 160–180 seconds prior to removing the sheath. Other options include a mechanical clamp or the use of a closure device. The two types of closure devices include those with collagen plugs and suture-mediated devices. Closure devices decrease the amount of time required for manual compression and the required time to remain supine after sheath removal, with perhaps a little as one hour required. The safety and efficacy of closure devices for arm access is not well established. A report of AngioSeal for brachial artery closure in 161 procedures reported an 11% complication rate.[7] Most large studies

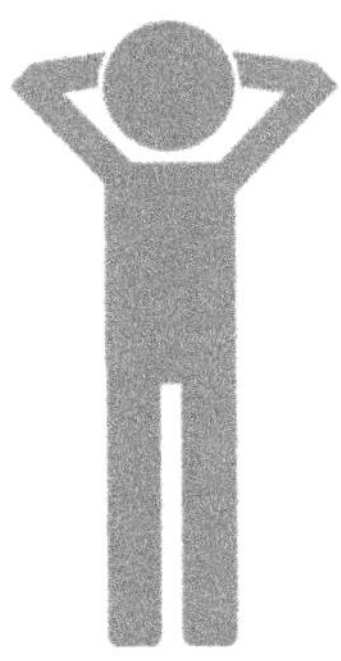

Figure 20-1. Optimal position for axillary artery percutaneous access.

of closure devices in the femoral artery have not been able to identify a benefit with regard to access complications. For percutaneous coronary interventions, closure devices may be associated with an increased risk of local complications including hematoma and pseudoaneurysm.[8,9]

It has been our standard for percutaneous access with <6F sheaths to control the access site with direct pressure followed by immobilizing the arm with an arm board for four to six hours. This approach is supported by a recent single-center study[2] describing a 10-year experience with a reported overall complication rate of less than 2%. In this study, sheath size varied from 4F to 7F, although the proportion of each was not reported. For procedures requiring >5F sheaths or for women or patients with increased risk of postprocedural bleeding, we favor an open approach with suture closure of the arteriotomy using 6-0 prolene sutures.

COMPLICATIONS

Complications can occur with any access location. The most common types of access-related complications are bleeding with resultant hematoma or pseudoaneurysm, vessel thrombosis, arteriovenous fistula, or infection.[1,10,11] Additionally, axillary and brachial access may be complicated by nerve compression and injury by even small hematomas. Rarely, athero-embolism can occur leading to distal embolization.

While femoral access is associated with a complication rate of 3%–6%, the overall complication rate for brachial access may be 6%–14%.[1,12,13] We compared brachial to femoral access in over 40,000 patients using national data extracted from the Society of Vascular Surgery Vascular Quality Initiative (SVS-VQI) data base,[1] and observed a higher rate of hematomas (7.2% vs. 3.0%; $P < 0.001$) as well as access site stenosis or occlusion (2.1% vs. 0.4%; $P < 0.001$) when comparing brachial to femoral access. For brachial access, complications occurred less frequently after arterial cutdown (4.1%) compared with either ultrasound-guided (11.8%) or fluoroscopically-guided percutaneous access (7.3%). Neither the surgeons' overall peripheral vascular intervention experience nor prior experience with brachial access predicted likelihood of adverse events. Independent factors associated with a lower likelihood of access complications included male sex (OR 0.48; 95% CI 0.28–0.84; $P < 0.01$) and arterial cutdown (OR, 0.25; 95% CI, 0.07–0.87; $P = 0.04$) (Table 20-1). Larger sheath sizes (>5F) were associated with increased risk of complications (OR, 2.19; 95% CI, 1.07–4.49; $P = 0.03$). Of note, neither smoking, dialysis, the use of antiplatelet agents, the use of heparin or protamine, body

TABLE 20-1. INDEPENDENT FACTOR ASSOCIATE WITH BRACHIAL ACCESS COMPLICATIONS

Increased Risk	Decreased Risk	No effect
Older age	Younger age	Body-mass index
Female sex	Male sex	Diabetes
Sheath size > 5F	Sheath size ≤ 5F	Preoperative antiplatelet agents
Ultrasound guidance*	Arterial cutdown	Heparin/protamine
		Closure device use

*Risk may be decreased with confirmation of access over bony prominence.

mass index, nor the use of a closure device had a significant effect on postoperative hematoma or vessel occlusion.

Estimated risk of access complications for ≥6F sheath for men and women was 2.9% and 5.6% with cutdown versus 7.2% and 13.2% for percutaneous access, respectively. For smaller sheaths estimated complications were 1.4% and 3.1% with cutdown versus 3.7% and 7.7% for percutaneous access, respectively (Table 20-2).

Hematoma Formation

Hematoma formation with brachial access can lead to median nerve compression which may take months to resolve. This compression may occur even with small volume of hematoma due to the constrained space of the brachial sheath. Brachial hematomas therefore must be observed carefully, and should be considered for early operative evacuation with signs of expansion or median nerve symptoms.

Arteriovenous Fistula

Arteriovenous fistula is rare after brachial access and may develop with through-and-through arterial access and decompression into an adjacent vein. Symptoms include a new bruit or thrill at the access site. Surgical repair is usually necessary as fistulae tend to enlarge with time.

Pseudoaneurysm

Pseudoaneurysms may occur in less than 2% of patients and are usually the result of inadequate manual compression after removal of the sheath. Other risk factors include sheath diameter, antiplatelet or anticoagulation treatment, obesity, and hemodialysis.[14–16] Treatment may include observation, thrombin injection, or surgical repair depending on it size, the presence of symptoms, and the anatomic considerations of the pseudoaneurysm neck.[2,15,17]

Arterial Thrombosis

Arterial thrombosis is rare and may occur slightly more often when the brachial approach is used. When it occurs surgical repair is mandated. Thrombosis may occur from vessel spasm, inadequate procedural anticoagulation, or excessive compression after sheath removal. However, vessel injury must be considered as a causative or contributing agent. As such, operative exploration must comprise thrombectomy, inspection of the vessel for intimal injury, and repair. Without vessel injury thrombectomy, primary repair and post-operative anti-platelet agents or anticoagulation will suffice.

TABLE 20-2. ESTIMATED RISK OF COMPLICATIONS WITH BRACHIAL ACCESS

Large Sheath (>5F)				Small Sheath (≤5F)			
Men		Women		Men		Women	
Cutdown	Percutaneous	Cutdown	Percutaneous	Cutdown	Percutaneous	Cutdown	Percutaneous
2.9%	7.2%	5.6%	13.2%	1.4%	3.7%	3.1%	7.7%

If an injury is identified, repair may include endarterectomy, patch angioplasty closure, or in the event of severe injury, bypass with autogenous vein reconstruction.

Atheroembolism

Physical trauma to the subclavian artery, aortic arch, or the descending aorta may rarely result in embolization of atheromatous debris. This type of injury can occur from the sheath itself or the wires and instrumentation required for the procedure. Embolism to the cerebral circulation can cause stroke, while that to the visceral vessels can cause mesenteric ischemia or renal infarction. It is important to assess the health of the approach vessels prior to consideration of brachial access, as the incidence of atheroembolism from brachial access for peripheral vascular interventions is unknown, but the consequences severe.

REFERENCES

1. Kret MR, Dalman RL, Kalish J, Mell M. Arterial cutdown reduces complications after brachial access for peripheral vascular intervention. *J Vasc Surg*. 2016;64(1):149–154.
2. Franz RW, Tanga CF, Herrmann JW. Treatment of peripheral arterial disease via percutaneous brachial artery access. *J Vasc Surg*. 2016;64(3):866–887.
3. Greenwood MJ, Della-Siega AJ, Fretz EB, et al. Vascular communications of the hand in patients being considered for transradial coronary angiography: is the Allen's test accurate? *J Am Coll Cardiol*. 2005;46(11):2013–2017.
4. Kotowycz MA, Dzavik V. Radial artery patency after transradial catheterization. *Circ Cardiovasc Interv*. 2012;5(1):127–133.
5. Barbeau GR, Arsenault F, Dugas L, Simard S, Lariviere MM. Evaluation of the ulnopalmar arterial arches with pulse oximetry and plethysmography: comparison with the Allen's test in 1010 patients. *Am Heart J*. 2004;147(3):489–493.
6. Hovagim AR, Katz RI, Poppers PJ. Pulse oximetry for evaluation of radial and ulnar arterial blood flow. *J Cardiothorac Anesth*. 1989;3(1):27–30.
7. Lupattelli T, Clerissi J, Clerici G, et al. The efficacy and safety of closure of brachial access using the AngioSeal closure device: experience with 161 interventions in diabetic patients with critical limb ischemia. *J Vasc Surg*. 2008;47(4):782–788.
8. Koreny M, Riedmuller E, Nikfardjam M, Siostrzonek P, Mullner M. Arterial puncture closing devices compared with standard manual compression after cardiac catheterization: systematic review and meta-analysis. *JAMA*. 2004;291(3):350–357.
9. Nikolsky E, Mehran R, Halkin A, et al. Vascular complications associated with arteriotomy closure devices in patients undergoing percutaneous coronary procedures: a meta-analysis. *J Am Coll Cardiol*. 2004;44(6):1200–1209.
10. Armstrong PJ, Han DC, Baxter JA, Elmore JR, Franklin DP. Complication rates of percutaneous brachial artery access in peripheral vascular angiography. *Ann Vasc Surg*. 2003;17(1):107–110.
11. Ortiz D, Jahangir A, Singh M, Allaqaband S, Bajwa TK, Mewissen MW. Access site complications after peripheral vascular interventions: incidence, predictors, and outcomes. *Circ Cardiovasc Interv*. 2014;7(6):821–828.
12. Alvarez-Tostado JA, Moise MA, Bena JF, et al. The brachial artery: a critical access for endovascular procedures. *J Vasc Surg*. 2009;49(2):378–385; discussion 385.
13. Stavroulakis K, Usai MV, Torsello G, et al. Efficacy and safety of transbrachial access for iliac endovascular interventions. *J Endovasc Ther*. 2016;23(3):454–460.
14. Katzenschlager R, Ugurluoglu A, Ahmadi A, et al. Incidence of pseudoaneurysm after diagnostic and therapeutic angiography. *Radiology*. 1995;195(2):463–466.

15. Krueger K, Zaehringer M, Strohe D, Stuetzer H, Boecker J, Lackner K. Postcatheterization pseudoaneurysm: results of US-guided percutaneous thrombin injection in 240 patients. *Radiology*. 2005;236(3):1104–1110.
16. Webber GW, Jang J, Gustavson S, Olin JW. Contemporary management of postcatheterization pseudoaneurysms. *Circulation*. 2007;115(20):2666–2674.
17. La Perna L, Olin JW, Goines D, Childs MB, Ouriel K. Ultrasound-guided thrombin injection for the treatment of postcatheterization pseudoaneurysms. *Circulation*. 2000;102(19):2391–2395.

21

Management of Complications after Invasive Upper Extremity Testing and Treatment

Katherine E. Hekman, MD, PhD and
Andrew W. Hoel, MD

The upper extremity arteries are routinely utilized for hemodynamic monitoring as well as for diagnostic and therapeutic interventions in the clinical setting. Ischemic complications of upper extremity arterial access are problematic and can result in severe morbidity. The broad use of upper extremity arterial access for hemodynamic monitoring and the increasing use of upper extremity arteries for vascular access procedures warrants review of this process. This chapter reviews the most common types of complications, as well as identified risk factors for these complications reported in the literature. We then discuss potential strategies for minimizing the risk of complications and current therapeutic options.

INCREASING USE OF UPPER EXTREMITY ARTERIAL ACCESS FOR ENDOVASCULAR THERAPIES

While use of radial artery access for hemodynamic monitoring has been increasingly routine since the 1960s,[1] advances in endovascular technology have rendered the upper extremity arteries also useful as access sites for diagnostic and therapeutic interventions. Since the RIVAL trial evaluating radial versus femoral access for coronary catheterizations, it has become a common access site for coronary interventions.[2]

More recently, vascular surgeons have also begun utilizing the radial and ulnar arteries as access sites. Sheathless radial and ulnar access for endovascular treatment of iliac artery disease was recently described. In 156 patients undergoing treatment,

151 were treated with transradial access and seven with transulnar access. Crossover rate from radial to brachial or femoral access due to technical failure was 3.8%.[3] In a series of 80 patients undergoing endovascular therapy via radial artery access, including peripheral interventions, mesenteric interventions, carotid interventions, and adjunctive interventions for aortic disease, all procedures via the radial artery utilized a 4-French or 5-French sheath.[4] In a series of 24 patients treated via radial access for iliac or femoral disease, the technical success rate was 91%, consistent with other reported success rates of 87.5%–100%.[5]

For the purposes of hemodynamic monitoring, there appears to be variation in the access site chosen depending on the medical specialty. In a series of 2119 with either a femoral, radial or brachial arterial line for hemodynamic monitoring in the ICU, complication rates of bleeding, infection, and ischemia were comparable among all three sites. Of note, the femoral artery was favored in the medical ICU and the radial in the surgical ICU.[6] This is corroborated by meta-analysis of papers published from 1978 to 2001 regarding complication rates from arterial line monitoring of the femoral, radial, and axillary artery. Complications in the radial artery ranged from 1% to 35% and were most commonly a temporary occlusion of the artery. Rates of complications were comparable among the three sites.[7]

HAND ARTERIAL ANATOMY AND HEMODYNAMIC CONSEQUENCES OF RADIAL ARTERY INSTRUMENTATION

The arterial supply to the hand is rich with collaterals, and variations away from this normal anatomy is thought to increase the risk of digital ischemia in the affected patients. The normal anatomy and most common variants are depicted in Figure 21-1.

Arterial access has a measurable effect on local blood flow dynamics, although not always clinically significant, ostensibly due to this extensive collateral network providing blood to the hand. In 1000 patients who underwent radial artery line placement for hemodynamic monitoring, 24 had evidence of diminution of flow, which resolved by two weeks after removal. Only two of these patients had complications.[1] While disturbances of flow dynamics may not be immediately clinically significant, the sequelae of radial artery instrumentation may become evident some time later following the periprocedural period. Critical ischemia of the upper extremity attributable to radial artery occlusion after instrumentation has been reported up to four months after radial artery access for coronary intervention.[9] Occlusion can occur soon after the procedure due to thrombus, or much later likely from neointimal hyperplasia.[10] When they do occur, ischemic sequelae can be devastating. In a case series reviewing eight patients with symptomatic radial artery occlusion from cannulation for hemodynamic monitoring, six of these had ongoing ischemic neurologic deficits or tissue loss. Only one of the eight had resolution of symptoms without sequelae.[11]

INCIDENCE

Complications from upper extremity arterial access can be mechanical (including hematoma, pseudoaneurysm, hemorrhage), infectious, thrombotic, or neurologic.

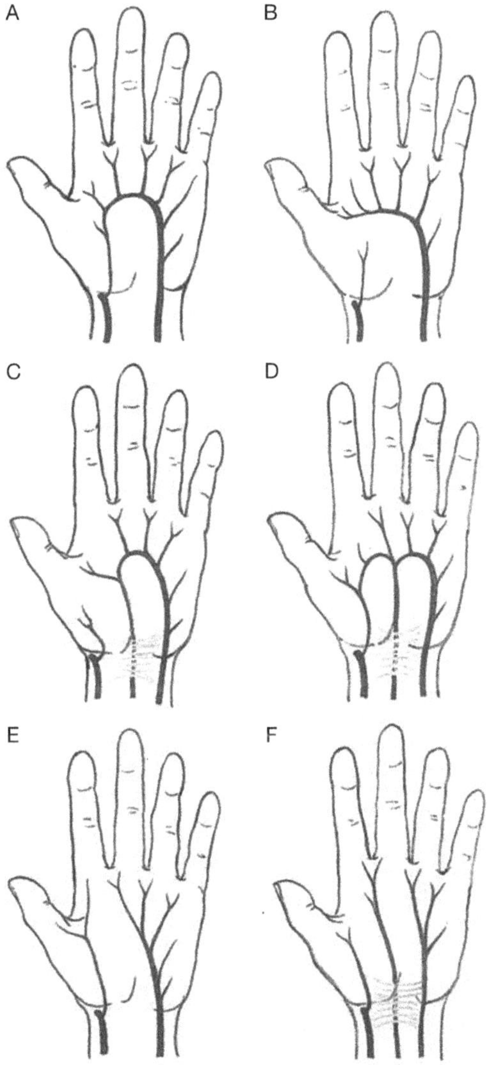

Figure 21-1. Variant arterial anatomy of the hand. (**A**) Complete arch (35%). (**B**) Complete arch formed by the ulnar artery (39%). (**C**) Complete arch via ulnar and median arteries (4%). (**D**) Complete arch via ulnar, radial, and median arteries (1%). (**E**) Incomplete arch (16%). (**F**) Digital arteries arising directly from ulnar, median, and radial artery branches (5%). Reprinted with permission from Strauch et al.[8]

Reported rates of complications vary widely by type of access as well as across institutions, likely attributable to variations in volume and experience (Table 21-1).

Arterial Line Complications

In a large retrospective review of 57,787 patients receiving arterial lines placed for hemodynamic monitoring, 21 had complications. These included asymptomatic arterial occlusions, symptomatic occlusions with focal pain, and ischemia.[12] Asymptomatic postprocedural radial artery occlusion is of uncertain significance, and reportedly ranges from 0.8% to 30%. It is often overlooked due to lack of clinical

TABLE 21-1. RATES OF ACCESS SITE COMPLICATIONS VARY BY INSTITUTION AND BY THE ARTERY ACCESSED

	N	Access Site Complication Rate
Endovascular Therapy		
Nasr[14]	57 brachial	0
Treitl[15]	150 brachial	14.0% minor, 2.7% major
Stavroulakis[16]	201 brachial	12.4%
Alvarez-Tostado[17]	323 brachial	6.5%
Kret[18]	732 brachial	9.0%
Armstrong[19]	1326 brachial	1.28%
Kumar[4]	80 radial	3.75%
Ruzsa[3]	151 radial, 7 ulnar	5.1% (all radial)
Hemodynamic monitoring		
Mandel[1]	1000 radial	40% minor, 0.2% major
Scheer[7]	19,617 radial	1%–35%
Nuttall[12]	57,787 radial	0.123%

features.[10] In this series, the radial artery appeared the safest site of placement, with a complication rate of only 2.7 per 10,000 patients compared with 9.0 per 10,000 for the femoral artery and 12.3 per 10,000 for the brachial artery. However, these differences were not statistically significant.[12]

Reported complications were also low among the early reports of routine arterial line placement for hemodynamic monitoring. In a retrospective case series of 1000 patients reported only two had major complications, one requiring an embolectomy and the other arterial reconstruction. Minor complications predominated, which included small hematomas and ecchymosis occurring at a rate of 40% overall, with increasing frequency the longer the line remained in place. No permanent damage occurred as a result of these minor complications.[1]

Fortunately, clinically significant infection from indwelling radial artery lines is relatively rare. In a series of 492 radial artery catheters, no local or systemic infections related to the arterial catheter were reported. Catheter tip cultures were positive in eight of 200 sampled, but none were of clinical significance.[13] In another large series, surveillance cultures detected 2.4 infections per 10,000 patients.[12] Arterial lines generally are well tolerated in most patients with low rates of complications, making them accessible as well as being of great utility. Specific groups of patients with potential for increased risk of complications are discussed later in this chapter.

Radial Artery Access for Endovascular Procedures

Less information is currently available regarding radial artery access for endovascular procedures. In a series of 80 patients undergoing radial artery access for endovascular therapies, there were only three complications, all of which were minor hematomas requiring no intervention. In this series, there were no cases of upper extremity ischemia from radial artery access.[4] In a series of 156 patients undergoing iliac endovascular interventions via a sheathless system through the radial and ulnar arteries, only eight patients had radial artery access site complications, mostly asymptomatic occlusions with one perforation treated with a stent.[3] In 24 patients treated endovascularly via left radial artery access for iliofemoral disease, the most common complication was transient arterial spasm. Only minor bleeding occurred but there was one case of a minor right hemispheric cerebrovascular accident.[5]

Brachial Artery Access for Endovascular Procedures

Complications from brachial artery access for endovascular therapies appear to carry a higher risk of complications compared to radial artery access, ranging from 1% to 14%, but reported complication rates vary. There were no complications related to brachial artery access in 57 cases performed a single institution from 2012 to 2013 for iliac artery endovascular revascularization. The majority (82%) were executed through a 6-French sheath, and the remainder through a 7-French sheath.[14]

In a prospective cohort of 150 patients undergoing brachial access for mesenteric or peripheral interventions, the rate of major complications was 2.7%, which included thrombotic occlusion of the access vessel in three cases and a subaponeurotic hematoma in one case, all of which required reoperation. Minor complications occurred at a rate of 14.0%, including 15 local hematomas not requiring intervention and six pseudoaneurysms treated with ultrasound-guided compression. The large majority of these interventions were conducted via a 6-French sheath (74.7%), with fewer via a 5-French (16.7%), a 4-French (3.3%), a 7-French (4%), or even an 8-French sheath (1.3%). The overall rate of successful access was 96.7%.[15]

In a retrospective review of 201 brachial access cases for iliac interventions, 25 had an access site complication. Nine had hematomas, with one requiring a transfusion. Eight had a pseudoaneurysm, six of which required surgical revision. Four had ongoing bleeding, and two had brachial artery thrombosis, all of which required surgical revision. No neurologic injury was reported. Similarly, most of these interventions were performed through a 6-French sheath (55%), followed by a 5-French sheath (29%), with few through a 4-French (14%) or a 7-French sheath (2%). The primary technical success rate was 81% via brachial access. An additional 11% required adjunctive femoral access to achieve success. Eight percent were unable to achieve technical success at all.[16]

In a slightly larger series, retrospective review of 323 brachial access cases from both peripheral and aortic cases revealed a 6.5% complication rate. Ninety-one percent were accessed percutaneously, while 9% were primarily achieved by open cut down, and there was no difference in complications between manual pressure or surgical repair for hemostasis. Pseudoaneurysm was the most common complication, occurring in eleven cases, five of which required surgical repair. Brachial artery thrombosis was the next most common, occurring in seven patients, all of which were women. None had neurological injury or tissue loss from ischemia. Most of these procedures were carried out via a 4- or 5-French sheath (61%), followed next by a 6- or 7-French sheath (31%). Few (8%) required an 8-French or larger size sheath. About half (44%) were short sheaths versus long sheaths.[17]

In the largest review of brachial access complications to date, from the Vascular Quality Initiative database from 2010 to 2014, there were 732 brachial artery only access cases for peripheral interventions. Compared to the 43,902 femoral artery only access cases from this same period, brachial cases were more likely to utilize protamine reversal, to be done under image guidance, and utilize a 5-French or smaller sheath. The brachial access cases had a higher overall complication rate of 9.0% versus 3.3% for femoral access cases. This bore out amongst individual types of complications, including hematomas (7.2% versus 3.0%) and access site stenosis or thrombosis (2.1% versus 0.4%). These complications were also more likely to require hospital admission. Most procedures (80.9%) utilized a sheath larger than 5 French.[18]

While reported rates of complications are variable, it is generally accepted that with appropriate precautions and vigilance, the brachial artery remains a viable and useful approach for endovascular procedures.

Repeat Brachial Access for Endovascular Procedures Appears Safe

Despite these reports of complications, among experienced practitioners repeat brachial access. In a series of 1326 angiograms via brachial artery access over 10 years, 111 had recurrent brachial access procedures, ranging from two to seven procedures per individual, and no complications were reported. For all comers in this series, the rate of all complications was low at only 1.28%.[19] The brachial artery, with appropriate precautions and experience, appears to be a safe site for access even for repeat procedures.

RISK FACTORS FOR COMPLICATIONS FROM UPPER EXTREMITY ARTERIAL ACCESS

Risk factors for complications have been suggested but the evidence remains conflicted. For radial artery lines for hemodynamic monitoring, a large retrospective review of 57,787 patients revealed that while female gender and preprocedure use of clopidogrel trended toward having increased rates of complications, no patient factors correlated with a statistically significant increase in complications. The only significant factor was the size of the arterial catheter, with the smallest 20-gauge catheter having the lowest rate of complications as compared with the larger catheters.[12]

For endovascular therapies conducted via brachial artery access, female gender is the most commonly cited risk factor for complications. In 111 cases of recurrent brachial access, complications were more common in women, including thrombosis (1.24% for women versus 0.28% for men) and failed access (2.1% versus 0).[19] The largest review of risk factors is from a review of the Vascular Quality Initiative data for 732 brachial access cases conducted from 2010 to 2014. In this study, univariate analysis demonstrated that age, BMI, female gender, and diabetes correlated with an increased risk of complications. In multivariate analysis, male gender and arterial cut down were protective factors, while sheath sizes larger than 5 French carried an increased risk of complications.[18]

Sheath size emerges as a risk factor in some studies, but not all. In a smaller series of 323 brachial access cases for peripheral and adjunctive aortic therapies at a single institution, longer but not larger sheath size correlated with an increased risk of complications.[17] In 201 brachial access cases for iliac interventions, female gender also did correlate with an increased risk of complications, particularly for pseudoaneurysm formation, but age, target lesion complexity, and sheath size did not.[16] Similarly, in a prospective cohort of 150 patients undergoing brachial access for mesenteric or peripheral interventions, there was no correlation between sheath size and complications.[15]

When compared with axillary access, the brachial artery appears to be a safer choice. Retrospective review of 266 cases of angiography or angioplasty in patients not eligible for femoral access compared brachial versus axillary artery access. Of 140 patients undergoing brachial artery access, five patients had a complication including two hematomas, one pseudoaneurysm, one arterial thrombosis, and one median nerve injury. Of the 126 axillary artery access cases, 13 patients had complications including six hematomas, one pseudoaneurysm, one arterial thrombosis, one venous thrombosis, and four ulnar or median nerve injuries. The overall complication rate for axillary artery access was significantly increased as compared with brachial artery access.[20]

In pediatric patients, risk factors for arterial obstruction are similar to those described for adults. In addition to the duration of cannulation, age is also a risk factor. In a cohort of 47 children undergoing radial artery cannulation for hemodynamic monitoring, 66% of children less than five years of age developed occlusion versus 34.1% of children 6 and older. Furthermore, cut down for access also correlated with an increased risk of arterial obstruction in children, with 71.4% of cut down cases resulting in obstruction as compared with 43.6% of percutaneous cases. None of these occlusions were clinically significant.[21]

Many additional widely accepted risk factors for radial artery cannulation induced hand ischemia can be gleaned from the medical history, including prior surgeries in the upper extremity, prior upper extremity trauma, congenital anomalies, peripheral vascular disease, diabetes, collagen vascular disorders, blood dyscrasias, active upper extremity infection, as well as current use of certain medications, especially vasopressors.[22] Therefore, while radial artery cannulation is safe and effective in most, patients with severe occlusive disease, particularly intrinsic hand disease and those with other acquired anatomic vascular abnormalities are likely at increased risk for complications and treated with caution.

STRATEGIES FOR PREVENTION OF COMPLICATIONS FROM UPPER EXTREMITY ARTERIAL ACCESS

Several factors have been suggested to help minimize the risk of access related complications in upper extremity arterial access. While often a firm tenet in the teaching of obtaining radial access, no high quality study has been performed to demonstrate that an Allen test prior to placement reduces ischemic hand complications.[23] A meta-analysis pooling studies that defined what constitutes an abnormal Allen test as well as correlations with outcomes demonstrated, there is wide variability in this definition and that an abnormal finding prior to radial artery cannulation did not correlate with hand ischemia. These authors conclude that an Allen test should not be considered the standard of care prior to radial artery cannulation in standard risk patients.[24]

A randomized trial comparing radial artery cannulation via ultrasound guidance versus by palpation in 60 patients demonstrated shorter time to successful cannulation with fewer cannulation attempts and fewer anatomical sites utilized. In fact, 37% of patients randomized to palpation had to cross over to ultrasound guidance in order to achieve successful cannulation. This did result in a lower incidence of hematoma, but no demonstrable effect on other types of complications was reported.[25]

In a meta-analysis, the optimal wrist angle for radial artery cannulation was determined from pooled data from five studies assessing 500 patients combined. A 45° angle was found to have the fastest cannulation time with the highest success rate, with a moderate degree of evidence limited by the heterogeneity of the angles used and the large proportion of young healthy volunteers assessed in the included studies. Of note, no reduction in complications could be reported with any angle in this meta-analysis.[26]

The PROPHET-II randomized controlled trial compared maintaining radial artery flow during hemostasis postradial artery access for coronary angiography via ipsilateral ulnar artery compression. In the 3000 randomized patients, treatment with ipsilateral ulnar artery compression significantly reduced the primary endpoint of 30-day radial artery occlusion (0.9% versus 3.0%, $P = 0.0001$) without compromising hemostasis. Risk factors for radial artery occlusion included female gender, diabetes, older age, and pain during compression.[27] This was described as a routine technique, in conjunction with a single dose of heparin, as an alternative for four weeks of low molecular weight heparin in order to restore flow in occluded radial arteries after transradial access for iliofemoral endovascular procedures.[6]

TREATMENT STRATEGIES

The most feared complication of upper extremity arterial access is ischemia, given the high morbidity with loss of upper extremity function. Once ischemia does occur from upper extremity arterial access, diagnosis and treatment must be prompt. Assessment for the precise location and extent of occlusion can be performed with duplex ultrasonography or with angiography. Active ischemia from radial artery injury secondary to cannulation necessitates revascularization. Invasive interventions include catheter-directed thrombolysis, thromboembolectomy or bypass revascularization. Noninvasive interventions include therapeutic anticoagulation, sympathetic block, warming of the affected extremity, limiting or eliminating medications that promote vasoconstriction (e.g., vasopressors), and immobilization of the affected area.[22]

Invasive therapies for ischemia can be minimally invasive or surgical. The mainstay of minimally invasive therapy is catheter-directed thrombolytic therapy. Focal thrombus may be best treated with a surgical thromboembolectomy. A limitation, particularly in the distal upper extremity, is that the smaller caliber arteries may not permit passage of the embolectomy catheters. In the event of severe arterial damage to the larger arteries, surgical reconstruction may be necessary in order to achieve revascularization. However, in well-selected patients, good results have been reported with thrombolysis for treating upper extremity ischemia secondary to arterial access.

Thrombolytic therapy is most effective in acute rather than chronic hand ischemia. Angiographic improvement has been reported to occur nearly 80% of the time. Amputations are rare, occurring less than 10% of the time, and typically only affecting the digital level.[28] Digital amputations have long-term sequelae for hand function, as well as having significant psychosocial ramifications. The thumb, in particular, is essential for the prehensile function of the hand, and is particularly vulnerable from radial artery ischemia.[29] The hand is a critical part of daily life and social interactions, and the psychological burden on amputees of their perceived disfigurement is significant, with much work ongoing to devise cosmetic prostheses for psychologic rehabilitation.[30]

With chronic ischemia of more than a couple weeks' duration, the rate of success is less favorable with little to no recanalization. Embolic phenomena similarly are composed of mature thrombus and less amenable to thrombolysis. Thrombolysis has also proven effective in treating distal embolization form hypothenar hammer syndrome, followed by arterial reconstruction.[28] Thrombolysis has even been used to treat hand ischemia after unintentional intra-arterial injections. In a case series of five patients, all had significant improvement in clinical symptoms, supported by improvement in digital pressures. One did progress to have necrosis of distal phalanges two to four of the affected hand, and another developed septic arthritis.[31]

Multihole microcatheters may be superior to small bore conventional diagnostic catheters for thrombolysis. In a series of three patients treated for acute hand ischemia secondary to intra-arterial injection (one) and trauma (two), thrombolysis resulted in the remission of acute symptoms in all. The two patients treated via a multihole microcatheter had superior angiographic results, while the patient treated with small bore diagnostic catheter had partial recanalization with evidence of distal spasm.[32]

For nonischemic injuries from upper extremity arterial access, including hematoma, infection and pseudoaneurysm, treatment modalities are varied. The most worrisome hematoma is that which occurs after brachial access as the brachial sheath has limited space. The hematoma quickly compresses the median nerve which can lead to permanent neurologic damage. Very small asymptomatic hematomas either after brachial or radial or ulnar access may be observed and will regress spontaneously over time. Symptomatic or expanding hematomas also require surgical washout, occasionally with arterial repair. These must be recognized and treated promptly particularly in the case of brachial sheath hematomas. Superficial infections may be treated with antibiotics alone. Deep infections and infected hematomas require surgical washout in addition to antibiotics. Fortunately, infected indwelling arterial lines are rare, with clinically insignificant line colonization being the most common finding.[12,13]

The optimal therapy for radial artery pseudoaneurysm at present is generally extrapolated from femoral artery pseudoaneurysm treatment. Pseudoaneurysm from arterial instrumentation appears to be relatively rare at a rate of 0.009% of all radial artery catheterizations. Retrospective review over a five-year period at three urban academic hospitals revealed eleven cases of catheter associated radial artery pseudoaneurysms. Five resulted from arterial line monitoring and six from cardiac catheterization. None of the three treated with ultrasound guided compression were successful. Of the four treated nonsurgically, three had patent radial arteries upon resolution. Seven were treated surgically for either symptoms or for a maximal diameter greater than 3 cm. Operative repair was comprised of pseudoaneurysm debridement or excision with reapproximation of the traumatic arteriotomy with simple stitches. One was coiled endovascularly. Five had complications, including median nerve numbness, digital ischemia (in the setting of vasopressor support and active malignancy), reoperation for wound breakdown or hematoma, and renal failure. No radial artery pseudoaneurysms ruptured in this series.[33]

One additional complication of radial artery access is asymptomatic occlusion. This is primarily a concern for future access or interventions, as it prevents utilization of that access site and increases the risk of future ischemia if recanalization does not occur. It is common practice to observe and not treat this complication. However, many occluded radial arteries will not recanalize of their own accord. In 488 consecutive catheterizations via the radial artery at a single institution, 51 (10.5%) demonstrated complete or partial radial artery occlusion one day postprocedure. Twenty patients had no symptoms. Thirty had symptoms and were treated with low molecular weight heparin, either prophylactically dosed if in conjunction with dual antiplatelet therapy, or therapeutically dosed if combined with single antiplatelet therapy. After four weeks, the patients receiving low molecular weight heparin had a higher rate of recanalization (86.7%) versus those receiving no therapy (19.1%, $P < 0.0001$).[34]

SUMMARY

Upper extremity arterial access is becoming increasingly common for endovascular procedures, in addition to its already relatively routine use in hemodynamic monitoring. Reported complications vary widely in frequency, but most commonly include minor complications such as small hematomas and ecchymosis. Risk factors for more serious complications include female gender for the brachial artery and possibly sheath size, with some studies supporting and others refuting this. Treatments for upper extremity ischemic complications frequently involve interventions including thrombolysis, particularly for small vessel territory ischemia, as well as thromboembolectomy and arterial reconstruction for larger vessels. Nonischemic complications such as hematoma and pseudoaneurysm formation also require surgical intervention with some frequency.

REFERENCES

1. Mandel M, Dauchot P. Radial artery cannulation in 1,000 patients: precautions and complications. *J Hand Surg*. 1977;2(6):482–485.
2. Jolly SS, Yusuf S, Cairns J, et al. Radial versus femoral access for coronary angiography and intervention in patients with acute coronary syndromes (RIVAL): a randomised, parallel group, multicentre trial. *Lancet*. 2011;377(9775):1409–1420.
3. Ruzsa Z, Tóth K, Nemes B, et al. Transradial and transulnar access for iliac artery interventions using sheathless guiding systems: a feasibility study. *Catheter Cardiovasc Interv*. 2016;88(6):923–931.
4. Kumar AJ, Jones LE, Kollmeyer KR, et al. Radial artery access for peripheral endovascular procedures. *J Vasc Surg*. 2017;66:820–825. doi:10.1016/j.jvs.2017.03.430.
5. Touma J, Coscas R, Ijaverliat I, et al. Radial access for endovascular ilio-femoral procedures. *J Cardiovasc Surg*. 2016;57(2):302–310.
6. Frezza EE, Mezghebe H. Indications and complications of arterial catheter use in surgical or medical intensive care units: analysis of 4932 patients. *Am Surg*. 1998;64(2):127.
7. Scheer BV, Perel A, Pfeiffer UJ. Clinical review: complications and risk factors of peripheral arterial catheters used for haemodynamic monitoring in anaesthesia and intensive care medicine. *Critical Care*. 2002;6(3):199.
8. Strauch B YH, Chen ZW, Liebling R. *Atlas of Microvascular Surgery: Anatomy and Operative Approaches*. New York, NY: Thieme Medical Publishers; 1993.
9. Rhyne D, Mann T. Hand ischemia resulting from a transradial intervention: successful management with radial artery angioplasty. *Catheter Cardiovasc Interv*. 2010;76(3):383–386.
10. Goswami R, Oliphant CS, Youssef H, Morsy M, Khouzam RN. Radial artery occlusion after cardiac catheterization: significance, risk factors, and management. *Curr Probl Cardiol*. 2016;41(6):214–227.

11. Valentine RJ, Modrall JG, Clagett GP. Hand ischemia after radial artery cannulation. *J Am Coll Surg*. 2005;201(1):18–22.
12. Nuttall G, Burckhardt J, Hadley A, et al. Surgical and patient risk factors for severe arterial line complications in adults. *Anesthesiology*. 2016;124(3):590–597.
13. Gardner RM, Schwartz R, Wong HC, Burke JP. Percutaneous indwelling radial-artery catheters for monitoring cardiovascular function: prospective study of the risk of thrombosis and infection. *N Engl J Med*. 1974;290(22):1227–1231.
14. Nasr B, Albert B, David CH, et al. Endovascular treatment of atherosclerotic iliac stenosis: local and systemic complications of the open brachial access. *Ann Vasc Surg*. 2016;33:45–54.
15. Treitl KM, Konig C, Reiser MF, Treitl M. Complications of transbrachial arterial access for peripheral endovascular interventions. *J Endovasc Ther*. 2015;22(1):63–70.
16. Stavroulakis K, Usai MV, Torsello G, et al. Efficacy and safety of transbrachial access for iliac endovascular interventions. *J Endovasc Ther*. 2016;23(3):454–460.
17. Alvarez-Tostado JA, Moise MA, Bena JF, et al. The brachial artery: a critical access for endovascular procedures. *J Vasc Surg*. 2009;49(2):378–385.
18. Kret MR, Dalman RL, Kalish J, Mell M. Arterial cutdown reduces complications after brachial access for peripheral vascular intervention. *J Vasc Surg*. 2016;64(1):149–154.
19. Armstrong PJ, Han DC, Baxter JA, Elmore JR, Franklin DP. Complication rates of percutaneous brachial artery access in peripheral vascular angiography. *Ann Vasc Surg*. 2003;17(1):107–110.
20. Tong Z, Gu Y, Guo L, et al. An analysis of complications of brachial and axillary artery punctures. *Am Surg*. 2016;82(12):1250–1256.
21. Miyasaka K, Edmonds J, Conn A. Complications of radial artery lines in the paediatric patient. *Can J Anesth/J can d'anesth*. 1976;23(1):9–14.
22. Wallach SG. Cannulation injury of the radial artery: diagnosis and treatment algorithm. *Am J Crit Care*. 2004;13(4):315–319.
23. Biondi-Zoccai G, Moretti C, Zuffi A, et al. Transradial access without preliminary Allen test—letter of comment on Rhyne et al. *Catheter Cardiovasc Interv*. 2011;78(4):662–663; author reply 664.
24. Barone JE, Madlinger RV. Should an Allen test be performed before radial artery cannulation? *J Trauma*. 2006;61(2):468–470.
25. Shiver S, Blaivas M, Lyon M. A prospective comparison of ultrasound guided and blindly placed radial arterial catheters. *Acad Emerg Med*. 2006;13(12):1275–1279.
26. Melhuish TM, White LD. Optimal wrist positioning for radial arterial cannulation in adults: a systematic review and meta-analysis. *Am J Emerg Med*. 2016;34(12):2372–2378.
27. Pancholy SB, Bernat I, Bertrand OF, Patel TM. Prevention of radial artery occlusion after transradial catheterization: the PROPHET-II randomized trial. *JACC: Cardiovas Interv*. 2016;9(19):1992–1999.
28. De Martino RR, Moran SL. The role of thrombolytics in acute and chronic occlusion of the hand. *Hand Clin*. 2015;31(1):13–21.
29. Emerson ETK, TJ, Greenwald DP. Anatomy, physiology, and functional restoration of the thumb. *Ann Plast Surg*. 1996;36:180–191.
30. Pereira BP, Kour AK, Leow E, Pho RWH. Benefits and use of digital prostheses. *J Hand Surg*. 1996;21(2):222–228.
31. Breguet R, Terraz S, Righini M, Didier D. Acute hand ischemia after unintentional intraarterial injection of drugs: is catheter-directed thrombolysis useful? *J Vasc Interv Radiol*. 2014;25(6):963–968.
32. Barbiero G, Cognolato D, Casarin A, Guarise A. Intra-arterial thrombolysis of acute hand ischaemia with or without microcatheter: preliminary experience and comparison with the literature. *Radiol Med*. 2011;116(6):919–931.
33. Tosti R, Özkan S, Schainfeld RM, Eberlin KR. Radial artery pseudoaneurysm. *J Hand Surg*. 2017;42(4):295.e291–295.e296.
34. Zankl A, Andrassy M, Volz C, et al. Radial artery thrombosis following transradial coronary angiography: incidence and rationale for treatment of symptomatic patients with low-molecular-weight heparins. *Clin Res Cardiol*. 2010;99(12):841–847.

22

Neurogenic and Vascular Quadrilateral Space Syndromes: A New Classification and Management

Arjun Jayaraj, MD and Peter Gloviczki, MD

The quadrilateral space (QS) is an area bound medially by the long head of triceps, laterally by the surgical neck of the humerus, inferiorly by the tendon of the teres major muscle, and superiorly by the teres minor muscle. Important structures crossing the QS include the axillary nerve and the posterior circumflex humeral artery (PCHA). Compression or repetitive trauma to these structures may result in neurogenic or vascular quadrilateral space syndrome (QSS). The term QSS was coined by Bernard Cahill in 1980 when he first reported the condition.[1] Cahill and Palmer published their experience as a case series, recounting the involvement of the axillary nerve in eighteen operated patients.[2] The QSS was originally described as a constellation of symptoms and signs that arise from repetitive trauma leading to fibrous tissue entrapment of the axillary nerve as it traverses the quadrilateral space. The syndrome has been primarily reported in individuals engaged in activity involving repetitive abduction and external rotation of the arm including volleyball, baseball and swimming. Multiple case reports and small series of the syndrome have been published since.[3-7] The importance of compression and injury to the PHCA was first recognized by the Northwestern group and first reported by McCarthy et al, in 1989[8] and later by Durham et al in 1995.[9] Other publications on athletes who presented with acute upper extremity ischemia due to axillary artery thrombosis or embolism due to involvement of the PCHA have also been reported.[10-21] While the etiology for arterial involvement is similar to the neurogenic involvement - repetitive trauma, the pathogenesis is different as noted below. In a recent publication that included nine patients, we have endeavored to combine the arterial and neurogenic types into a single entity: QSS with arterial and neurogenic forms to reflect common etiology.[22] This chapter describes the two forms of the syndrome in the process laying out the case for a unified classification.

ETIOLOGY

The etiology responsible for arterial and neurogenic forms of the syndrome is similar – repetitive trauma that occurs during abduction and external rotation (AER) of the affected arm. In the arterial form, such trauma to the posterior humeral circumflex artery may lead to intimal or medial injury. In the neurogenic form, entrapment of the axillary nerve occurs due to fibrous bands. Space occupying lesions that compress the nerve and subject it to repetitive trauma during AER can also cause similar symptom complex and is included in the etiology. Such lesions include hypertrophy of the muscular boundaries, atypical course of the axillary nerve, bone spikes, or space-occupying lesions, such as glenoid labral cysts, paralabral cysts, ganglia, fracture hematoma, and humeral osteochondroma.[2, 23-29] Demographically, there is a preponderance of quadrilateral space syndrome as a whole in men, particularly in competitive athletes. The syndrome has been frequently observed in volleyball players, in overhead or "throwing" athletes, in baseball players and swimmers.[22] The neurogenic form appears to be more prevalent than its vascular counterpart.[22]

PATHOGENESIS

In vascular QSS, the repetitive mechanical stress that occurs on the PHCA during repetitive abduction and external rotation leads to intimal injury and wall weakness. Additional stretching of the vessel that occurs as it traverses the tight QS leads to turbulent flow and shear stress, intimal and medial injury, arterial dissection and pseudoaneurysm formation with subsequent thrombosis and thromboembolism to the arm and hand. In some patients, intimal hyperplasia may also lead stenosis and post stenotic dilation or frank aneurysm formation of the PCHA. These aneurysmal changes eventually lead to thrombus development (Figure 22-1). Such thrombus is then squeezed retrograde back into the axillary artery during AER and results in embolism to the arteries of the arm and hand.

Fibrous bands that represent the primary etiology of the neurogenic form of the syndrome are typically located between the teres major muscle and the long head of the triceps.[30] External rotation at the shoulder reduces the cross-sectional area of the QS, in the process concentrating overt or occult repetitive microtrauma to connective tissue in the QS leading to fibrous band/scar tissue formation. Chronic fixed nerve compression permanently displaces internal nerve contents in transverse and longitudinal dimensions, leading to long-term damage of axons and myelin.[31-32] The stretch trauma that causes the vascular QSS does not appear to cause axillary nerve injury per se since the nerve can tolerate such excursions.

CLINICAL FEATURES

Clinical signs of vascular QSS arise from thrombosis of the PCHA and in a retrograde fashion, the axillary artery, leading to micro or macroembolism to the arm and hand arteries. Symptoms include cold intolerance, coolness, pallor, and cyanosis of the upper extremity and digit(s), although severe limb and hand threatening

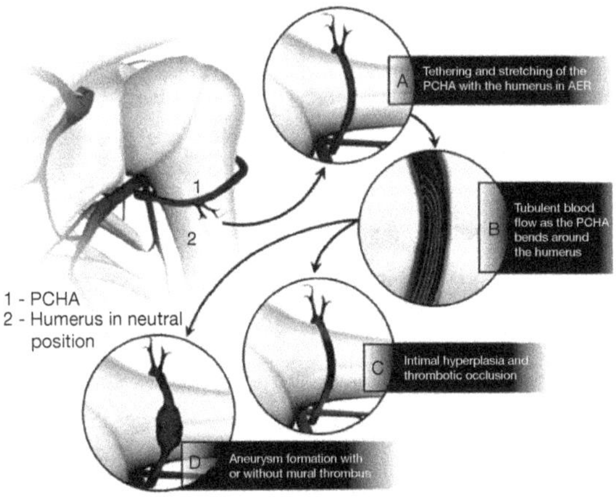

Figure 22-1. Possible mechanism for PCHA aneurysmal degeneration and thrombosis (From Brown et al.[22]; reprinted with permission from the Mayo Foundation).
AER — Abduction and External Rotation; PCHA — Posterior Circumflex Humeral Artery
A - The posterior humeral circumflex artery stretches around the neck of the humerus leading to intimal injury and weakening of the vessel wall
B - The repetitive pulley movement likely leads to turbulent blood flow within the "bend" of the PCHA around the humeral neck
C - Vessel injury from these changes leads to intimal hyperplasia
D - Aneurysmal degeneration sets in with subsequent thrombus development over time

acute ischemia can also develop. Differential diagnosis for Vascular QSS can mimic other neurovascular disorders that involve thrombosis or aneurysm formation in other more proximal branches of the axillary artery or involvement of the subclavian artery due to arterial thoracic outlet syndrome (TOS). Additionally conditions that involve repetitive arterial trauma also constitute differential diagnosis including hypothenar hammer hand syndrome where the ulnar artery is injured by repeated impact against the hamate bone at the wrist. Both these conditions can cause intimal damage, aneurysm formation, thrombotic occlusion, and distal embolization of thrombus with ischemia of the hand. Other causes of ischemic fingers such as emboli from the heart, scleroderma, vasculitis, atherosclerosis, and thromboangiitis obliterans should also be considered as part of the differential diagnosis.

Neurogenic QSS patients present with paresthesia, poorly localized shoulder pain and/or tenderness over the anterior, lateral, or posterior shoulder, corresponding to deltoid and teres minor muscle fibers.[20,22,33] Radiating paresthesias to the arm and/or forearm in a non-dermatomal distribution can also be seen. Additionally, fasciculation of the long head of the triceps has also been identified.[7] Differential diagnosis for nQSS includes C5 and/or C6 radiculopathy, suprascapular nerve entrapment, complex regional pain syndrome and overt shoulder trauma.

DIAGNOSIS

Patients presenting with clinical features suggestive of vascular QSS should undergo an arterial duplex of the upper extremity to evaluate inflow in neutral position and in abduction - external rotation. Compression of the PHCA during AER can occur in normal individuals. In fact, in two separate studies 16% and 80% of asymptomatic volunteers exhibited PCHA stenosis during AER on ultrasound and magnetic resonance angiogram (MRA) respectively.[35,36] Following duplex exam, computerized tomographic arteriogram (CTA) or direct contrast arteriogram following selective catheterization of the subclavian artery can be done to delineate the anatomy in normal and in AER positions. Catheter arteriogram can be followed by catheter directed thrombolysis if needed. High index of suspicion and imaging the PHCA during arteriogram usually reveals the diagnosis of QSS.

For neurologic QSS, in symptomatic patient's initial work up includes shoulder x-ray to evaluate for trauma related pathology. Magnetic Resonance Imaging (MRI) of the affected shoulder will help identify Teres Minor injury/atrophy in addition to any space occupying lesion. EMG helps characterize the nature of the injury including reduced amplitude motor changes of the axillary nerve and decreased recruitment in both the deltoid and teres minor muscle. Confirmation can be obtained by arteriogram of the affected extremity that demonstrates compression of the posterior humeral circumflex humeral artery with abduction and external rotation. Symptom relief obtained from local anesthetic injection of the teres minor muscle helps to confirm the diagnosis and predicts potential relief from surgery.[22,37]

TREATMENT

For patients who present with acute upper extremity ischemia due to arterial QSS, catheter directed thrombolysis should be considered up to 14 days from onset of symptoms. Treatment of subacute or chronic thrombosis or thromboembolism can be attempted using percutaneous or surgical thromboembolectomy, but the results are less predictable. Definitive treatment requires proximal and distal ligation of the PHCA to prevent recurrent thrombosis and thromboembolism. Any associated injury to the axillary artery must be repaired, usually with vein patch or interposition vein graft to avoid recurrence. Endovascular exclusion of the aneurysmal PCHA using coils has also been described.[17,18] Postoperative anticoagulation is recommended for a period of at least 3 months.

Once diagnosis of Neurogenic QSS is confirmed, treatment involves use of anti-inflammatory agents, physical therapy and when not responsive surgical decompression. The latter involves neurolysis, excision of fibrous bands and removal of any space occupying lesion if found.

The following are two case reports previously published documenting our experience with both forms of QSS.[22]

Case report (vascular QSS)

A 20-year-old female volleyball player presented with a 2-week history of purplish discoloration, coolness, pain and severe paresthesias involving multiple digits of her dominant right hand. Her past medical history was unremarkable and she was a non-smoker without any known personal or family history of thrombophilia. Physical exam revealed a pale, cool right hand with splinter hemorrhages and non-palpable radial and ulnar pulses. Doppler arterial signals at the wrist were weak and monophasic. There was no sensory loss above the wrist and she had no motor loss.

CTA revealed multi-segment occlusion of the right ulnar and common interosseous arteries with distal reconstitution. Additionally, a long-segment occlusion of the right radial artery was also present. No evidence of alternate pathology including thoracic outlet arterial compression or a more proximal embolic source was identified. She was promptly placed on therapeutic heparin drip and was taken to the operating room for a percutaneous right transfemoral arch aortogram with right upper extremity runoff (Figures 22-2 and 22-3). The latter confirmed the CTA findings in addition to revealing a thrombosed PCHA. Cather directed thrombolysis was pursued and continued for 48 hours. She continued to have significant hand ischemia and surgical exploration was pursued. Exposure of the distal axillary artery revealed aneurysmal degeneration of the PHCA with fresh thrombus. Thrombectomy was carried out and the PCHA ligated. Additionally, embolectomy of the radial, ulnar, and interosseous arteries was performed. She had an uneventful recovery, but at 3 months required patch angioplasty of the right common femoral artery during which time intimal injury to the site of femoral access for prior arteriogram was successfully repaired. By 6 months, she had returned to volleyball training and at 2 years she is asymptomatic and playing volleyball regularly.

Case Report (Neurogenic QSS)

A twenty seven year old male sailor presented with a 6-month history of position-dependent shoulder pain and upper arm twitching in the dominant right upper extremity. Lifting the arm overhead and complete flexion of the arm above the shoulder brought on his symptoms. Prior history of trauma was present that had occurred during fly dumbbell weight-lifting exercises. On exam there was no atrophy of the shoulder muscles, but tenderness on palpation in the right posterior shoulder and decreased strength with shoulder abduction was present.

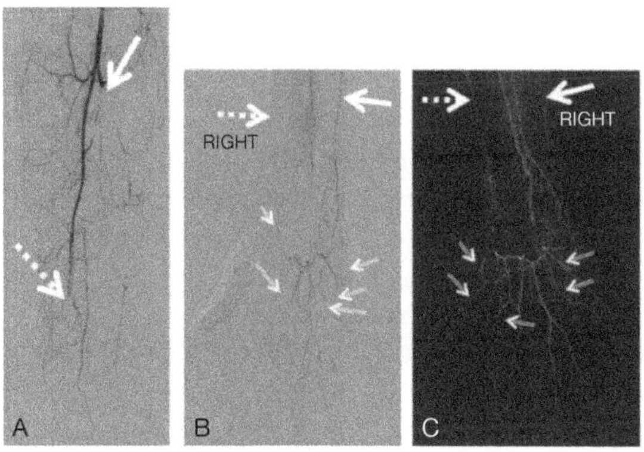

Figure 22-2. Angiography of the right hand for case report - vascular QSS (From Brown et al.[22]; reprinted with permission from the Mayo Foundation).

A – Initial angiogram of the right forearm demonstrates occlusion of the proximal ulnar artery (solid arrow) and proximal interosseous arteries with distal reconstitution. The radial artery occlusion (dashed arrow) begins in the mid forearm.

B – Initial angiogram of right hand demonstrates poor/absent contrast filling of the ulnar (solid arrow) and radial (dashed arrow) arteries, as well as common digital arteries (smaller double arrows) due to embolization.

C – Post embolectomy angiogram demonstrates overall improved flow into the hand with partial revascularization of the ulnar (solid arrow) and radial (dashed arrow) arteries, as well as digital arteries (smaller double arrows).

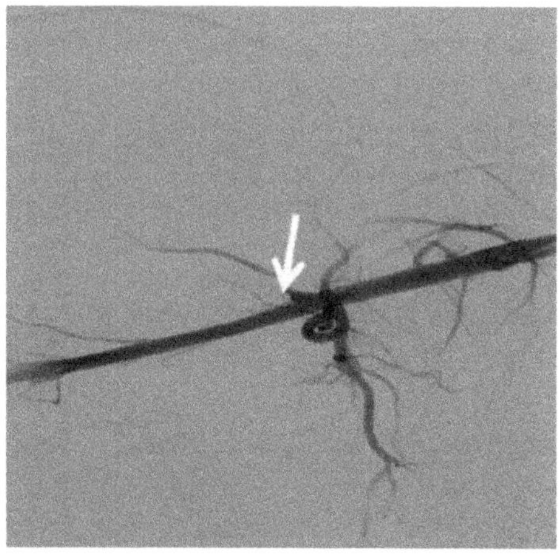

Figure 22-3. Angiography of the axillary artery for case report—vascular QSS.

Angiography of the right shoulder showing abrupt occlusion of the posterior circumflex humeral artery caused by thrombus burden in the aneurysmal artery. (From Brown et al.[22]; reprinted with permission from the Mayo Foundation.)

Magnetic resonance imaging (MRI) of the right shoulder was unrevealing of pathology including space occupying lesions of the QS. Electromyography of the right upper extremity revealed old denervation to the right posterior deltoid. Right upper extremity arteriogram revealed dynamic PCHA occlusion during abduction of the shoulder. Ultrasound-guided local anesthetic injection of the QS relieved symptoms. Secondary to his symptoms and relief obtained with local anesthetic injection, operative intervention was pursued. Abundant scar tissue was noted to entrap the axillary nerve on exploration of the QS. Neurolysis was carried out and he patient went on to recover and at 12 months post-intervention he had returned to full activity with complete resolution of symptoms.

DISCUSSION

Quadrilateral space syndrome is a clinical condition-affecting individuals, usually competitive athletes, who are engaged in repetitive abduction and external rotation of the upper extremity leading to trauma to PHCA or the axillary nerve in the QS. The etiology of the injury to the PHCA and the axillary nerve are similar in that they both pass through the QS and that the injury arises from repetitive trauma. In this regard we have used the nomenclature of arterial and neurogenic quadrilateral space syndrome. However the actual pathophysiology leading to clinical manifestations is different. In arterial QSS the PHCA is injured, it becomes aneurysmal or develops intimal injury, both leading to a nidus for thrombus development. Retrograde extension of the thrombus into the axillary artery leads to embolism to arteries of the arm and hand. In neurogenic QSS the axillary nerve is compressed and injured due to entrapment caused by fibrous bands or other space occupying lesions. Since both vascular and neurogenic forms are rare, a high degree of suspicion is required to establish the diagnosis in individuals engaged in activities involving repetitive abduction and external rotation of the upper extremity. Such suspicion will enable early diagnosis and treatment and thereby preservation of the full function of the affected limb. An algorithm for such assessment is provided in Table 22-1. Additionally, a demographic breakdown of the experience from the Mayo Clinic (REF) and review of literature published is recounted in Table 22-2. With early diagnosis and prompt intervention or surgical treatment, patients with both arterial and neurogenic QSS can expect to recover and return to full activity, including competitive sports.

CONCLUSION

Quadrilateral space syndrome is a rare condition afflicting individuals, usually athletes, engaged in repetitive activity that involves abduction and external rotation of the upper extremity. Both vascular and neurologic forms of the disease exist and must be considered as having a common etiology but different pathophysiology. To establish the diagnosis of QSS a high index of suspicion and exclusion of other pathologies is needed. Early diagnosis and prompt treatment will frequently result in full functional recovery.

TABLE 22-1. WORK-UP AND TREATMENT ALGORITHM OF PATIENT WITH QUADRILATERAL SPACE SYNDROME[a]

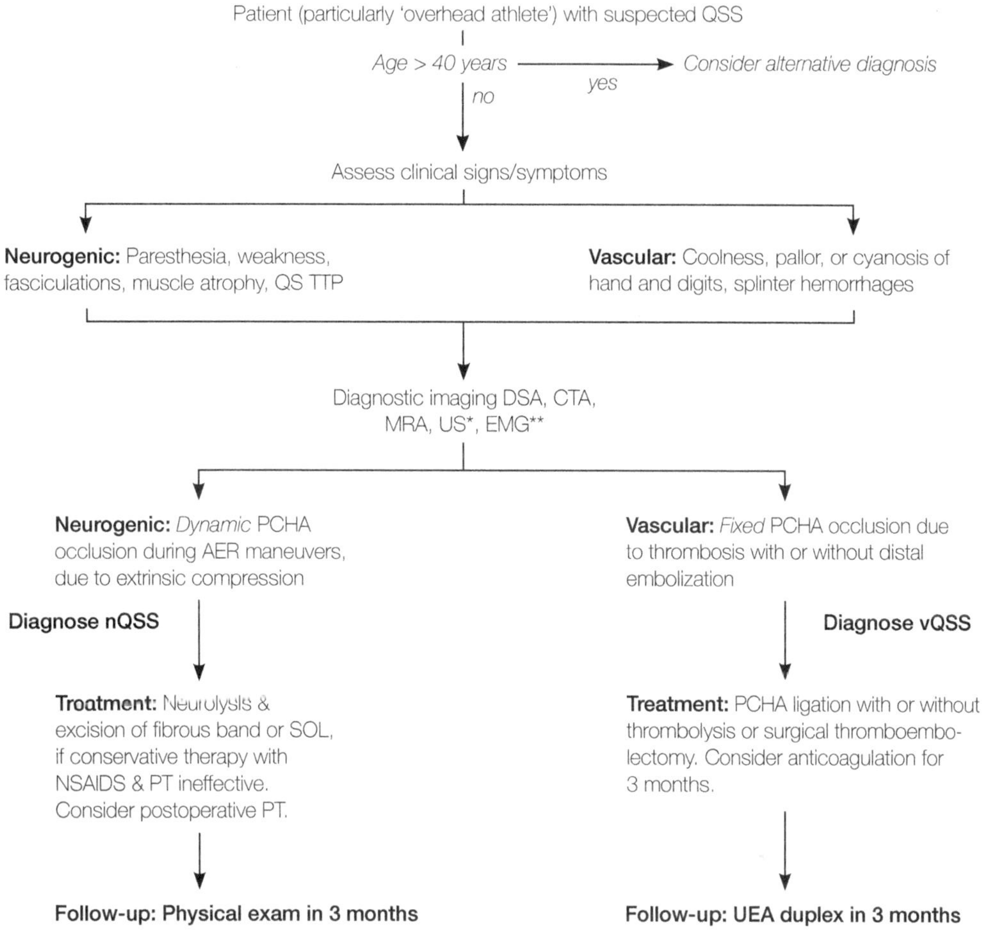

[a]From Brown et al.[22]; reprinted with permission from the Mayo Foundation.

Abbreviations: QS TTP, tenderness to palpitation QSS, Quadrilateral Space Syndrome; QS, Quadrilateral Space; DSA, Digital Subtraction Angiography; CTA, Computerized Tomographic Angiogram; MRA, Magnetic Resonance Angiogram; US, Duplex Ultrasound; EMG, Electromyography; PHCA, Posterior Humeral Circumflex Artery; nQSS, neurogenic QSS; vQSS, vascular QSS; SOL, Space Occupying Lesion; NSAIDS, Non-Steroidal Anti-inflammatory agents; PT, Physical Therapy; UEA, Upper Extremity Arterial.

TABLE 22-2. DEMOGRAPHIC BREAKDOWN OF PUBLISHED LITERATURE ON QUADRILATERAL SPACE SYNDROME (NEUROGENIC and VASCULAR)[a]

Demographic characteristic	The Mayo experience (n=9)	Reviewed/previously published (n=76)
Year		
1980–1989	0 (0)	22 (29)
1990–1999	0 (0)	24 (32)
2000–2014	9 (100)	30 (39)
Neurogenic	6 (67)	46 (61)
Sex		
Female	6 (67)	6 (13)

(Continued)

TABLE 22-2. *(Continued)*

Demographic characteristic	The Mayo experience (n=9)	Reviewed/previously published (n=76)
Male	3 (33)	18 (39)
Unknown	0 (0)	22 (48)
Etiology		
Structural	6 (100)	44 (96)
Not reported	0 (0)	2 (4)[b]
Overhead athletes		
Baseball	0 (0)	2 (4)
Swimmer	0 (0)	1 (2)
Triathlete	0 (0)	1 (2)
Vascular	3 (33)	30 (39)
Sex		
Female	3 (100)	0
Male	0 (0)	26 (87)
Unknown	0 (0)	4 (13)
Etiology		
Mechanical	3 (100)	30 (100)
Overhead athletes[c]		
Volleyball	3 (100)	16 (53)
Baseball	0 (0)	12 (40)
Trapeze	0 (0)	1 (3)
Yoga	0 (0)	1 (3)

[a]represents Values are N (%)
[b]Two neurogenic case did not report surgical exploration to assess for structural causes.
[c]Overhead athletes = any patient engaged in elite, collegial, professional, or dedicated sport or activity involving repetitive abduction and external rotation of the arm above the head.
Source: From Brown et al.[22]; reprinted with permission from the Mayo Foundation.

REFERENCES

1. Cahill BR. Quadrilateral space syndrome. In: Omer GE Jr. Spinner M, eds. *Management of Peripheral Nerve Problems*. Philadelphia: WB Saunders; 1980:602-606.
2. Cahill BR, Palmer RE. Quadrilateral space syndrome. *J Hand Surg Am*. 1983;8(1):65-69.
3. Cormier PJ, Matalon TA, Wolin PM. Quadrilateral space syndrome: a rare cause of shoulder pain. *Radiology*. 1988;167:797–798.
4. Redler MR, Ruland LJ III, McCue FC III. Quadrilateral space syndrome in a throwing athlete. *Am J Sports Med*. 1986;14:511–513.
5. Chautems RC, Glauser T, Waeber-Fey MC, Rostan O, Barraud GE. Quadrilateral space syndrome: case report and review of the literature. *Ann Vasc Surg*. 2000;14:673–676.
6. Hoskins WT, Pollard HP, McDonald AJ. Quadrilateral space syndrome: a case study and review of the literature. *Br J Sports Med*. 2005;39:e9.
7. McClelland D, Hoy G. A case of quadrilateral space syndrome with involvement of the long head of the triceps. *Am J Sports Med*. 2008;36:1615–1617.

8. McCarthy WJ, Yao JS, Schafer MF, et al. Upper extremity arterial injury in athletes. *J Vasc Surg*. 1989;9:317–327.
9. Durham JR, Yao JS, Pearce WH, Nuber GM, McCarthy WJ 3rd. Arterial injuries in the thoracic outlet syndrome. *J Vasc Surg*. 1995 Jan;21(1):57-69.
10. van de Pol D, Kuijer PP, Langenhorst T, Maas M. High prevalence of self-reported symptoms of digital ischemia in elite male volleyball players in the Netherlands: a cross-sectional national survey. *Am J Sports Med*. 2012;40:2296–2302.
11. Vlychou M, Spanomichos G, Chatziioannou A, Georganas M, Zavras GM. Embolisation of a traumatic aneurysm of the posterior circumflex humeral artery in a volleyball player. *Br J Sports Med*. 2001;35:136–137.
12. Stänz K, Wedler V, Köpfli P, Künzi W, Pfammatter T. Compression syndrome of the arteria circumflexa humeri posterior in a volleyball player. [in German] *Vasa*. 2001;30:229–232.
13. Atema JJ, Unlü C, Reekers JA, Idu MM. Posterior circumflex humeral artery injury with distal embolisation in professional volleyball players: a discussion of three cases. *Eur J Vasc Endovasc Surg*. 2012;44:195–198.
14. Seinturier C, Blaise S, Maufus M, Magne JL, Pasquier B, Carpentier PH. A rare cause of embolic ischemia of the hand: an isolated aneurism of a branch of the axillary artery. [in French] *J Mal Vasc*. 2008;33:225–228.
15. Rohrer MJ, Cardullo PA, Pappas AM, Phillips DA, Wheeler HB. Axillary artery compression and thrombosis in throwing athletes. *J Vasc Surg*. 1990;11:761–768 (discussion 768-769).
16. Arko FR, Harris EJ, Zarins CK., Olcott C IV. Vascular complications in high-performance athletes. *J Vasc Surg*. 2001;33:935–942.
17. Reekers JA, Koedam N. Re: Volleyball-related ischemia of the hand. *Cardiovasc Intervent Radiol*. 1998;21:261.
18. Reekers JA, den Hartog BM, Kuyper CF, Kromhout JG, Peeters FL. Traumatic aneurysm of the posterior circumflex humeral artery: a volleyball player's disease?. *J Vasc Interv Radiol*. 1993;4:405–408.
19. Nuber GW, McCarthy WJ, Yao JS, Schafer MF, Suker JR. Arterial abnormalities of the shoulder in athletes. *Am J Sports Med*. 1990;18:514–519.
20. Reutter D, Hunziker R, Husmann M. Computed angiogram of the upper extremities for diagnosing a rare cause of brachial arterial embolism: the "Pitcher Syndrome". *Eur Heart J*. 2010;31:2782.
21. Duwayri YM, Emery VB, Driskill MR, et al. Positional compression of the axillary artery causing upper extremity thrombosis and embolism in the elite overhead throwing athlete. *J Vasc Surg*. 2011;53:1329–1340.
22. Brown SA, Doolittle DA, Bohanon CJ, et al. Quadrilateral space syndrome: the Mayo Clinic experience with a new classification system and case series. *Mayo Clin Proc*. 2015 Mar;90(3):382-94.
23. Friend J, Francis S, McCulloch J, et al. Teres minor innervation in the context of isolated muscle atrophy. *Surg Radiol Anat*. 2010;32:243–249.
24. Amin MF, Berst M, el-Khoury GY. An unusual cause of the quadrilateral space impingement syndrome by a bone spike. *Skeletal Radiol*. 2006;35:956–958.
25. Robinson P, White LM, Lax M, Salonen D, Bell RS. Quadrilateral space syndrome caused by glenoid labral cyst. *AJR Am J Roentgenol*. 2000;175:1103–1105.
26. Molina Granados JF, Domínguez Franjo E. Quadrilateral space syndrome with complete denervation of the deltoid and teres minor muscles. ([in Spanish]) *Radiologia*. 2010;52:373–374.
27. Ishima T, Usui M, Satoh E, Sakahashi H, Okamura K. Quadrilateral space syndrome caused by a ganglion. *J Shoulder Elbow Surg*. 1998;7:80–82.
28. Cirpar M, Gudemez E, Cetik O, Uslu M, Eksioglu F. Quadrilateral space syndrome caused by a humeral osteochondroma: a case report and review of literature. *HSS J*. 2006;2:154–156.
29. Sanders TG, Tirman PF. Paralabral cyst: an unusual cause of quadrilateral space syndrome. *Arthroscopy*. 1999;15:632–637.

30. McClelland D, Paxinos A. The anatomy of the quadrilateral space with reference to quadrilateral space syndrome. *J Shoulder Elbow Surg*. 2008;17:162–164.
31. Topp KS, Boyd BS. Structure and biomechanics of peripheral nerves: nerve responses to physical stresses and implications for physical therapist practice. *Phys Ther*. 2006;86:92–109.
32. Georgeu GA, Walbeehm ET, Tillett R, et al. Investigating the mechanical shear-plane between core and sheath elements of peripheral nerves. *Cell Tissue Res*. 2005;320:229–234.
33. Chen H, Onishi K, Zhao X, Chang EY. Neuromuscular ultrasound application to the electrodiagnostic evaluation of quadrilateral space syndrome. *PM R*. 2014;6:845–848.
34. Brestas PS, Tsouroulas M, Nikolakopoulou Z, Malagari K, Drossos C. Ultrasound findings of teres minor denervation in suspected quadrilateral space syndrome. *J Clin Ultrasound*.
35. Mochizuki T, Isoda H, Masui T, et al. Occlusion of the posterior humeral circumflex artery: detection with MR angiography in healthy volunteers and in a patient with quadrilateral space syndrome. *AJR Am J Roentgenol*. 1994;163:625–627.
36. Robinson DJ, Marks P, Schneider-Kolsky M. Occlusion and stenosis of the posterior circumflex humeral artery: detection with ultrasound in a normal population. *J Med Imaging Radiat Oncol*. 2011;55:479–484.
37. Chen H, Narvaez VR. Ultrasound-guided quadrilateral space block for the diagnosis of quadrilateral syndrome. *Case Rep Orthop*. 2015;2015:378627. doi: 10.1155/2015/378627. Epub 2015 Jan 20.

23

Surgical Approaches to Thoracic Outlet Syndrome: Supraclavicular Versus Transaxillary

Robert W. Thompson, MD

Thoracic outlet syndrome (TOS) represents several different clinical conditions affecting the upper extremity, which occur most commonly in young, active, otherwise healthy individuals.[1,2] Each type of TOS is caused by extrinsic compression of neurovascular structures within the thoracic outlet, which may be considered to extend from the inter-scalene triangle in the supraclavicular space, through the costoclavicular space, and to the axillary neurovascular bundle underneath the pectoralis minor muscle, in the infraclavicular (subcoracoid) space. The three forms of TOS are distinguished by the principal structure involved and the characteristic clinical manifestations that are produced: (1) neurogenic TOS, caused by compression of the brachial plexus nerve roots, which is characterized by arm, shoulder and/or neck pain, numbness and paresthesia, and functional disability; (2) arterial TOS, caused by chronic compression of the subclavian artery in association with a congenital or acquired bony abnormality, which typically leads to either occlusive lesions or post-stenotic aneurysm formation and thromboembolism; and (3) venous TOS, caused by compression of the central subclavian vein, which underlies the development of the effort thrombosis (Paget-Schroetter) syndrome.

Surgical treatment has an important role in the management of patients with all three forms of TOS. However, there remains considerable controversy regarding optimal patient selection for operation, timing of surgical interventions, and the specific surgical techniques to be used.[1,2] Current indications for surgery in TOS include the following: (1) patients with persistently disabling neurogenic TOS who have failed to achieve sufficient improvement with a conservative management program directed by a physical therapist with appropriate expertise in this condition; (2) patients with arterial TOS with any evidence of aneurysmal degeneration or a symptomatic occlusive lesion of the subclavian artery at the level of the first rib; and (3) patients with symptomatic venous TOS and/or recent subclavian vein effort thrombosis, usually following initial treatment with catheter-directed thrombolysis.

Operations performed for neurogenic TOS are designed to decompress the anatomic structures considered responsible for clinical symptoms.[3] This may include removal of the first rib, anomalous cervical ribs, the anterior and middle scalene muscles, aberrant muscles, ligaments or fascial bands, and perineural or perivascular fibrosis, all of which require open operative procedures. In the treatment of vascular forms of TOS, these operative procedures may also include arterial or venous reconstruction, either by direct open approaches or in combination with endovascular techniques (e.g., balloon angioplasty). The most commonly performed procedures for neurogenic TOS are conducted through either the transaxillary or supraclavicular approaches, with each approach having distinct advantages and disadvantages. In this chapter, the specific operative techniques used in the transaxillary and supraclavicular approaches to TOS are described, focusing on the treatment of patients with neurogenic TOS.

TRANSAXILLARY APPROACH

The primary advantages of the transaxillary approach for neurogenic TOS include a relatively limited field of operative dissection, a cosmetically placed skin incision, and sufficient exposure to reliably accomplish first rib resection.[4-7] This approach also makes it possible to achieve at least partial resection of the anterior scalene muscle, as well as identification and removal of most anomalous ligaments and fibrous bands that may be associated with TOS. The disadvantages of the transaxillary approach include incomplete exposure of the structures comprising the scalene triangle, inability to achieve complete anterior and middle scalenectomy or brachial plexus neurolysis, and the necessity for first rib resection in all cases. This approach is also limited when vascular reconstruction is needed, where repositioning of the patient and addition of a separate incision are required.

Under general anesthesia, the patient is positioned supine with the back of the table raised about 30 degrees. A small towel pack is placed behind the shoulder to elevate the affected side. The arm is prepped circumferentially and wrapped in stockinette, and the sterile field includes the neck, upper chest, and posterior shoulder to the scapula. The arm is not placed on a table or crossbar; rather, it is held and positioned by a reliable, flexible and sturdy assistant.

A transverse skin incision is made at the lower border of the axillary hairline, extending from the anterior border of the latissimus dorsi muscle to the lateral edge of the pectoralis major muscle. This incision is carried through the subcutaneous tissues directly to the chest wall, with blunt dissection used to establish a plane extending to the apex of the axilla. The long thoracic, thoracodorsal, and second intercostobrachial nerves are identified near the chest wall to avoid direct injury. Excessive elevation of the arm (unique to transaxillary exposure) is a potential mechanism of injury to the second intercostobrachial cutaneous nerve, resulting in postoperative pain and numbness along the medial aspect of the upper arm. The first rib is typically palpable at the upper reaches of the areolar tissue plane along the chest wall. Using a Deaver retractor to gently lift the subcutaneous tissues and axillary contents away from the chest wall, the first rib is more clearly exposed in the upper aspect of the wound. It is necessary to carefully lift the arm to facilitate this exposure, both at this stage and throughout the remainder of the procedure, and the operating surgeon should use a fiberoptic headlight to properly illuminate the operative field.

Exposure obtained during the transaxillary approach is generally limited to the operating surgeon. It is therefore important that the surgeon be constantly aware of how the assistants and retractors are positioned with respect to the nerve roots and blood vessels. In order to avoid serious injury, the blades of the retractors must not apply excess traction to the neurovascular structures visible above the first rib. In addition to the nerve roots of the brachial plexus, proper attention must be given to avoid traction on the long thoracic nerve, which exits the plane of the middle scalene muscle before coursing over the first rib to the serratus anterior muscle.

Once the first rib is sufficiently exposed, the subclavian vein and subclavian artery are identified along with the intervening anterior scalene muscle. These structures are carefully dissected such that the anterior scalene tendon can be encircled with a right-angle clamp just above its insertion onto the scalene tubercle of the first rib, which is typically palpable as a slight bony prominence. The anterior scalene muscle is exposed over several centimeters superior to the first rib, and while taking care to avoid the phrenic nerve, the muscle is divided with a scissors at the highest level feasible. The importance of resecting a portion of the scalene muscle, rather than simply dividing it at the level of the first rib itself, has been underscored by analysis of the factors causing recurrent TOS.

The soft tissues attaching to the inferior and medial borders of the first rib are progressively divided with scissors, beginning with the attachments medial to the subclavian vein (the subclavius muscle tendon and the costosternal and costoclavicular ligaments). A periosteal elevator is used along the inferior border of the rib, extending underneath the rib from the vantage point of the exposure used. The intercostal muscle is fully separated from the bone and the parietal pleura is pushed away from the deep aspect of the rib by blunt dissection. The middle scalene muscle is detached from the superior surface of the rib, posterior to the brachial plexus nerve roots. Although the proximal aspect of the long thoracic nerve is not directly visualized during this maneuver, injury to this nerve is prevented by keeping the periosteal elevator directly upon the rib during scalene muscle detachment, avoiding any tendency to stray laterally. Once the posterior surface of the first rib is exposed and the T1 nerve root is protected under direct vision, a bone-cutting instrument is carefully applied across the neck of the rib. The lateral portion of the divided rib is pulled downward and its anterior aspect is cut in a similar fashion, just medial to the subclavian vein at the costochondral junction. The first rib is then fully detached and removed from the operative field. A bone rongeur is used to trim the remaining ends of the bone to smooth surfaces well beyond the neurovascular structures.

Any additional soft tissue bands found to be crossing the brachial plexus nerve roots are sought and carefully divided, particularly those that may insert upon Sibson's fascia, the thickened aspect of the apical pleural surface. After hemostasis is achieved, the wound is irrigated and the lung is inflated to detect any breaks in the pleural lining. If small air bubbles are observed during positive-pressure ventilation or if the irrigation fluid appears to be lost into the pleural space, a small chest tube may be placed through a separate wound. The incisional wound is closed in two layers after placing a small closed suction drain in the operative field.

SUPRACLAVICULAR APPROACH

The supraclavicular approach to thoracic outlet decompression carries the major advantages of wider exposure of all of the relevant anatomical structures.[8-13] This allows complete resection of the anterior and middle scalene muscles, as well as brachial plexus neurolysis with direct visualization of all five nerve roots. In some cases, symptomatic relief of neurogenic TOS can be achieved by scalenectomy without the need for first rib resection, an option provided by the supraclavicular approach. This approach also allows for resection of cervical ribs, anomalous first ribs, or the normal first rib. A further advantage is that all forms of vascular reconstruction can also be accomplished through supraclavicular exposure; although removal of the anteromedial portion of the first rib and distal vascular control may require addition of a second (infraclavicular) incision, this is performed without the need for repositioning the patient.

Under general anesthesia, the patient is positioned supine with the head of the bed elevated 30 degrees. The hips and knees are flexed and the neck is extended and turned to the opposite side. The neck, upper chest and upper extremity are prepped into the field, with the arm wrapped in stockinette and held comfortably across the abdomen. This allows access to the hand if needed during the procedure and for arm movement through an extended range of motion. A transverse skin incision is made two fingerbreadths above the clavicle, beginning at the lateral border of the sternocleidomastoid muscle. This incision is then carried through the platysma muscle layer to expose the scalene fat pad.

The scalene fat pad is mobilized beginning at the lateral border of the internal jugular vein and the omohyoid muscle is resected. As this tissue plane is entered, the fat pad is progressively dissected off the anterior surface of the anterior scalene muscle and reflected laterally. The phrenic nerve is identified coursing in a lateral to medial direction within the investing fascia of the muscle, where gentle manipulation may produce a diaphragmatic startle ("dartle") response. Lateral retraction of the scalene fat pad then permits exposure of the underlying roots of the brachial plexus, the middle scalene muscle, and long thoracic nerve. The scalene fat pad is held in position with several retaining sutures and a self-retaining Henley retractor is put in place, with the middle blade along the edge of the sternocleidomastoid muscle. Thus, the critical view to be obtained in this initial dissection includes the internal jugular vein, the anterior scalene muscle and phrenic nerve, the brachial plexus and subclavian artery, and the middle scalene muscle and long thoracic nerve, all within the same operative field.

The insertion of the anterior scalene muscle is dissected taking special effort to avoid traction on the phrenic nerve. After circumferential mobilization of the anterior scalene muscle, a finger is passed behind it and the muscle is sharply divided at its site of attachment to the first rib using a curved scissors. Additional slips of muscle or tendon may also need to be divided more posteriorly, including direct attachments of the muscle to the thickened pleural lining behind the rib itself. The anterior scalene muscle is lifted superiorly to detach it from the additional structures underneath including the pleural apex, the subclavian artery and the brachial plexus nerve roots. This dissection is carried superiorly and the muscle is passed underneath the phrenic nerve to its medial side, to allow easier exposure of the anterior scalene muscle origin on the transverse process of the sixth cervical vertebrae. The muscle origin is sharply divided while avoiding injury to the upper brachial plexus, and the entire anterior scalene muscle is then removed, weighed, and sent to the neuromuscular pathology laboratory.

The brachial plexus and middle scalene muscle are then separated from each other by a combination of sharp and bunt dissection, to expose the inner curve of the first rib and to locate the C8 and T1 nerve roots at the posterior aspect of the first rib, where they join to form the lower trunk of the brachial plexus. While the middle scalene muscle lies posterior to the roots of the brachial plexus, in some cases its insertion upon the first rib may occur as far anteriorly as the scalene tubercle (the site of attachment of the anterior scalene muscle). The brachial plexus is retracted medially and the insertion of the middle scalene muscle on the posterolateral first rib is exposed as the long thoracic nerve is displaced laterally. Braches of the transverse cervical artery and vein, which pass through the brachial plexus, are ligated just lateral to the first rib. The attachment of the middle scalene muscle is divided from the first rib using the cautery and a periosteal elevator, extending to a point posterior to the brachial plexus nerve roots. Middle scalene muscle tissue anterior to the long thoracic nerve is divided with the nerve in direct view, then the remaining middle scalene muscle is resected and removed from the operative field.

First rib resection is readily accomplished given the exposure achieved at this stage of the operation. The brachial plexus nerve roots are displaced medially to expose the posterior neck of the rib, and using a periosteal elevator, any remaining muscle fibers of the middle scalene muscle are detached from their insertion on the top of the posterior first rib. While the C8 and T1 nerve roots are protected with a fingertip, a Stille rib cutter is inserted around the neck of the isolated first rib and applied. A Kerrison bone rongeur is used to resect additional amounts of bone as needed to ensure that the end of the rib will not impinge upon the lower nerve roots and to create a smooth surface on the posterior stump of the first rib. Using a fingertip, the pleural membrane is bluntly dissected away from the inferior aspect of the first rib. Intercostal muscle attachments to the first rib are divided using a periosteal elevator, to relieve the posterior and lateral aspects of the first rib of all soft tissue attachments, and any remaining attachments are divided along the anterolateral aspect of the rib up to the scalene tubercle. A small Richardson retractor is used to gently elevate the clavicle and the proximal portion of the rib is displaced inferiorly to further open the anterior costoclavicular space. With the subclavian artery and brachial plexus displaced posterolaterally, a Still bone cutter is inserted around the first rib at a level immediately medial to the scalene tubercle. The first rib is then divided and extracted from the operative field, and the proximal end of the rib is remodeled to a smooth surface with a bone rongeur.

Following scalenectomy and first rib resection, each of the nerve roots contributing to the brachial plexus are identified and meticulously dissected free of any postinflammatory fibrous scar tissue. Moderately dense fibrotic tissue encasing the nerve roots is not uncommon in patients with neurogenic TOS and may contribute to nerve root compression, irritation and neurogenic symptoms; thus, failure to perform an adequate neuroloysis may be one cause of persistent symptoms. This aspect of the operation is not complete until each nerve root from C5 to T1 is completely dissected and mobilized throughout its course in the operative field. Upon completion of the operation, the brachial plexus nerves are wrapped with an absorbable polymer film, to help suppress postoperative formation of perineural adhesions. A closed-suction drain is placed into the supraclavicular field with its tip extending into the open pleural space, and the scalene fat pad is reapproximated over the brachial plexus prior to wound closure.

DISCUSSION

It is now generally accepted that neurogenic TOS may arise from compression of the brachial plexus nerve roots at several different levels and by different etiologic factors, not solely as a consequence of bony deformation by the first rib.[2,3] Numerous soft tissue anomalies within the thoracic outlet have been described and classified, each of which can give rise to symptomatic neural compression. Significant factors playing a role in this process appear to include scalene muscle injury with fibrosis and sustained spasm, associated with pathologic changes in the scalene musculature, and fibrotic postinflammatory reactions surrounding the brachial plexus nerve roots. Current approaches to the surgical treatment of neurogenic TOS must take each of these potential contributing factors into account, in selecting the optimal treatment for individual patients.[14-16]

With regard to the selection of operative approach, the transaxillary approach allows the surgeon to reliably accomplish partial first rib resection through a relatively limited operative dissection and a cosmetically placed skin incision. In a large proportion of patients, this will provide satisfactory early results with regard to a low incidence of complications and markedly improved symptoms, with a reasonably low incidence of recurrence over time.[17] Nonetheless, there are some patients with neurogenic TOS who will not achieve satisfactory improvement after transaxillary first rib resection, due to brachial plexus compression involving the upper nerve roots, which is not fully addressed by this approach.[16,18,19] The incidence of recurrent neurogenic TOS after transaxillary first rib resection may also be considerable (and under-reported), due in large part to reattachment of incompletely resected scalene muscles and perineural fibrosis, as well as instances when there has been incomplete first rib resection.[18,19] In this light there are distinct advantages of the supraclavicular approach for neurogenic TOS, including more direct anatomic exposure to permit complete scalene muscle resection and brachial plexus neurolysis with direct visualization of all five nerve roots. With experience, operations utilizing the supraclavicular approach can also be performed with a low incidence of postoperative complications, a substantial rate of improved symptoms, and longer-term recurrence rates that are probably lower than those with the transaxillary approach.[20] Supraclavicular exposure is also ideal for reoperations performed after previous operations by either transaxillary first rib resection or supraclavicular decompression.[21] After accumulating considerable experience with the surgical management of neurogenic TOS, these factors have led our group to conclude that operative strategies based on supraclavicular exposure and its variations provide the most versatile, comprehensive, and safe approach to the treatment of neurogenic and other forms of TOS.[3,13,20]

REFERENCES

1. Sanders RJ. *Thoracic Outlet Syndrome: A Common Sequelae of Neck Injuries.* Philadelphia: J. B. Lippincott Company; 1991.
2. Illig KA, Thompson RW, Freischlag JA, Donahue DM, Jordan SE, Edgelow PI, editors. *Thoracic Outlet Syndrome.* London: Springer-Verlag; 2013.
3. Thompson RW, Driskill M. Thoracic outlet syndrome: neurogenic. In: Cronenwett JL, Johnston KW, editors. *Rutherford's Vascular Surgery.* 7th ed. Philadelphia: Elsevier; 2010. pp. 1878–98.

4. Roos DB. Transaxillary approach for first rib resection to relieve thoracic outlet syndrome. *Ann Surg*. 1966;163:354–8.
5. Machleder HI. Transaxillary operative management of thoracic outlet syndrome. In: Ernst CB, Stanley JC, editors. *Current Therapy in Vascular Surgery*. 2nd ed. Philadelphia: BC Decker; 1991. pp. 227–30.
6. Thompson RW, Petrinec D. Surgical treatment of thoracic outlet compression syndromes: diagnostic considerations and transaxillary first rib resection. *Ann Vasc Surg*. 1997;11:315–23.
7. Arnaoutakis GJ, Reifsnyder T. Surgical techniques: operative decompression using the transaxillary approach for NTOS. In: Illig KA, Thompson RW, Freischlag JA, Donahue DM, Jordan SE, Edgelow PI, editors. *Thoracic Outlet Syndrome*. London: Springer-Verlag; 2013. pp. 201–8.
8. Reilly LM, Stoney RJ. Supraclavicular approach for thoracic outlet decompression. *J Vasc Surg*. 1988;8:329-334.
9. Hempel GK, Shutze WP, Anderson JF, et al. 770 consecutive supraclavicular first rib resections for thoracic outlet syndrome. *Ann Vasc Surg*. 1996;10:456–63.
10. Thompson RW, Petrinec D, Toursarkissian B. Surgical treatment of thoracic outlet compression syndromes: supraclavicular exploration and vascular reconstruction. *Ann Vasc Surg*. 1997;11:442–51.
11. Sanders RJ, Hammond SL. Supraclavicular first rib resection and total scalenectomy: technique and results. *Hand Clin*. 2004;20:61–70.
12. Illig KA. Surgical techniques: operative decompression using the supraclavicular approach for NTOS. In: Illig KA, Thompson RW, Freischlag JA, Donahue DM, Jordan SE, Edgelow PI, editors. *Thoracic Outlet Syndrome*. London: Springer-Verlag; 2013. pp. 209–16.
13. Thompson RW, Vemuri C. Neurogenic thoracic outlet syndrome exposure and decompression: supraclavicular. In: Mulholland MW, Hawn MT, Hughes SJ, Albo D, Sabel MS, Dalman RL, editors. *Operative Techniques in Surgery*. Philadelphia: Wolters Kluwer Health; 2015. pp. 1848–61.
14. Cikrit DF, Haefner R, Nichols WK, et al. Transaxillary or supraclavicular decompression for the thoracic outlet syndrome: a comparison of the risks and benefits. *Am Surg*. 1989;55:347–52.
15. Sanders RJ, Pearce WH. The treatment of thoracic outlet syndrome: a comparison of different operations. *J Vasc Surg*. 1989;10:626–34.
16. Green RM. Controversies in NTOS: transaxillary or supraclavicular first rib resection in NTOS? In: Illig KA, Thompson RW, Freischlag JA, Donahue DM, Jordan SE, Edgelow PI, editors. *Thoracic Outlet Syndrome*. London: Springer-Verlag; 2013. pp. 315–17.
17. Rochlin DH, Gilson MM, Likes KC, et al. Quality-of-life scores in neurogenic thoracic outlet syndrome patients undergoing first rib resection and scalenectomy. *J Vasc Surg*. 2013;57:436–43.
18. Ambrad-Chalela E, Thomas GI, Johansen KH. Recurrent neurogenic thoracic outlet syndrome. *Am J Surg*. 2004;187:505–10.
19. Altobelli GG, Kudo T, Haas BT, et al. Thoracic outlet syndrome: pattern of clinical success after operative decompression. *J Vasc Surg*. 2005;42:122–8.
20. Caputo FJ, Wittenberg AM, Vemuri C, et al. Supraclavicular decompression for neurogenic thoracic outlet syndrome in adolescent and adult populations. *J Vasc Surg* 2013;57:149–57.
21. Cheng SW, Stoney RJ. Supraclavicular reoperation for neurogenic thoracic outlet syndrome. *J Vasc Surg*. 1994;19:565–72.

24

Patency after Limited Venoplasty and Anticoagulation following First Rib Resection for Venous Thoracic Outlet Syndrome

Gabriela Velazquez-Ramirez, MD and Julie A. Freischlag, MD

INTRODUCTION

Venous thoracic outlet syndrome (vTOS) has been thoroughly studied and is well understood; however, treatment strategies can vary, and several algorithms have been developed in order to standardize care and improve functional outcomes. Controversies regarding the timing of surgical treatment, use of thrombolysis, anticoagulation, venoplasty, and the need for first rib resection have been all debated.

vTOS is defined by compression of the subclavian vein by the first rib, the clavicle, and subclavius tendon. Only 3% of patients with thoracic outlet syndrome have its venous form, this is the second most common kind after neurogenic TOS This is also known as axillary-subclavian vein effort thrombosis or Paget-Schroetter syndrome. There is definitely a consensus when it comes to being aggressive with surgical decompression rather than conservative treatment with anticoagulation alone. When treated with anticoagulation alone, residual symptoms and chronic disability in the arm becomes quite challenging, directly affecting patient's quality of life; most patients presenting with this problem are young, active, and otherwise healthy.

The most important outcome for vTOS is long-term patency and functional recovery. Prompt detection and aggressive treatment has led to the improvement of patency rates and recovery. Contemporary reports indicate that a comprehensive approach to vTOS has consistently resulted in better outcomes. As more patients are diagnosed and treated, referral patterns have increased to centers of excellence and this becomes of the essence when developing processes to better serve these patients and return them to their daily activities as soon as possible.[1] The aim of this chapter is to provide a comprehensive review of vTOS focusing on outcomes following limited venoplasty and anticoagulation as well as an overview of treatment controversies.

PATHOPHYSIOLOGY, CLINICAL PRESENTATION, AND SURGICAL APPROACH

Patients presenting with vTOS suffer from compression of the axillo-subclavian vein which ultimately results in thrombosis. It occurs after a mechanical abnormality at the costoclavicular portion of the axillo-subclavian vein. Most commonly, acute thrombosis occurs in an area of chronic compression and stricture, usually between the hypertrophied scalene or subclavius tendon and the first rib (Figure 24-1).

Special consideration is given to those patients with cervical ribs. In the general population, the incidence is only 0.5%; however, in population studies of TOS patients, the incidence is higher. In these patients, both the cervical and the first rib must be removed. Most ribs can be resected from a transaxillary approach.[2]

Presentation of vTOS is acute; it can initially be asymptomatic, involving compression injury that will eventually form scar tissue, fibrosis, wall thickening, and contraction outside the vein. This will lead to acute thrombosis within the injured subclavian/axillary

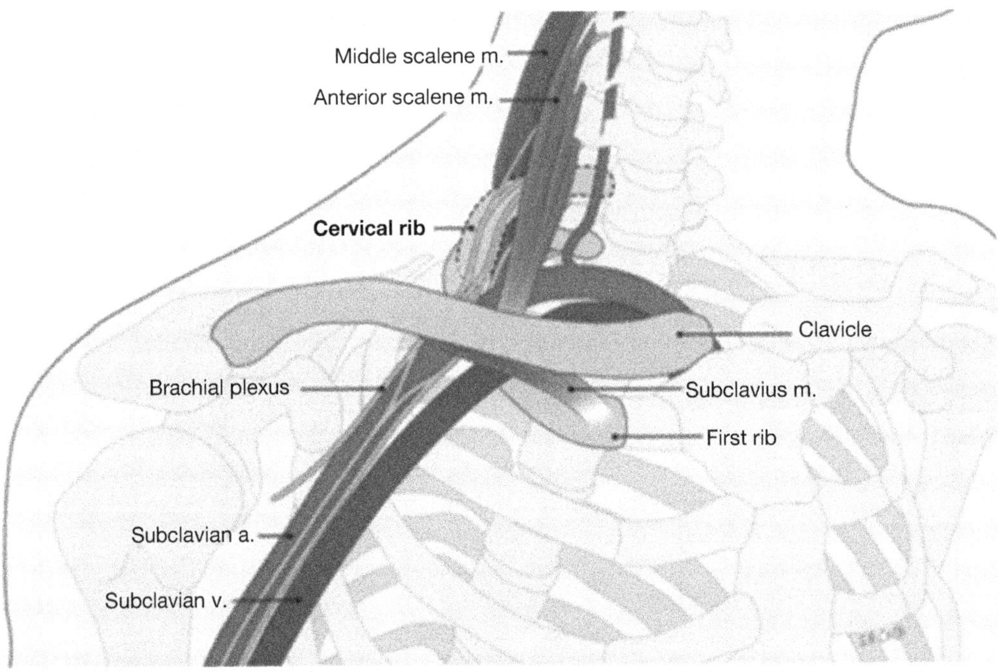

Figure 24-1. Common stricture location: shows the hypertrophied scalene and subclavius tendon and the first rib. Position of cervical rib is also shown. Drawing by Sarah Chen, UC Davis.

vein. Propagation of the thrombus results in further obstruction of collateral veins that will then present with worsening arm swelling, rubor or cyanosis, pain and/or heaviness.

When left untreated, arm swelling will usually resolve over time as a venous collateral networks develops, however, patients will have significant limitations when performing physical activities. In the long term, this will result in venous hypertension and postthrombotic syndrome. Due to the potential long-term disability, early diagnosis and prompt treatment are essential. Diagnosis is mostly based on history and symptoms in the presence of upper extremity venous thrombosis/occlusion and this is first suspected with venous duplex. Catheter-based venogram or magnetic resonance can further confirm the diagnosis. It is important to note that positional maneuvers with arms at rest and elevated reveal more details on the effects of position on the subclavian vein (Figures 24-2–24-4).

There are two surgical approaches for the treatment of vTOS: transaxillary and supraclavicular. Both are safe and equal in terms of outcomes. The main goal is to remove the whole rib as well as cutting the subclavius tendon (Figure 24-5). We strongly believe that if the whole rib is not removed, it will lead to recurrent symptoms in the future and increase the likelihood of undergoing re-do operations long term. We favor the transaxillary approach for all initial rib resection and the supraclavicular approach for re-do interventions for vTOS.[3]

TREATMENT ALGORITHMS

As the treatment of vTOS becomes more standardized, more extensive data is now available to evaluate the efficacy and outcomes of these algorithms as well as evolution of treatment.

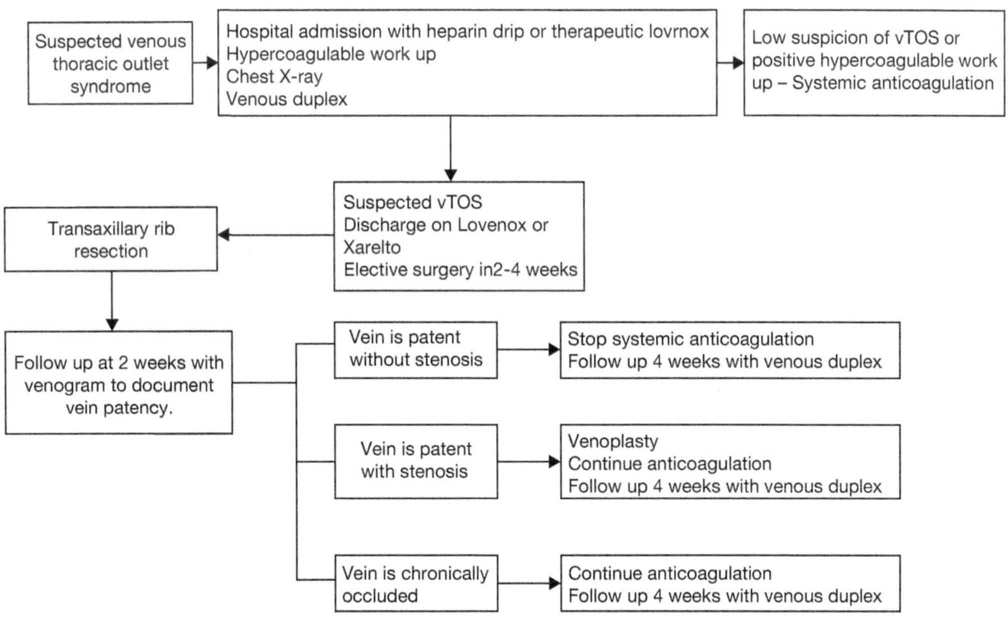

Figure 24-2. Venous thoracic outlet syndrome protocol.

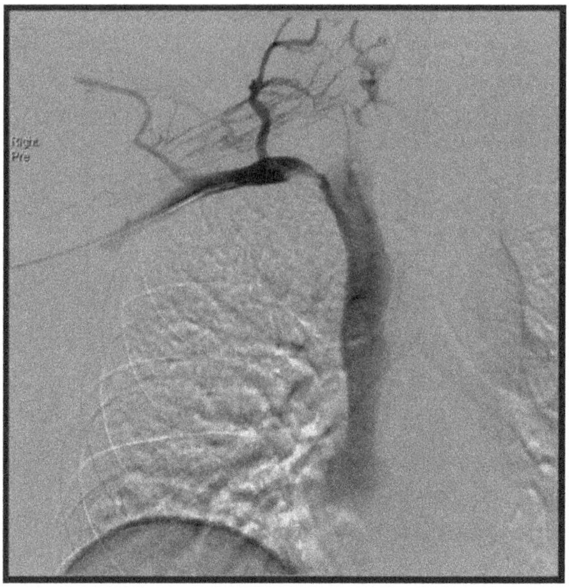

Figure 24-3. Venogram prevenoplasty.

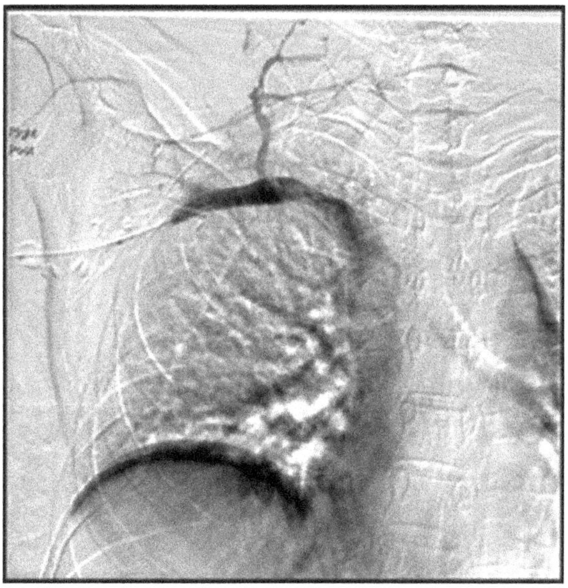

Figure 24-4. Venogram postvenoplasty.

As reported previously, practice patterns can be standardized with the use of algorithms; in our case, those patients who present with suspected vTOS are admitted with heparin infusion, chest radiograph, hypercoagulable work up and duplex ultrasound. Of those, patients with positive hypercoagulable work up or low suspicion for vTOS receive long-term anticoagulation. The group of patients suspected to have vTOS are

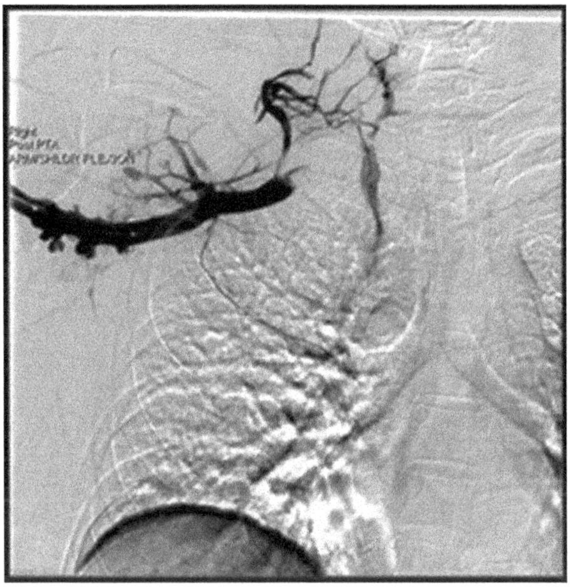

Figure 24-5. Venogram postvenoplasty with arm elevated.

discharged on therapeutic anticoagulation with lovenox or xarelto (rivaroxaban) and scheduled for outpatient surgery within two to four weeks. All of our patients undergo transaxillary rib resection. Two weeks after thoracic outlet decompression they undergo venogram. If the subclavian vein is patent, anticoagulation is stopped and follow-up in four weeks. If the subclavian vein is patent with residual stenosis, venoplasty is performed; anticoagulation is continued and follow-up in four weeks with a venous duplex if vein is patent, anticoagulation is stopped. If the vein is chronically occluded, the patient continues therapeutic anticoagulation and follow-up in four weeks, anticoagulation is continued up to six months or until vein is patent on venous duplex. (Figure 24-6)

Following the principles of our algorithm, in the authors experience most patients will fit into one of four treatment pathways depending on their presentation.[4] This protocol has proved successful and 95% of patients using this algorithm were patent and symptom-free at 10-month follow-up.[3,4] (Table 24-1)

Other centers of excellence have also developed their own protocols and flow diagrams with reported outcomes of patent subclavian vein, asymptomatic, and without the need for long-term anticoagulation in 96% of their patients.[5]

FUNCTIONAL OUTCOMES

Patients who undergo successful treatment for vTOS are able to return to their daily activities typically symptom-free within six months without long-term anti coagulation. It is now well established that patients undergoing surgical treatment for vTOS have better functional outcomes than those treated with anticoagulation only, prompt surgical treatment has shown to be superior when compared to delayed management with respect to rethrombosis and functional outcome.[6]

The use of short form 12 (SF-12) and Disability of the Arm, Shoulder, and Hand (DASH), validated patient-reported quality of life instruments, have been of extreme

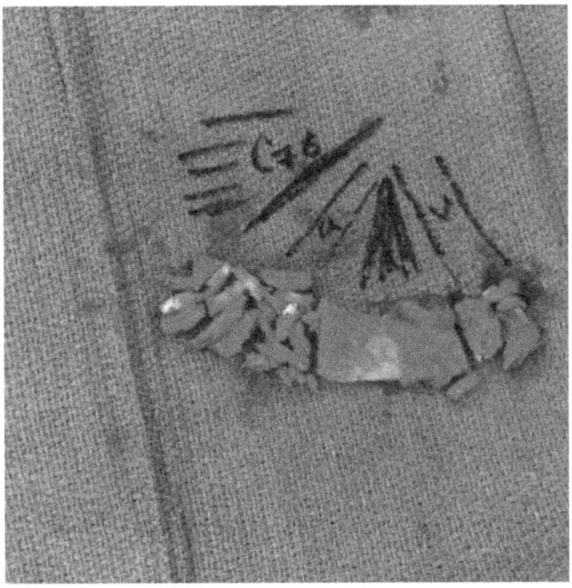

Figure 24-6. Rib removed entirely.

TABLE 24-1. MULTIPLE TREATMENT ALGORITHMS BASED ON CLINICAL PRESENTATION, DURATION OF SYMPTOMS AND OUTCOMES[3,4]

Group 1	Group 2	Group 3	Group 4
Acute thrombosis, initially treated with venous lysis	Symptomatic subclavian vein stenosis transferred from outside institution (initial event at varied times, not acute) average 22 weeks	Intermittent occlusion but did not have thrombosis; lifestyle limiting symptoms.	Patients with occluded subclavian veins months or years postinitial event
Early transaxillary rib resection and discharge with therapeutic lovenox	Rib resection and therapeutic lovenox	Rib resection and no anticoagulation was started unless duplex demonstrated stenosis or thrombosis	Transaxillary rib resection and therapeutic lovenox
Follow-up two weeks with venogram and venoplasty as needed	Follow-up two weeks with venogram and venoplasty as needed	Venogram and venoplasty for patients who had persistent symptoms or stenosis (25%)	Follow up two weeks with venogram
Anticoagulation continued until vein patency achieved	Anticoagulation continued until vein patency achieved	Anticoagulation for those treated with venoplasty until patency achieved	Anticoagulation continued until vein patency achieved
Long-term follow-up (seven months) all veins were patent	One third of patients had patent subclavian vein at time of venogram; two-thirds required venoplasty, 92% were patent at three months; anticoagulation stopped.	All patients were symptom free on long-term follow-up	At six months, 80% of patients had a patent subclavian vein

help in determining functional outcomes after intervention. It has been stated that surgical intervention is associated with significant improvement in the quality of life for TOS patients. Specifically for vTOS, they improved physical and mental function in a shorter time than neurogenic counterparts and they were able to go back to work by 6 months. vTOS patients improved physical and mental function in shorter times than neurogenic counterparts. Patient factors such as comorbid pain syndromes, narcotic use and smoking, are more predictive of long-term scores than relief from scalene block.[7] Thrombolysis and surgery has been reported to be superior to delayed management with respect to rethrombosis and functional outcomes.[6]

PATENCY OUTCOMES AND CONTROVERSIES

Extensive data exists on the safety of thrombolysis as the initial treatment to a staged multidisciplinary approach ending in rib resection. This has been overall widely used, but has also been modified by other practices. Most large studies arise from centers of excellence, single institutions which are in favor of a particular surgical approach or algorithm.

Other points of discussion exist regarding the optimal management of axillo-subclavian veins postoperatively. Post-FFRs (post-fractional flow reserves) stenting after inadequate venoplasty, adjunctive arteriovenous fistula, and venous bypass have all been reported and have shown poor patency rates of these venous adjunctive procedures.[8,9]

As mentioned previously, vein patency is one of the most important outcomes after treatment of vTOS; routine venography following transaxillary first rib resection and scalenectomy (FRRS) for subclavian vein thrombosis showed excellent outcomes and vein patency. Chang et al. assessed the role of routine postoperative venography in patients who have undergone FRRS by evaluation of long-term patency using imaging by duplex scan. Venography is performed two weeks after thoracic outlet decompression. The subclavian vein was dilated if there is a >50% stenosis and those patients were anticoagulated. If stenosis is not appreciated, anticoagulation is then stopped. If the vein was occluded, anticoagulation was continued for six months or until the vein recanalized. Eighty-four patients were included within a six-year period, the average age was 32 years old and average time from thrombosis to FRRS was six months (one week to two years). At the time of venography, 21 patients had widely patent veins and remained patent in the postoperative period and long-term follow-up (18 months). For those patients who had stenotic veins, 47 underwent venoplasty, three had acute thrombus and were lysed, two thrombosed after venogram and were anticoagulated. The average period of anticoagulation was two months, follow-up was 18 months. For those patients who had occluded veins, 16 had chronically occluded veins by venogram and all received systemic anticoagulation for an average period of 3 months. Fourteen of these patients recanalized within the first six months, follow-up was for 15 months. Five patients in the venoplasty group had either symptomatic restenosis or late vein occlusion. The authors concluded routine venography directs individual treatment plans for the patient, which includes vein dilatation, anticoagulation, and duplex scanning only within the first year.

Long-term patency was achieved in >90% of the patients using this treatment protocol.[10,11] To further validate these findings, long-term outcomes were later reported following the same protocol, in this study median follow-up was 13 months for 159 patients. All underwent FRRS. Postoperative complications in the entire cohort included 22% pneumothoraces, 3% hematomas requiring reoperation and one wound infection. At the time of the two-week venography, there were 42 patent, 72 stenotic, and 44 occluded veins with no perioperative complications. Most stenotic and occluded veins were treated with venoplasty; nineteen of the occluded veins could not be crossed. In the entire cohort, the three-year primary patency and primary assisted patency of venoplasty was 75% and 93%, respectively. The three-year overall secondary patency was 97%. This specific treatment algorithm, FRRS with routine postoperative venography and without preoperative endovascular intervention affords excellent long-term results. Limited venoplasty without over dilatation in those veins that could be crossed, and prolonged anticoagulation for occluded veins that cannot be crossed are associated with excellent long-term functional outcome without the need for adjunctive stenting or venous reconstruction.[12]

Given the success with FRRS, anticoagulation, and postoperative venogram/venoplasty, another prospective study was performed to compare this treatment strategy with preoperative endovascular intervention. A total of one hundred patients with vTOS were included, and 110 FRRS were performed. Seven of these patients had contralateral vTOS. The average age was 31 years and eight of these patients had documented hypercoagulable disorders. Forty-one percent of the patients had preoperative endovascular intervention prior to FRRS, the reminder of the cohort was managed with systemic anticoagulation alone prior to FRRS. Of those patients who had preoperative endovascular intervention, 91% were patent without symptoms at follow-up, of those that had anticoagulation alone prior to FRRS, 91% were patent without symptoms at follow-up. When comparing the need for venoplasty after FRRS, 49% in the preoperative endovascular intervention group and 59% in the anticoagulation only group required venoplasty at two weeks follow-up venogram. Preoperative thrombolysis did not have a meaningful impact on the need for further venoplasty after FRRS. In this case, preoperative endovascular intervention offered no benefit over anticoagulation alone prior to FRRS since the use of thrombolysis before elective operative decompression, regardless of the need for postoperative venoplasty, had little impact on overall rates of patency and patient symptom relief. Optimal treatment may be anticoagulation alone prior to operative decompression via FRRS and postoperative endovascular intervention. Multicenter, randomized trials will be needed to validate this potential change in treatment.[13]

Other groups strongly advocate the use of endovascular treatment and thrombolysis prior to thoracic outlet decompression, which provides prompt reduction in subclavian vein thrombus and success, can often be obtained within the first treatment. These particular groups support the use of continues infusion of thrombolytic agent over 24 to 48 hours with monitoring in an intensive care unit.[14–16]

Other endovascular techniques utilized prior to first rib resection include balloon angioplasty of the subclavian vein, although initially can improve venous flow and improve symptoms, this will likely recur due to the chronic mechanical compression of the vein and residual scar tissue. Two things most vTOS experts agree on, is against the use of systemic anticoagulation as the sole treatment of vTOS as well as the use of subclavian vein stents on patients who have not undergone thoracic outlet decompression. These are known to be at very high risk for deformation and thrombosis, both these options hinder symptom relief as well as risk for long-term disability.[17,18] However, earlier reports suggest that the use of subclavian venous stents may be safely used in those patients with short-segment venous strictures after successful lysis and thoracic outlet decompression.[19]

Points of discussion exist regarding the optimal management of axillo-subclavian veins postoperatively. Post-FFRS stenting after inadequate venoplasty, adjunctive arteriovenous fistula, intraoperative angioplasty, and venous bypass have all been reported, some have shown poor patency rates of these venous adjunctive procedures.[8,9,20]

Timing to surgical resection is highly varied among institutions. Advocacy for a three-month delay in surgery was instituted to allow for intimal healing, although used by a wide variety of institutions others continued to perform same admission surgical intervention with preoperative thrombolysis. Most reports try to avoid long delays prior to thoracic outlet decompression. Although excellent results have been reported for all of these surgical approaches, the best published outcomes have consistently been with approaches that involve direct reconstruction of the subclavian vein at the time of decompression surgery.[21,17]

More recently, outcome trends when treating vTOS have been performed using the American College of Surgeons (ACS) National Surgical Quality Improvement Program (NSQIP) to evaluate current practices and perioperative outcomes across the nation with institutions registered on NSQIP. These studies included all patients treated for TOS, we report those findings related to vTOS. Both studies had 176 and 141 patients respectively, median age was 34 for both and they both had similar operative time, length of stay as well as perioperative complications which was <3% (bleeding, surgical site infection, and DVT). In Reinhardt's study, strong predictors to influence 30-day reoperation, readmission, or both were patient's ASA Physical Status Classification and a nonneurogenic (vascular) indication for thoracic outlet decompression.[1,22] None of these studies reported functional outcomes.

OTHER CONSIDERATIONS

Hypercoagulability is a rare finding in those patients who present with Paget-Schroetter syndrome. It should be considered in those patients who present with lack of activity leading to the thrombosis, especially if they are female, to identify the need for long-term anticoagulation. Patients identified with hypercoagulability do as well with FRRS for subclavian venous thrombosis as those without. Keeping this in mind, judicious testing will yield improved outcomes and prevent future venous thromboembolic events in this subset of patients.[23]

Another point of consideration is the need for bilateral FRRS for patients with vTOS. In a cohort of 53 patients undergoing bilateral FRRS with a mean follow-up of 11 months, 26 of the patients had vTOS. Time between operations should be at least one year to facilitate favorable outcomes. Bilateral FRRS was deemed safe and effective for symptomatic and prophylactic treatment of vTOS; this set of patients often includes younger, competitive athletes and must be monitored closely postoperatively for recurrent stenosis and thrombosis.[24]

Patients rarely present with edema of the upper extremity without evidence of thrombosis, known as McCleery's syndrome. This is due to intermittent compression of the subclavian vein from the subclavius and anterior scalene muscles. In this particular population, FRRS alone has been effective in relieving symptoms. A postoperative venogram is not always needed as long as symptoms do not persist or in those patients who present with venous duplex evidence of chronic thrombus.[25]

CONCLUSIONS

- Treatment algorithms are extremely important in the treatment of vTOS. Standardizing care and follow-up leads to improved long-term vein patency and functional outcomes.
- Both transaxillary and supraclavicular approaches are equal and effective for decompression of the thoracic outlet. The most important principle is to completely remove the rib and subclavius tendon to prevent recurrent symptoms and need for reintervention.
- Documenting vein patency is essential after surgical intervention, because this will determine the need for further interventions such as venoplasty, a longer duration of anticoagulation, and follow-up with venous duplex.
- The utilization of a national vascular registry for thoracic outlet syndrome will allow for the identification of regional and institutional trends as well as the standardization of care, treatment algorithms, and follow-up with the goal of improving long-term vein patency and functional outcomes.

REFERENCES

1. Rinehardt EK, Scarborough JE, Bennett KM. Current practice of thoracic outlet decompression surgery in the United States. *J Vasc Surg*. 2017;66:858–865.
2. Freischlag JA, Chang K, Gurkar M, Reifsnyder T, Davis K. Cervical ribs—a rare entity but clinically significant. *J Vasc Surg*. 2010;52:805.
3. Propper BW, Freischlag JA. Venous thoracic outlet syndrome: best practice. In: Eskandari MK, Pearce WH, Yao JSTY, eds. *Current Vascular Surgery 2012*, Sheldon, CT: PMPH-USA; 2013:551–559.
4. de León RA, Chang DC, Hassoun HT, et al. Multiple treatment algorithms for successful outcomes in venous thoracic outlet syndrome. *Surgery*. 2009;145:500–507.
5. Vemuri C, Salehi P, Benarroch-Gampel J, McLaughlin LN, Thompson RW. Diagnosis and treatment of effort-induced thrombosis of the axillary subclavian vein due to venous thoracic outlet syndrome. *J Vasc Surg Venous Lymphat Disord*. 2016;4:485–500.
6. Taylor J, Telford R, Kinsella D, Watkinson A, Thompson J. Long term clinical and functional outcome following treatment for Paget–Schroetter syndrome. *Br J Surg*. 2013;100:1459–1464.
7. Chang DC, Rotellini-Coltvet LA, Mukherjee D, De Leon R, Freischlag JA. Surgical intervention for thoracic outlet syndrome improves patient's quality of life. *J Vasc Surg*. 2009;49:630–637.
8. Spivack A, Troutman D, Dougherty M, Calligaro K. Changing strategies to treat venous thrombotic occlusions of the upper and lower extremities secondary to compressive phenomena. *Vasc Endovasc Surg*. 2013;47:274–277.
9. Melby SJ, Vedantham S, Narra VR, et al. Comprehensive surgical management of the competitive athlete with effort thrombosis of the subclavian vein (Paget-Schroetter syndrome). *J Vasc Surg*. 2008;47:809–820. e803.

10. Chang KZ, Likes K, Demos J, Black III JH, Freischlag JA. Routine venography following transaxillary first rib resection and scalenectomy (FRRS) for chronic subclavian vein thrombosis ensures excellent outcomes and vein patency. *Vasc Endovasc Surg*. 2012;46:15–20.
11. Orlando MS, Likes KC, Lum YW, Freischlag JA. Utilization of venous duplex scanning and postoperative venography in patients with subclavian vein thrombosis. *J Vasc Surg Venous Lymphat Disord*. 2015;3:173–177.
12. Abularrage CJ, Rochlin DH, Selvarajah S, Lum YW, Freischlag JA. Limited venoplasty and anticoagulation affords excellent results after first rib resection and scalenectomy for subacute Paget-Schroetter syndrome. *J Vasc Surg Venous Lymphat Disord*. 2014;2:297–302.
13. Guzzo JL, Chang K, Demos J, Black JH, Freischlag JA. Preoperative thrombolysis and venoplasty affords no benefit in patency following first rib resection and scalenectomy for subacute and chronic subclavian vein thrombosis. *J Vasc Surg*. 2010;52:658–663.
14. Thompson RW. Comprehensive Management of Subclavian Vein Effort Thrombosis. *Semin Intervent Radiol*. March 2012;29(1):44–51.
15. Doyle A, Wolford HY, Davies MG, et al. Management of effort thrombosis of the subclavian vein: today's treatment. *Ann Vasc Surg*. 2007;21:723–729.
16. Schneider DB, Curry TK, Eichler CM, Messina LM, Gordon RL, Kerlan RK. Percutaneous mechanical thrombectomy for the management of venous thoracic outlet syndrome. *J Endovasc Ther*. 2003;10:336–340.
17. Urschel HC, Patel AN. Surgery remains the most effective treatment for Paget Schroetter syndrome: 50 years' experience. *Ann Thorac Surg*. 2008;86:254–260.
18. Illig KA, Doyle AJ. A comprehensive review of Paget-Schroetter syndrome. *J Vasc Surg*. 2010;51:1538–1547.
19. Kreienberg PB, Chang BB, Darling RC. 3rd, et al. Long-term results in patients treated with thrombolysis, thoracic inlet decompression, and subclavian vein stenting for Paget-Schroetter syndrome. *J Vasc Surg*. 2001;33:100–105.
20. Schneider DB, Dimuzio PJ, Martin ND, et al. Combination treatment of venous thoracic outlet syndrome: open surgical decompression and intraoperative angioplasty. *J Vasc Surg*. 2004;40:599–603.
21. Orlando MS, Likes KC, Mirza S, et al. A decade of excellent outcomes after surgical intervention in 538 patients with thoracic outlet syndrome. *J Am Coll Surg*. 2015;220:934–939.
22. Nejim B, Alshaikh HN, Arhuidese I, et al. Perioperative outcomes of thoracic outlet syndrome surgical repair in a nationally validated database. *Angiology*. 2017;68:502–507.
23. Likes K, Rochlin D, Nazarian SM, Streiff MB, Freischlag JA. Females with subclavian vein thrombosis may have an increased risk of hypercoagulability. *JAMA Surg*. 2013;148:44–49.
24. Rochlin DH, Likes KC, Jacobs C, Yu B, Freischlag JA. Should thoracic outlet syndrome patients ever undergo bilateral first rib resection and scalenectomy? *J Vasc Surg*. 2013;57:61S.
25. Likes KC, Rochlin D, Freischlag JA. McCleery's syndrome: incidence, etiology, and treatment in 2011. *J Vasc Surg*. 2012;56:882.

25

Cervical Ribs and Arterial Thoracic Outlet Syndrome

Kaj H. Johansen, MD, PhD

INTRODUCTION

That a supernumerary rib occasionally arises off the seventh cervical vertebra—a cervical rib—has been known since the time of Galen in the second century AD, and the relationship of such extra supraclavicular ribs to the development of subclavian artery abnormalities—arterial thoracic outlet syndrome (TOS)—has been evident since reports by Halsted a century ago.[1] Such subclavian (and more peripheral upper extremity) arterial abnormalities are an ongoing although an uncommon aspect of contemporary vascular surgical practice. The recent publication of reporting standards for various forms of TOS[2] encourages a revisiting of the relationship between cervical ribs (and other bony abnormalities at the thoracic outlet) and upper extremity arterial disease.

ANATOMY AND PATHOPHYSIOLOGY

The embryologic development of the cervical rib arises from extension of the bony anlage of the transverse process of the seventh cervical vertebra. Anatomic nomenclature dictates that the presence of an articulation with the C7 transverse process distinguishes a cervical rib: The absence of such an articulation indicates an extended C7 transverse process. Consonant with a longstanding classification,[2] the extent to which the cervical rib extends beyond the lateral aspect of the transverse process of the first thoracic vertebra, and whether the distal end of the cervical rib articulates (or "pseudoarticulates") on the first rib, defines the type (I through IV) of the cervical rib (Figure 25-1). Upon rare occasions, a cervical rib has been reported to extend down to articulate upon the second thoracic rib. Arterial complications are thought to occur only with long, well-developed [types III and IV[2]] cervical ribs.

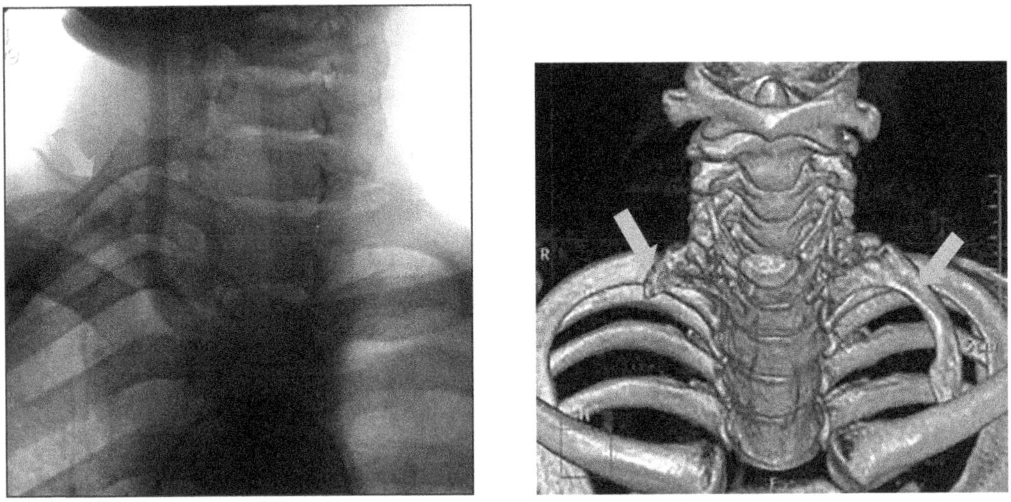

Figure 25-1. **(Left)** chest roentgenogram displaying a complete (type IV) right cervical rib, and **(right)** CT reconstruction exhibiting a small type II right and a large type IV left cervical rib.

When present, a cervical rib is commonly accompanied by a series of bands extending in various directions off the tip of the rib downward toward the first (or occasionally the second) thoracic rib.[1,2]

Other bony abnormalities relevant to the development of arterial TOS may include atrophic or dysplastic first thoracic ribs, fused first and second thoracic ribs or abnormalities of the clavicle, most commonly callus formation following fracture. Unusually, development of arterial abnormalities consequent to operative fixation of a prior clavicle fracture—i.e., an "iatrogenic" arterial TOS—has been reported.[3]

The subclavian artery exits the upper mediastinum over the first rib and passes through the scalene triangle, after which it transits the costoclavicular and subpectoralis spaces. In the presence of a cervical rib (or other bony abnormalities listed above) the position of the subclavian artery can be distorted—most commonly by sharp angulation over the top of the extra rib or its associated bands. It is theorized, as elsewhere in the body, that this sharp angulation or distortion of the subclavian artery, combined with its recurrent pulsations, over the top of the cervical rib initiates a focal neointimal hyperplasia which may develop into an actual stenosis, beyond which poststenotic dilation is known to develop.[4]

The resulting endoluminal narrowing or arterial dilatation (which may become truly aneurysmal), of the subclavian artery may initiate the deposition of mural thrombus (Figure 25-2, top), leading to peripheral (or, rarely, central) artery-to-artery embolization (Figure 25-2, lower). Upon rare occasions, the patient may present with a pulsatile mass in the supraclavicular region which represents a previously-undiagnosed subclavian artery aneurysm (Figure 25-3).

Most embolization from a stenotic or aneurysmal subclavian artery in arterial TOS occurs distally into the small digital arteries of the hand or, alternatively, into the brachial artery or its branch vessels. But stroke (or lesser forms of central nervous system embolization) has also been reported as a rare but catastrophic complication of arterial TOS.[5,6] The underlying pathophysiology appears to relate to subclavian artery thrombus which propagates retrograde toward the vertebral or (right) common

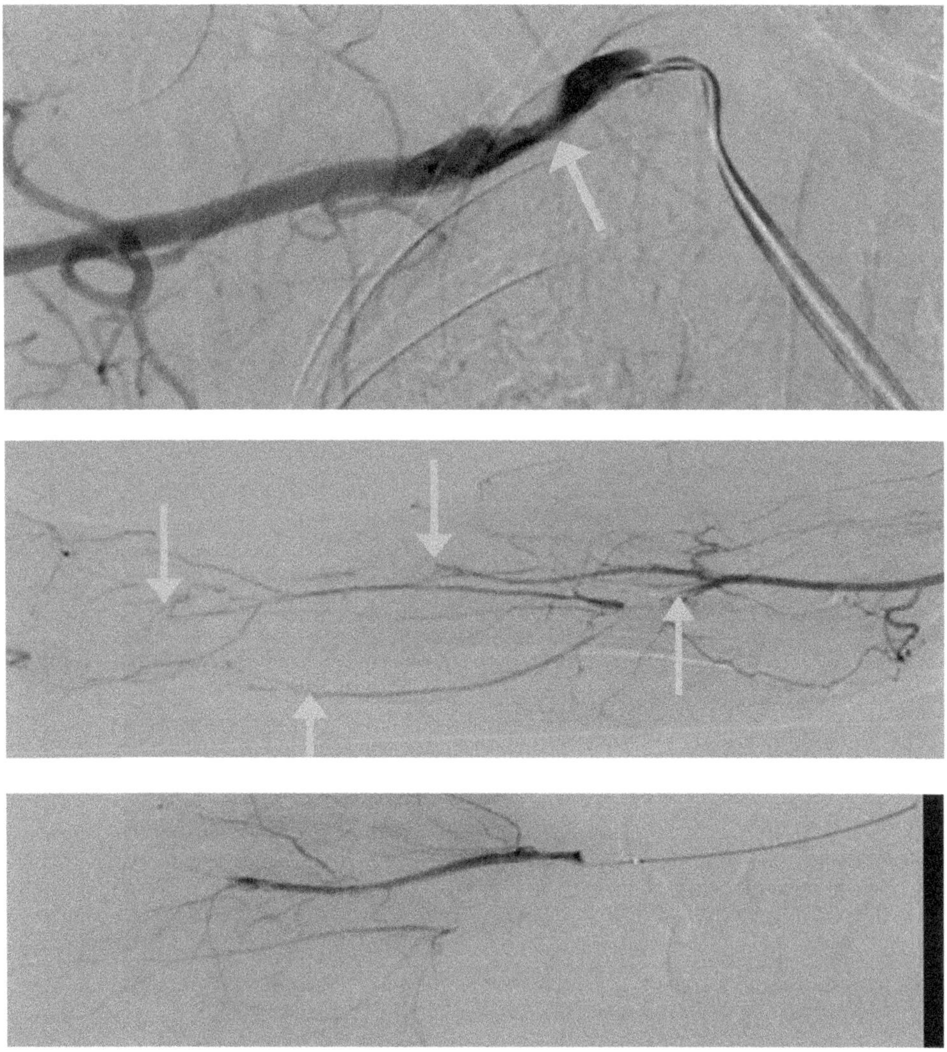

Figure 25-2. (Top) endothelial damage within the right subclavian artery due to an underlying cervical rib (not shown) resulted in deposition of mural thrombus (arrow) **(Middle)** eventuating in distal embolic occlusion at multiple levels (arrows) in the forearm arteries **(Bottom)** requiring treatment by catheter-directed thrombolysis.

carotid arteries: embolization into the intracranial circulation results from the occasional positional cessation or even reversal of subclavian artery flow when elevation of the arm results in extrinsic compression and transient occlusion of the artery in the costoclavicular space.

The pathophysiology resulting from peripheral embolization of thrombus within the subclavian artery in arterial TOS revolves predominantly around the development of peripheral ischemia, including upper extremity muscular fatigue or claudication or, rarely, critical limb ischemia, including rest pain or rest numbness or actual tissue loss (usually evidenced by digital ulcerations). This is consequent to varying degrees of embolization either to the brachial artery and its outflow radial and ulnar branches (Figure 25-2) or, alternatively, into the small arteries of the fingers and hand. This

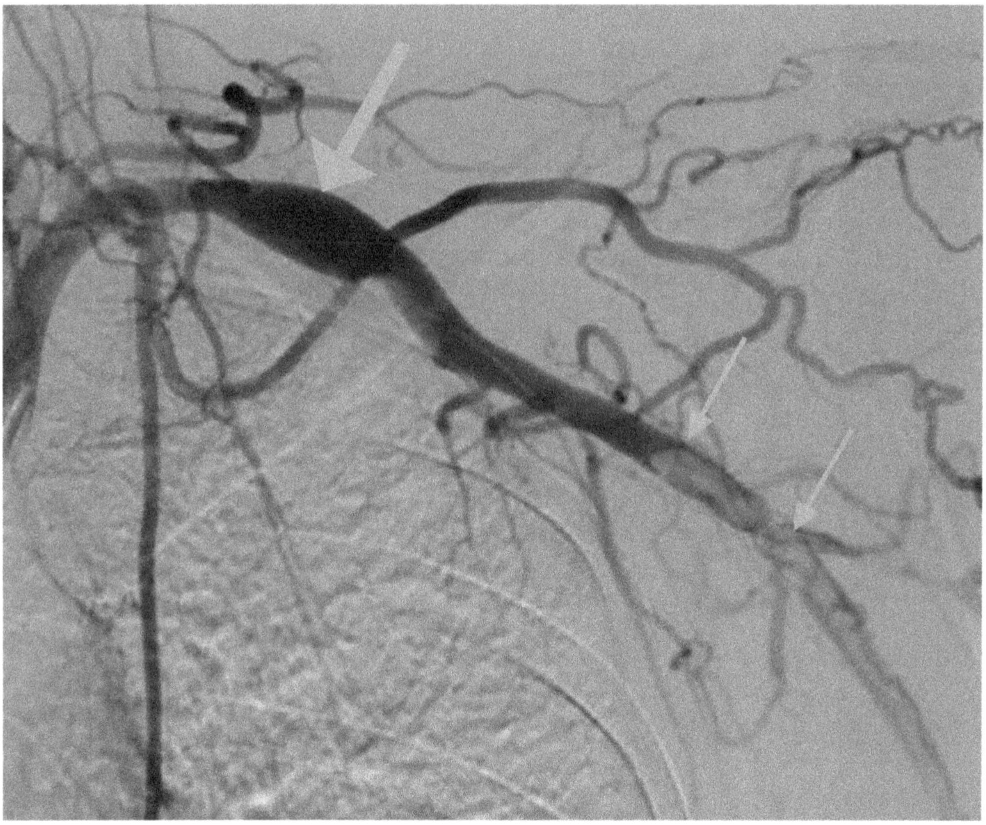

Figure 25-3. A left subclavian artery aneurysm (large arrow) accompanying an underlying complete left cervical rib resulting in thromboembolic occlusion of the distal subclavian and axillary arteries (narrow arrows).

latter phenomenon may initially be silent, and when ultimately discovered may be—analogous to the chronic arterial embolization that occurs distal to a popliteal artery aneurysm[7]—difficult to resolve. However, *unlike* the consequences of neglected or untreated embolization distal to a lower extremity aneurysm, where limb loss is a substantial likelihood, upper extremity amputation due to embolization from an abnormal subclavian artery damaged by a cervical rib is extremely rare—likely because of the lower blood supply requirements as well as the robust collateral reserve present in the upper extremities.

The same structural deformation which results in pathophysiologic changes in the subclavian artery in the presence of a cervical rib may also distort the contiguous brachial plexus leading to symptoms and signs of a form of neurogenic TOS. Indeed, brachial plexus compression or deformation by an underlying cervical rib (or its associated bands), resulting in symptoms and signs of neurogenic TOS (Figure 25-4), is a much more common presentation for a cervical rib than that of arterial TOS (cervical ribs account for 4%–8% of patients operated upon for neurogenic TOS). Clinically, such patients may display florid evidence for brachial plexus compression, including the development of intrinsic hand muscle atrophy with clawing (Gilliatt-Sumner hand).[8] Histologic examination demonstrates epineural and perineural fibrosis, vascular hyalinization, mucinous degeneration, and nodular intraneural collagen deposition in this setting.[9]

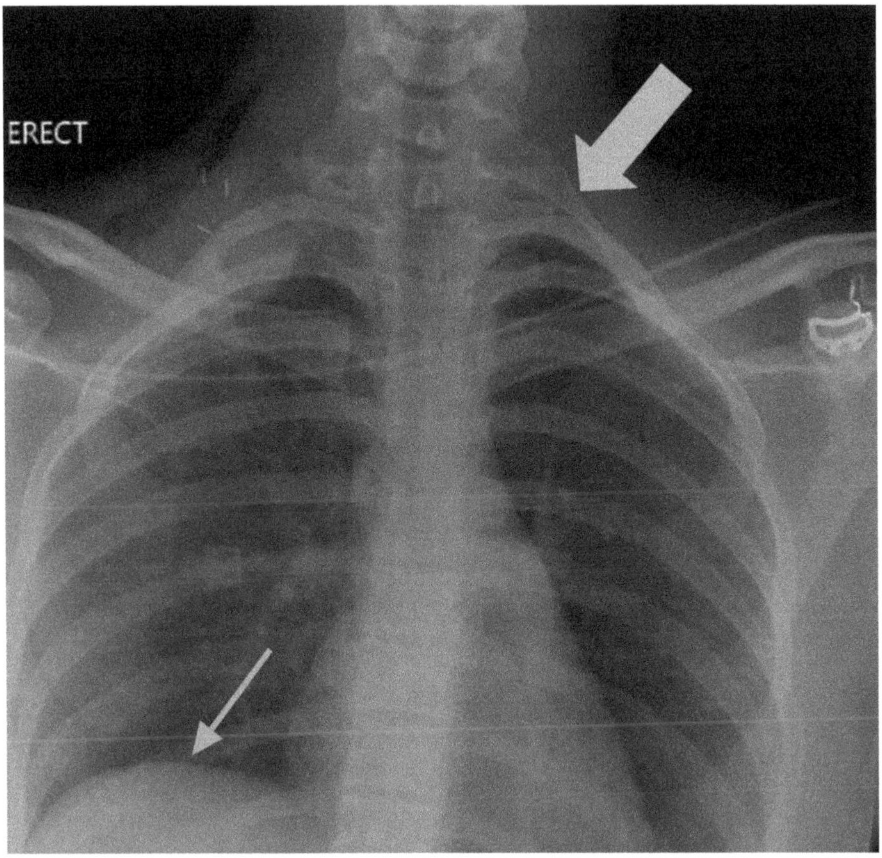

Figure 25-4. A 23-year-old dental student who had just undergone excision of a right cervical rib (note supraclavicular hemostatic clips) to treat incapacitating symptoms and dysfunction (preoperative QuickDASH score 84) of *neurogenic* thoracic outlet syndrome (it is not this surgeon's practice to remove the first rib to treat neurogenic thoracic outlet syndrome). The right-sided operation was successful (QuickDASH score at 18 months is 0) but operation on the patient's equally-symptomatic left cervical rib (large arrow) was delayed for 15 months because a phrenic nerve palsy and diaphragmatic paresis resulted from the prior right cervical rib excision (narrow arrow).

EPIDEMIOLOGY

Standard teaching has suggested that 0.5%–1% of humans have a cervical rib—0.5% of males and 1% of females. About 40% of the time, such extra ribs are bilateral. Older studies, derived from chest roentgenograms,[10] have recently been updated: the Hopkins neuroradiology group assessed 3400 cervical CT scans and their dictated reports and provide more contemporaneous data suggesting that cervical ribs are present in as much as 2.0% of the population.[11] This study also documented neuroradiologists' significant under-reporting (75% of the time!) of the presence of cervical ribs. There appear to be racial differences as well: cervical ribs are more common in African Americans and in individuals from the Levant.[11]

Arterial TOS is extremely rare compared to neurogenic and venous TOS. Series of operated patients in the literature from various vascular centers generally demonstrate the relative proportion of types of TOS as follows: neurogenic TOS 90%–95%, venous TOS 5%–8%, and arterial TOS only 1%–2%, the last including only scattered numbers of patients accumulated over many years' time.[12–14] The average vascular surgeon has been involved with the management of only a few such patients (the Author has treated 12 arterial TOS patients in a 40-year vascular surgical career).

CLINICAL PRESENTATION

Cervical Ribs

Cervical ribs are commonly asymptomatic. They may upon occasion be palpated, on a careful physical examination, as a hard mass in the medial supraclavicular region, but most commonly are discovered during an imaging assessment for neck, shoulder, and upper extremity pain, usually in pursuit of a diagnosis of cervical spine or shoulder abnormalities or of neurogenic or arterial TOS. Apical lordotic chest x-rays or, better, A-P cervical spine x-rays (Figure 25-1, left), commonly display these structures. As noted previously, such structures can also be discovered on CT (Figure 25-1, right) or MR studies of the cervical spine. Similar such imaging evaluations may reveal alternative skeletal abnormalities—dystopic or hypoplastic first and/or second ribs, callus from clavicular or first rib fractures—potentially resulting in neurogenic or arterial TOS.

Arterial TOS

Arterial TOS may be discovered consequent to the palpation of a pulsatile mass representing an ectopic or aneurysmal subclavian artery in the supraclavicular space. More commonly, patients present with ischemic symptoms and signs—upper extremity claudication, rest pain or numbness in the hands, trophic changes in the fingers (or—rarely—stroke or transient ischemic attack)—due to embolization from the stenotic or dilated (or both) subclavian artery. Unilateral development of finger and hand symptoms consistent with Raynaud syndrome may represent subtle digital arterial embolization due to an ipsilateral cervical rib. Upon occasions, this presentation may be sudden, as in acute limb ischemia: an immediate effort at revascularization by disobliteration of the occluded peripheral arteries—by thrombolysis (Figure 25-2), or by open surgical embolectomy—becomes obligatory (see "Surgical Approaches" below). More commonly, the patient presents with chronic upper extremity fatigue or claudication and is found to have an ipsilateral pulse deficit: on upper extremity vascular evaluation (most commonly duplex sonography) partial or complete occlusion of the brachial and/or more peripheral arteries will be discovered, a finding subsequently confirmed on upper extremity arteriography.

SURGICAL APPROACHES

It is generally accepted that a cervical rib, just by its presence, is not invariably associated with the development of *neurogenic* TOS; a large majority of patients harboring a cervical rib remain asymptomatic throughout their lives. Instead, sustaining a small degree of trauma is thought to set in motion the process which results in neurogenic

TOS in such individuals. And the development of *arterial* TOS due to a cervical rib (or other bony abnormality) is even less likely. However, it is important to note that recent studies assessing the subclavian arteries of patients with cervical ribs but no symptoms of arterial TOS have suggested a high proportion of silent intraluminal abnormalities.[15] The natural history of these asymptomatic subclavian artery abnormalities is not known but raises concerns that silent but progressive subclavian arterial degeneration occurs as long as the cervical rib is intact, and raising the possibility that preemptive excision of a cervical rib might be considered in order to halt such progressive deformation and extrinsic compression of the subclavian artery by the underlying osseous structure.

As intimated previously, the presence of symptoms and signs of acute upper extremity ischemia warrant an aggressive diagnostic and therapeutic approach. As for the lower extremities, most patients will undergo initiation of catheter-directed thrombolysis at the time of their diagnostic upper extremity arteriogram (Figure 25-2). Because chronic artery-to-artery embolization into the upper extremity may have occurred over a prolonged period of time, thrombolysis may be less than completely successful (the prior analogy to efforts at thrombolysis of chronically occluded tibial arteries distal to a popliteal artery aneurysm[7] is instructive in this regard).

Proceeding to open arterial embolectomy, at the antecubital fossa and at the wrist, is the next therapeutic step and may often be successful; if not, case reports in such settings suggest that revascularization by bypass grafting (prosthetic or biologic conduits or reversed great saphenous vein) maybe required.[16,17]

Resolution of the cause of the underlying bony problem, repair or ligation of the damaged subclavian artery, and distal revascularization are commonly undertaken in sequence. Via a supraclavicular approach, the diseased subclavian artery can be ligated or replaced. The bypass graft is anastomosed to the proximal subclavian artery or, occasionally, to the ipsilateral common carotid artery, then commonly (but not exclusively) passed through the costoclavicular space, usually anteromedial to the native subclavian artery, with distal anastomosis to the axillary, brachial, or (if necessary) the wrist arteries. In the Author's opinion, in view of the chronically damaged upper extremity arterial outflow in this setting (and the relative youth of many of these patients), use of an autogenous bypass graft should be emphasized. Similarly, long-term postoperative anticoagulation may be prudent.

Despite occasional case reports and small series[18] contemporary endovascular reconstructive procedures have not yet taken hold to any significant degree in the management of arterial TOS, likely because open surgery is already required, at a minimum, for rib resection: graft or bypass treatment for the damaged subclavian artery is more durable and is thus a better choice in this particular clinical setting.

Excision of a cervical rib can be carried out via diverse approaches. The transaxillary approach is cosmetically most acceptable, and also permits removal of the first thoracic rib, felt by many to provide maximal decompression of the thoracic outlet.[19] It also may have a lesser likelihood of intraoperative nerve traction injuries (Figure 25-3). A lateral intermuscular approach is said to provide access to the cervical rib with less risk to the brachial plexus and the phrenic and long thoracic nerves.[20] In unusual circumstances, such as the presence of a tumor of the first rib resulting in neurogenic TOS, the transaxillary approach may not provide adequate access for decompression, and a high posterolateral thoracotomy[21] or a posterior trapezius-splitting approach[22] may be required.

COMMENTS

Cervical ribs are not uncommon, and recent studies suggest that they likely have a higher prevalence than conventionally reported. They are not associated with the development of significant symptomatology a majority of the time; when they are symptomatic, most commonly the problem relates to the development of a form of *neurogenic* TOS. Cervical rib resulting in *arterial* TOS is significantly less common. Anatomic deformation of the subclavian artery over a cervical rib (or a similar bony abnormality) is almost always the underlying cause.

Management of symptomatic arterial TOS, while sometimes technically challenging, is straightforward from a decision-making perspective: the source of the presenting problem—the damaged subclavian artery—is repaired or replaced; the underlying cause—the cervical rib or other bony abnormality—is removed; and distal disease—occluded peripheral arteries and accompanying ischemia—is treated.[2] Similarly, neurogenic symptoms and signs arising from cervical ribs are generally resolved in straightforward fashion by thoracic outlet decompression including cervical rib excision.[19]

However, recent studies[15,19] demonstrating the presence of intraluminal subclavian artery abnormalities on duplex sonography or other imaging studies in asymptomatic patients with cervical ribs raises the possibility that these arteries may indeed be at risk for the development of the intraluminal or poststenotic dilatory abnormalities recognized as the progenitors for symptomatic arterial TOS. Are all patients with complete cervical ribs at risk for eventually developing subclavian artery damage and arterial TOS? Should cervical ribs be removed even when entirely asymptomatic?

While recent data do not—yet—support the conclusion that such asymptomatic and frequently subtle imaging abnormalities predictably progress to arterial TOS, these recent studies seem compelling enough that, at the least, it seems prudent to carry out ultrasonographic surveillance of the subclavian arteries in patients with cervical ribs (or equivalent osseous anomalies) to assure that there is no evidence for ongoing arterial disease in these patients. Post-operative surveillance of the subclavian arteries of patients who have undergone cervical rib excision for neurogenic TOS might be instructive in this regard as well.

REFERENCES

1. Halsted WS. An experimental study of circumscribed dilation of an artery immediately distal to a partially occluding band, and its bearing on dilation of the subclavian artery observed in certain cases of cervical rib. *J Exp Med*. 1916;24:217–286.
2. Illig K, Donahue D, Duncan A, et al. Reporting standards of the society for vascular surgery for thoracic outlet syndrome: executive summary. [Review]. *J Vasc Surg*. 2016;64:797–802.
3. Burnand K, Lagocki S, Lahiri R, et al. Persistent subclavian artery stenosis following surgical repair of non-union of a fractured clavicle. *Grand Rounds*. 2010;10;55–58.
4. Roach M. Post-stenotic dilatation in arteries. In: Bergel DH, ed. *Cardiovascular Fluid Dynamics*. Vol 2. London, England: Academic Press; 1972:111–139.
5. Sharma S, Kumar S, Joseph L, Singhal V. Cervical rib with stroke as the initial presentation. *Neurol India*. 2010;58:645–647.
6. Bearn P, Patel J, O'Flynn R. Cervical ribs: a cause of distal and cerebral embolism. *Postgrad Med J*. 1993;69:65–68.

7. Dorigo W, Pulli R, Alessi Innocenti A, et al. A 33-year experience with surgical management of popliteal artery aneurysms. *J Vasc Surg*. 2015;62:1176–1182.
8. Tender G, Thomas A, Thomas N, Kline D. Gilliatt-Sumner hand revisited: a 25-year experience. *Neurosurgery*. 2004;55:883–890.
9. Tubbs RS, Louis RG, Wartmann CT, et al. Histopathological basis for neurogenic thoracic outlet syndrome: laboratory investigation. *J Neurosurg Spine*. 2008;8:347–351.
10. Brewin J, Hill M, Ellis H. The prevalence of cervical ribs in a London population. *Clin Anat*. 2009;22:331–336.
11. Viertel V, Intrapiromkul J, Maluf J, et al. Cervical ribs: a common variant overlooked in T imaging. *Am J Neuroradiol*. 2012;33:2191–2194.
12. Chang K, Likes K, Davis K, Demos J, Freischlag J. The significance of cervical ribs in thoracic outlet syndrome. *J Vasc Surg*. 2013;57:771–775.
13. Durham JR, Yao JST, Pearce W, Nuber G, McCarthy III W. Arterial injuries in the thoracic outlet syndrome. *J Vasc Surg*. 1995;21:57–70.
14. Marine L, Valdes F, Mertens R, et al. Arterial thoracic outlet syndrome: a 32-year experience. *Ann Vasc Surg*. 2013;27:1007–1013.
15. Criado E, Berguer R, Greenfield L. The spectrum of arterial compression at the thoracic outlet. *J Vasc Surg*. 2010;52:406–411.
16. Bae M, Chung W, Chung S, Choi J, Kim M. Bypass surgery in arterial thoracic outlet syndrome. *Korean J Thorac Cardiovasc Surg*. 2015;48:146–150.
17. Vemuri C, McLaughlin L, Abuirqeba A, Thompson R. Clinical presentation and management of arterial thoracic outlet syndrome. *J Vasc Surg*. 2017;65:1429–1439.
18. Malliet C, Fourneau I, Daenens K, Maleux G, Nevelsteen A. Endovascular stent-graft and first rib resection for thoracic outlet syndrome complicated by an aneurysm of the subclavian artery. *Acta Chirurgica Belgica*. 2005;105:194–197.
19. Likes K, Rochlin D, Call D, Freischlag J. Coexistence of arterial compression in patients with neurogenic thoracic outlet syndrome. *JAMA Surg*. 2014;149:1240–1243.
20. Chauhan A, Ray M, Kumar S, Sabui K. Lateral intermuscular approach to cervical rib—Is it safe? *J Med Soc*. 2015;29:113–115.
21. Kemp C, Rushing G, Rodic N, McCarthy E, Yang. S. Thoracic outlet syndrome caused by fibrous dysplasia of the first rib. *Ann Thorac Surg*. 2012;93:994–996.
22. Molina JE, D'Cunha J. The vascular component in neurogenic-arterial thoracic outlet syndrome. *Int J Angiol*. 2008;17:83–87.

26

Upper Extremity Trauma and the Advanced Surgical Skills Exposures for Trauma (ASSET) Course

Col. (ret.) Mark W. Bowyer, MD, FACS, DMCC

Vascular trauma is a leading cause of morbidity and mortality worldwide, and rapid identification and control of hemorrhage is essential to survival. It is imperative that surgical trainees be proficient in the management of traumatically injured patients to include operative exposure and control of bleeding. Surgical training and vascular surgery training in particular face a number of significant current and future challenges. The introduction of work hour restrictions in the United States, the United Kingdom, and the European Union has led to dramatically decreased opportunities for exposure to clinical material.[1–8] The full impact of work hour restrictions has yet to be fully assessed. However, a recent study by the Royal College of Surgeons of England suggests that the quality of patient care has sharply declined because of the lack of continuity of care and further suggests that operative exposure is insufficient to ensure competency in a range of adequate procedures for independent practice.[9] The introduction of increasing complex procedures to include endovascular techniques has placed additional strain on the ability to ensure that competence and proficiency are achieved during the course of a residency or fellowship program.

In addition to the above, there has also been an increasing trend towards nonoperative management of trauma patients which has resulted in significant decrease in exposure by trainees to surgical experience with trauma.[10–13] The increasing specialization of vascular surgeons and their training has also diluted the available training cases for general surgery residents with the majority of open vascular cases being done by vascular surgeons and vascular residents/fellows to the detriment of general surgery trainees.[14–16] In spite of vascular surgery still being considered an integral part of general surgery training there has been a decreasing experience with vascular trauma among graduating residents. Over the last ten years the average number of major vascular repairs for trauma (includes repair of thoracic aorta, innominate, subclavian, neck vessels, abdominal aorta, peripheral and other vascular injuries) reported by graduating chief residents to the American Board of Surgery decreased from 4.7 in 2003–2004 to 2.3 in 2013–2014 over the course of a residency in general surgery (see Table 26-1).[17] It is important to bear in mind that the numbers reported are averages and as such there are significant numbers of trainees who have zero experience with caring for major vascular trauma. The exposure to vessels to the upper extremity either electively or in the management of trauma is likewise very limited. The Accredited Council of Graduate Medical Education (ACGME) case logs do not specifically report axillary artery exposures, but do list axillary-peripheral bypass which is an adequate surrogate for axillary artery exposure.[17] As seen in Table 26-1, axillary-femoral and other axillary-peripheral bypass procedures done by surgical residents over a residency have averaged between 0.6 and 0.9 with a trend towards decreasing performance. Brachial artery exposures for trauma were not tracked by the ACGME until the 2009–2010 reporting period and have averaged a dismal 0.0 to 0.1 since that time (Table 26-1). Experience with elective exposure of the brachial artery may be postulated from the tracked entry "Upper Extremity Bypass, Endarterectomy, or Repair"; which has an average over the last 10 years of 0.6 to 0.9 (Table 26-1). Additional experience with exposure of the vessels of the upper arm (brachial, radial, and ulnar arteries) can be postulated from the ACGME tracked entry "Vascular Access: Arterio-Venous fistulas and grafts," which averaged between 33.7 and 38.4 over the last decade (Table 26-1). Though only recently added to the case logs, reported experience with fasciotomy by graduating residents was similarly scant with a reported average of 1.5 in 2009–2010, with a decrease each subsequent year to 0.8 in 2013–2014 (Table 26-1).[17] This category does not describe which extremity the fasciotomy was done on, and it is likely that the average experience with fasciotomy of the upper extremity is closer to 0.0.

TABLE 26-1. AVERAGE NUMBER OF SELECTED CASES OVER DURATION OF TRAINING REPORTED BY GRADUATING SURGICAL CHIEF RESIDENTS SUPPLIED AS PART OF CASE LOGS SUBMITTED TO THE AMERICAN BOARD OF SURGERY FROM 2004 TO 2014

Report Year	04–05	05–06	06–07	07–08	08–09	09–10	10–11	11–12	12–13	13–14
Major Vascular Cases (trauma)	4.7	4.6	4.7	4.4	4.7	3.2	2.1	2.9	2.4	2.3
Ax-Fem, Axillary Peripheral Bypass	0.9	0.9	0.9	0.9	0.8	0.7	0.6	0.6	0.6	0.6
Brachial Artery Exposure	X	X	X	X	X	0.1	0.0	0.1	0.1	0.1
UE Bypass, Endarterectomy or repair	0.7	0.8	0.8	0.8	0.8	0.9	0.8	0.7	0.6	0.6
Vascular Access: AV fistulas/ grafts	36.4	38.4	37.9	36.3	36.3	36.2	35.2	36.3	34.2	33.7
Fasciotomy for Injury	X	X	X	X	X	1.5	1.2	1.0	0.8	0.8

Note: Numbers represent the mean for each procedure, and if missing (X), that procedure was not requested during that particular data collection year. Data collated from http://www.acgme.org/acgmeweb/tabid/274/DataCollectionSystems/ResidentCaseLogSystem/CaseLogsStatisticalReports.aspx.

Abbreviations: Ax-Fem = Axillo-Femoral; UE= Upper Extremity; AV = Arterio-Venous.

On the basis of the numbers presented, it is clear that general surgery residents in the United States have, on average, a suboptimal experience with the surgical management of vascular trauma, in spite of it being an integral part of general surgery training. In Canada, vascular surgery has been removed from the Canadian general surgery training objectives. In a recent survey of 29 Canadian surgical residents, 90% reported an intention to perform vascular procedures after training though they reported being inadequately trained in 10 of 13 procedures surveyed.[18] The authors of this study concluded that current trainees may lack the skills and abilities to deal with vascular emergencies. In spite of the growing prevalence of specialist trained vascular surgeons, there are still many areas in the world (developed and developing) where the primary surgeon may not always be a vascular surgical specialist. He or she may have had limited previous exposure to vascular surgery (which is becoming more limited with the specialization of training) and not be practicing the skills set regularly.

While it may be argued that the solution to this is to ensure that a fully trained vascular surgical specialist is available for every trauma case, this is not practical at the present time in many situations outside major centers and certainly in most areas of military and humanitarian surgical practice. Thus the need to train competent practitioners who can handle vascular trauma is universal.[19–21]

In the developed world, vascular trauma is being managed to a greater extent by trauma surgeons and vascular specialists than it has in the past.[20] In spite of this concentration, outside of major urban trauma centers with high percentages of penetrating trauma the experience in vascular trauma is also surprisingly limited for this group as well. As can be seen in Table 26-2, the numbers of major vascular repairs for trauma (thoracic, neck, abdomen, and peripheral vessels) reported to the ABS by vascular surgery fellows though significantly greater than reported by graduates of general surgery residencies, is limited with an average number of cases in the last decade reported between 8.7 and 12.5 during a vascular fellowship.[17] The experience with repair of peripheral vessels (included in the major vascular repairs cited above) averaged 7.2 to 9.0, and exposure of the axillary artery (Axillary-distal bypass) had an average range of 3.4 to 4.4 over the same period (Table 26-2). Experience with brachial

TABLE 26-2. AVERAGE NUMBER OF SELECTED CASES OVER DURATION OF TRAINING REPORTED BY VASCULAR FELLOWS DURING FELLOWSHIP SUPPLIED AS PART OF CASE LOG SUBMITTED TO THE AMERICAN BOARD OF SURGERY FROM 2004 TO 2014

	04–05	05–06	06–07	07–08	08–09	09–10	10–11	11–12	12–13	13–14
Major Vascular Cases (trauma)	8.7	10.9	10.6	10.9	12.5	11.3	10.8	10.7	11.2	12.2
Repair Peripheral Vessels	7.8	8.0	8.2	8.4	9.0	8.3	7.6	7.4	7.2	8.2
Ax-Fem, Axillary Peripheral Bypass	3.5	3.3	3.5	3.4	3.9	3.7	3.9	4.0	3.9	4.4
Brachial Artery Exposure	X	X	X	0.1	0.1	0.3	0.3	0.2	0.4	0.3
Vascular Access: AV fistulas/ grafts	16.6	20.0	21.6	22.2	25.5	28.1	31.1	34.7	34.6	38.7
Fasciotomy for Injury	1.2	1.0	1.2	1.0	1.4	1.4	1.4	2.0	2.0	2.3

Note: Numbers represent the mean for each procedure, and if missing (X), that procedure was not requested during that particular data collection year. Data collated from http://www.acgme.org/acgmeweb/tabid/274/DataCollectionSystems/ResidentCaseLogSystem/CaseLogsStatisticalReports.aspx.

Abbreviations: Ax-Fem = Axillo-Femoral; UE= Upper Extremity; AV = Arterio-Venous.

artery exposure (average 0.1 to 0.4) and fasciotomy, not specified by extremity (1.0 to 2.3) was also remarkably low, and the experience with AV fistulas and grafts (surrogate of elective exposure to brachial, radial, and ulnar arteries was similar if not somewhat less than surgical residents averaging between 16.6 and 38.7 (Table 26-2).[17]

When looking at the practice of specialist vascular surgeons in the United States who recertify in vascular surgery, the number of cases of vascular trauma experience is also quite low. Only 46% of vascular surgeons reported a vascular trauma experience (a one-year experience prior to taking the recertification exam) of greater than zero with a mean average of 4.0 for the remainder in 2003, and in 2009 only 23% reported a vascular trauma experience of greater than zero with a mean of 4.0 for the remainder.[22]

Though it is difficult to judge proficiency and competence by numbers alone, it is clear that the experience of trainees is anything but uniform and that we are graduating specialists with a surprisingly wide spectrum of abilities who when called upon to care for vascular trauma may or may not have the requisite skill set to ensure optimal outcomes. Likewise, a minority of practicing vascular surgeons report having the management of vascular trauma as even a small part of their clinical practice. As such there is a critical need to improve the way we train and maintain the skills of the surgeon caring for vascular trauma in the future.

THE ASSET COURSE

In recognition of these significant training gaps, the American College of Surgeons (ACS) Committee on Trauma (COT) leadership established a Surgical Skills Committee in 2005. This committee was charged with developing a standardized, skills-based cadaver course designed to teach surgical exposure of vital structures that are most likely to pose an immediate threat to life or limb when injured.[23,24] The result of this effort was the development of the Advanced Surgical Skills for Exposure in Trauma (ASSET) course.

The ASSET course is a one-day, case-based, scenario-driven dissection course using unpreserved (fresh) human cadavers, emphasizing surgical exposure of extremity, neck, chest, abdomen, and pelvic vasculature, with additional instruction in fasciotomies and pelvic packing. The target audience of this course is senior surgical residents, trauma fellows, and practicing surgeons who care for victims of trauma. The course is done entirely in the lab with a student to faculty ratio of 4:1. The skills included in the course were culled from a comprehensive list of all possible exposures needed for trauma and a modified Delphi approach was utilized to choose 59 separate skills deemed relevant to the management of trauma for inclusion in the course.[23,24] The committee subsequently developed a course manual, narrated videos of selected procedures, faculty manual, lab slides, and assessment tools, all of which were subjected to review by subject matter and educational experts. A demonstration course was conducted at the Uniformed Services University of the Health Sciences in March of 2008, followed by three additional beta courses, during which the course was further refined prior to final approval and released of the course as an ACS-branded continuing medical education course in March of 2010.[23,24] Since that time the course has been widely adopted, and there are now over 80 approved sites throughout the United States and Canada,[25] as well as sites in Thailand, the United Kingdom, Norway, France, Germany, and Sweden that have conducted more than 300 courses to date.

Additionally, the ASSET course has become the de facto cadaver training course for predeployment training of U.S. military surgeons.

The skills taught in the ASSET course relevant to the upper extremity (UE) include exposure of the axillary artery, the brachial artery, and the ulnar and radial arteries in the forearm. Additionally, fasciotomy of the forearm and hand is taught in the course as well. The course is accompanied by a richly illustrated manual that describes the detailed steps of the exposures in a bullet point format. Examples of the photos used in the text (shot by the author but not included in the ASSET manual) can be found in Figures 26-1 and 26-2.

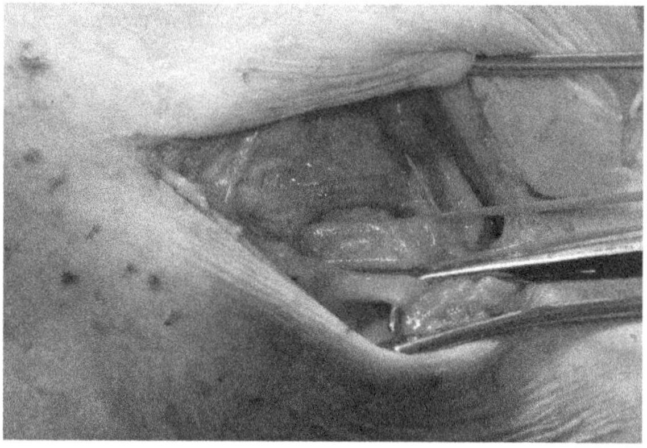

Figure 26-1. Representative photo of the step by step exposure of the axillary artery taught in the ASSET course. The photo is oriented with the right neck to the left lower corner. An infra-clavicular incision has been made, the pectoralis major muscle split, and the pectoralis minor muscle divided to demonstrate (from top to bottom) the axillary vein, axillary artery (with red vessel loop), and the brachial plexus (retracted upwards by right-angle clamp)

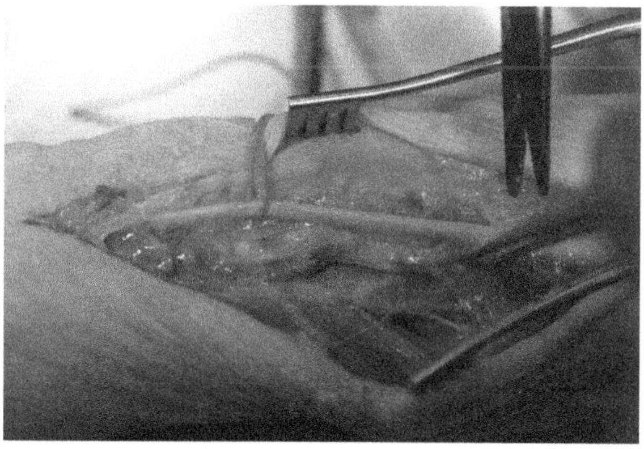

Figure 26-2. Representative photo of the step-by-step exposure of the brachial artery taught in the ASSET course. The photo depicts the right arm of a fresh cadaver with the radial aspect of the arm superior and the wrist to the left of the photo. The median nerve is tagged with a red vessel loop, and the brachial artery is seen immediately inferior to the nerve.

The course has been well received and prior reviews of the course effect have shown significant improvements over base line for both surgical trainees and practicing surgeons for all of the procedures taught in the course. In a review of the first 25 courses, Bowyer et al. found that for 214 participants, significant improvements over baseline self-reported efficacy or comfort level (on a 5-point Likert scale) for exposure of the axillay artery (2.95 vs. 4.19; $P < 4.2 \times 10^{-37}$); exposure of the brachial artery (3.35 vs. 4.27; $P < 1.7 \times 10^{-27}$); and for the performance of forearm fasciotomy (2.76 vs. 4.05; $P < 2.7 \times 10^{-32}$).[15] The ASSET course is currently undergoing a validation study in which surgical trainees who have not taken the course (novices) are asked to perform both axillary and brachial artery exposures (among others) in a fresh cadaver without coaching, while being scored with rigidly developed metrics both in real time and by blinded experts reviewing videos of their performance. In this ongoing validation study, senior surgical trainees were noted in this study to have significantly more confidence in their both the ability to expose the axillary and brachial arteries and their knowledge of anatomy required to perform these exposures than did expert evaluators.[27] This study highlighted significant gaps in anatomical knowledge and the preparation of surgical trainees to care for vascular injuries to the upper extremity, and should serve as a wake-up call for surgical educators.

CONCLUSIONS

Current graduates of general surgical residencies and vascular fellowships are in general ill-prepared to care for vascular injuries to the upper extremities. The reasons behind this are multi-factorial as outlined above, and the solution will need to be multi-modality as well. Increased emphasis on anatomy and broad operative experience with exposure and repair of blood vessels is needed and will require augmentation with specifically designed curricula such as the ASSET course to fill the gaps.

DISCLAIMER

The views, opinions and/or findings contained in this publication are those of the author and do not necessarily reflect the views of the Department of Defense and should not be construed as an official DoD/Army/Air Force position, policy, or decision unless so designated by other documentation. No official endorsement should be made.

REFERENCES

1. Lamont PM, Scott DJ. The impact of shortened training times on the discipline of vascular surgery in the United Kingdom. *Am J Surg*. 2005;190:269–72.
2. Pellegrini CA, Warshaw AL, Debas HT. Residency training in surgery in the 21st century: a new paradigm. *Surgery*. 2004;136:953–65.
3. Bell RH Jr, Banker MB, Rhodes RS, Biester TW, Lewis FR. Graduate medical education in surgery in the United States. *Surg Clin North Am*. 2007;87:811–23.
4. Ferguson C, Kellog K, Hutter M, Warshaw A. Effect of work-hour reforms on operative case volume of surgical residents. *Curr Surg*. 2005;62:535–8.
5. De Martino RR, Brewster LP, Kokkosis AA, et al. The perspective of the vascular surgery trainee on new ACGME regulations, fatigue, resident training and patient safety. *Vasc Endovascular Surg*. 2011;45:697–702.
6. Sadababa JR, Urso S. Does the introduction of duty-hour restrictions in the United States negatively affect the operative volume of surgical trainees? *Interact Cardiovasc Thorac Surg*. 2011;13:316–319.
7. Damadi A, Davis AT, Saxe A, Apelgren K. ACME duty-hour restrictions decrease resident operative volume: a 5-year comparison at an ACGME-accredited university general surgery residency. *J Surg Educ*. 2007;64:256–9.
8. Drake FT, Van Eaton EG, Huntington CR, et al. ACGME case logs: surgery resident experience in operative trauma for two decades. *J Trauma Acute Care Surg*. 2012;73:1500–6.
9. Thomas RL, Karanja N. Comparison of SHO surgical log books a generation apart. *Ann R Coll Surg Eng*. 2009;9(suppl):356–9.
10. Bulinski P, Bachulis B, Naylor DF, et al. The changing face of trauma management and its impact on surgical resident training. *J Trauma*. 2003;54:161–3.
11. Bittner JG 4th, Hawkins ML, Medeioros RS, et al. Nonoperative management of solid organ injury diminishes surgical resident operative experience: is it time for simulation training? *J Surg Res*. 2010;163:179–85.
12. Brigham RA, Salander JM. Lack of a significant exposure to trauma by residents. *Mil Med*. 1989 Nov;154(11):581.
13. Gaarder C, Skaga NO, Eken T, et al. The impact of patient volume on surgical trauma training in a Scandinavian trauma centre. *Injury*. 2005;36:1288–92.

14. Joels CS, Langan EM 3rd, Cull DL, Kalbaugh CA, Taylor SM. Effects of increased vascular surgical specialization on general surgery trainees, practicing surgeons, and the provision of vascular surgical care. *J Am Coll Surg.* 2009 May;208(5):692–7.
15. Grabo DJ, DiMuzio PJ, Kairys JC, et al. Have endovascular procedures negatively impacted general surgery training? *Ann Surg.* 2007;246:472–7.
16. Cronenwett JL. Vascular surgery training: is there enough case material? *Semin Vasc Surg.* 2006;19:187–90.
17. Accreditation Council for Graduate Medical Education. http://www.acgme.org/acgmeweb/tabid/274/DataCollectionSystems/ResidentCaseLogSystem/CaseLogsStatisticalReports.aspx. Accessed June 5, 2015.
18. Boutros J, Sekhon M, Webber E, et al. Vascular surgery training, exposure, and knowledge during general surgery residency: implications for the future. *Am J Surg.* 2007;193:561–6.
19. van Bockel JH, Bergqvist D, Cairols M, et al. European Section and Board of Vascular Surgery of the European Union of Medical Specialists. Education in vascular surgery: critical issues around the globe-training and qualification in vascular surgery in Europe. *J Vasc Surg.* 2008 Dec;48(6 Suppl):69S–75S.
20. Burkhardt GE, Rasmussen TE, Propper BW, et al. A national survey of evolving management patterns for vascular injury. *J Surg Educ.* 2009 Sep-Oct;66(5):239–47.
21. Eckert M, Cuadrado D, Steele S, et al. The changing face of the general surgeon: national and local trends in resident operative experience. *Am J Surg.* 2010 May;199(5):652–6.
22. Eidt JF, Mills J, Rhodes RS, et al. Comparison of surgical operative experience of trainees and practicing vascular surgeons: a report from the Vascular Surgery Board of the American Board of Surgery. *J Vasc Surg.* 2011 Apr;53(4):1130–9.
23. Kuhls DA, Risucci DA, Bowyer MW, Luchette FA. Advanced surgical skills for exposure in trauma: A new surgical cadaver course for residents and fellows. *J Trauma Acute Care Surg.* 2013;74:664–70.
24. Kuhls DA, Risucci DA, Bowyer MW, Luchette FA. ASSET: An effective educational experience for practicing surgeons. *Bull Am Coll Surg.* 2012;97:31–5.
25. Ali J, Sorvari A, Haskin D, Luchette F, Bowyer M. Potential role of the Advanced Surgical Skills for Exposure in Trauma (ASSET) course in Canada. *J Trauma.* 2011;71:1491–3.
26. Bowyer MW, Kuhls DA, Haskin D, et al. Advanced Surgical Skills for Exposure in Trauma (ASSET): the first 25 courses. *J Surg Res.* 2013;183:553–8.
27. Bowyer MW, Shackelford SA, Garofalo E, Pugh K, Mackenzie CF. Perception does not equal reality for resident vascular trauma skills. *J Surg Res.* 2015 Apr 1. pii: S0022-4804(15)00347-9. doi: 10.1016/j.jss.2015.03.082. [Epub ahead of print.]

27

Management of Upper Extremity Arterial Civilian Trauma

Nicole Toscano, MD and Michael Stoner, MD

Upper extremity arterial civilian injury is a complex problem that requires coordinated surgical care to minimize risk of morbidity and mortality. A majority of the knowledge regarding diagnosis and management strategies of upper extremity vascular trauma has evolved from combat experience during World War II. Many studies have emphasized the importance of prompt diagnosis to prevent massive blood loss and tissue ischemia to maximize opportunities for limb salvage and preserve limb function.

Literature suggests the annual incidence of upper extremity vascular injury to be approximately 30-40%.[1] In both the civilian and military setting a majority of these injuries result from penetrating trauma with blunt trauma resulting in significant morbidity and mortality. Both mechanisms can result in concomitant injuries involving neighboring bone, veins, and nerves causing significant morbidity and mortality.

INITIAL ASSESSMENT AND EVALUATION

Evaluation of patients with upper extremity vascular trauma should follow a systematic approach as defined by the American College of Surgeons Advanced Trauma Life Support, by first performing a primary survey.[2] Rapid assessment of airway patency, breathing and ventilation, circulatory status, and neurologic status allows providers to quickly determine patient stability, begin resuscitation, and prioritize injury management.[2] Evidence of active bleeding requires immediate hemorrhage control, which is most effectively provided with direct pressure at the bleeding site or at the most proximal artery. Resuscitation should allow for permissive hypotension with goal systolic blood pressures of 90 mmHg to prevent excessive bleeding. Ongoing assessment with a secondary survey should involve careful assessment for pulse discrepancies between extremities, neurologic deficits, and identification of fractures or bony deformities. If patient stability permits, a brief history can be taken focusing on key factors including time of injury, mechanism of injury, estimated blood loss in the pre-hospital setting, as well as the type of weapon that may have been used.

Diagnosis of vascular injury begins with a thorough physical examination for the presence of hard and soft signs of injury. Hard signs include witnessed active arterial bleeding, pulse deficit, expanding hematoma, evidence of distal ischemia, presence of bruit or thrill, or ankle brachial index < 1.0. Soft signs of injury include trauma in close proximity to a major vessel, presence of a neurologic deficit, history of hemorrhage at the scene, or non-expanding hematoma. Unstable patients or patients with hard signs of arterial injury warrant immediate operative intervention and repair without further diagnostic imaging.

Clinically stable patients with suspected vascular injury should undergo imaging to define anatomy and direct treatment options. There are a number of imaging modalities that can be utilized to aid in diagnosis including duplex ultrasound, magnetic resonance imaging, and axial computed tomography. However, catheter-directed arteriography is the most effective and reliable method of diagnosis and can be safely pursued in the unstable patients transported immediately to the operating room. Additional imaging with x-ray and computed tomography can be obtained to rule out presence of concomitant injuries including fractures, thoracic, mediastinal, and intra-abdominal injuries.

COMMON PRESENTING INJURIES

Arterial trauma of the upper extremity is defined as injury to the vasculature distal to the lateral border of the first rib, which includes the axillary, brachial, radial and ulnar arteries.[3] Injury to the brachial artery is the most commonly reported arterial injury to the upper extremity followed by the radial and ulnar artery in the forearm. Some institutions have reported an incidence of brachial artery trauma of 28%.[4] The superficial nature of this artery makes it highly susceptible to injury. Evidence of supracondylar fractures or posterior elbow dislocation should prompt providers to investigate for potential injury to the brachial artery.[4–5]

Trauma to the subclavian and axillary artery are rare and only account for 3% to 9% of all civilian vascular trauma.[6-10] Modern studies have estimated morbidity and mortality rates from axillosubclavian injuries of 5% to 39%.[8,11–13] Although relatively rare in occurrence, these injuries can have significant morbidity and mortality secondary to hemorrhagic shock and brachial plexus injuries. Patients with axillosubclavian injuries commonly present with hemodynamic instability and first rib, clavicle, or humerus fractures. On physical examination supraclavicular swelling may be present with resultant respiratory distress secondary to tracheal compression. Basic imaging studies may reveal the presence of a hemopneumothorax on chest X-ray. It is also important to remember that while patients may present with a number of concomitant injuries that may also present with a mixed pattern of vascular injury and multiple arterial vascular injuries may be identified.

TIMING OF REPAIR

Revascularization of the upper extremity should be pursued within 4 to 6 hours of injury. Studies suggest critical ischemic times for more proximal injuries are shorter, measuring only four hours. However, these times may be extended up to 12 hours in the setting of injuries distal to the brachial artery.[14] Significant delay in hemorrhage control and restoration of inline flow may result in loss of function and increases risk of limb amputation. These patients are at significant risk for interval development of compartment syndrome. Patients should undergo immediate fasciotomy or be monitored closely for signs and symptoms of increased compartment pressures including pain with passive range of motion, pallor, and motor or sensory deficits. Failure to perform fasciotomy in these patients can result in irreversible limb ischemia, neurologic deficits or limb loss.[15] If direct repair is not immediately possible, various strategies such as shunting may be utilized to promote limb salvage.

In the setting of concurrent vascular, orthopedic, and soft tissue injuries there is much controversy regarding what is the most appropriate sequence of repair. Historically, there was concern that without bony stabilization initially, vascular repairs would be at risk for disruption while other studies demonstrated significant concern for prolonged ischemia with delay in revascularization.[16-22] Current literature suggests that prompt revascularization should not be delayed for bony repair or soft tissue reconstruction if there is evidence of limb ischemia to ensure limb salvage.[23] In general, orthopedic fractures and dislocations should be reduced with external fixation or traction ideally prior to diagnostic imaging or revascularization. Diligent pulse assessment is essential with extremity manipulation. Once revascularization and bony stabilization have been achieved timing and consideration of soft tissue coverage can be discussed.

OPEN REVASCULARIZATION

Arterial injury to the thoracic outlet and upper extremity can be especially challenging to manage given surrounding bony anatomy as well the presence of concomitant injuries. Patients should be prepped and draped in a manner that facilitates proximal and distal control of the vascular injury and need for distal fasciotomy at the conclusion of the procedure. The surgeon should have a complete knowledge of exposure multiple exposure techniques (Table 27-1). Consideration should be made to prep the lower extremity for potential saphenous vein harvest as an autologous conduit. Longitudinal incisions overlying the potential arterial injury should be made with incisions extended to facilitate proximal and distal control. With injuries of the thoracic outlet median sternotomy may be required to ensure proximal control. Endoluminal balloon occlusion can be considered if there is difficulty with hemorrhage control. Once the injury is identified the artery should be debrided to healthy intima. The type of repair ultimately performed is directed by the extent of arterial injury as well as location of the injury. Small lacerations to the vessel, typically less than 2cm, can undergo primary repair. If primary repair cause significant luminal narrowing patch angioplasty with either vein or prosthetic graft should be considered. Arteries that have been completely transected will likely require interposition grafts with autologous conduit or prosthetic grafts. Literature and current guidelines suggests that prosthetic grafts such as polytetrafluoroethylene (PTFE) graft may be utilized in the setting of contaminated fields.[24] However, this should be a temporary solution to facilitate prompt revascularization and limb salvage with consideration for interval autologous reconstruction.[25] Non-viable soft tissue should be debrided. Soft tissue coverage of graft material is essential to minimize

TABLE 27-1. SURGICAL APPROACH AND CONSIDERATIONS OF THE UPPER EXTREMITY ARTERIAL TREE

Artery	Approach	Considerations
Right Subclavian	Median Sternotomy	Good central aortic exposure, can still expose distal extremity
Left Subclavian	Anterolateral thoracotomy	Proximal control good, limited mid-distal exposure
	Trapdoor thoracotomy	Allows more radical exposure
Axillary	Infraclavicular	First portion
	Lateral	Second and third portions, positioning may limit distal arm and forearm repairs
	Deltapectoral	All portions of artery
Brachial	Medial approach	Wide incision allows excellent exposure of neurovascular structures
Brachial Bifurcation	Transverse or S-shaped antecubital	Likely prefer S-shaped to allow proximal and distal extension
Radial	Lateral volar	Variable radial nerve
Ulnar	Medical volar	Nerve in close proximity in the proximal forearm

risk of infection and pseudoaneurysm. Post-operatively patients may require anticoagulation or antiplatelet agents if prosthetic grafts are utilized.

Following distal revascularization patients are at high risk for interval development of compartment syndrome of the upper extremity. Compartment syndrome develops secondary to a rapid rise in pressure within an osteofascial compartment secondary to tissue ischemia.[26–28] The forearm compartments are at higher risk of reperfusion injury compared to the upper arm. After inline flow is established to the distal upper extremity, performing a forearm fasciotomy should be considered prior to leaving the surgical suite. Typically, patients within 4 to 6 hours of critical ischemic time, should undergo prophylactic fasciotomy. Compartment syndrome is a clinical diagnosis, which can be made in the setting of pain out of proportion to injury, pain with passive range of motion, paralysis, and sensory deficitis.[28] Patients that are unable to participate in physical examination can be assessed using a Stryker needle to measure intra-compartment pressures, with pressures greater than 30mmHg suggestive of compartment syndrome.[29] Patient's diagnosed with compartment syndrome should undergo fasciotomy performed via a single volar incision to decompress the three major compartments of the forearm.[30] Fasciotomy incisions can undergo delayed primary closure, healing by secondary intention facilitated by placement of a negative pressure healing system, as well as skin grafting.

Non-operative management can be considered in patients with low-velocity injuries and intact distal circulation. These patients require close follow-up within one to two weeks as they may require elective repair.

Venous injuries to the upper extremity should be addressed briefly. Management of venous injuries in the upper extremity remains a controversial topic with some advocating for repair and others, ligation.[31–32] Small lacerations can be repaired primarily or with vein patch or interposition graft. However, complex venous reconstruction should not be attempted and significant venous injury should be controlled with ligation.

ENDOVASCULAR REPAIR

Conventional vascular repairs of the upper extremity are technically challenging. Recent literature has suggested utilization of a more minimally invasive approach through endovascular interventions. These approaches while appealing require proper patient selection. Endovascular repair should be considered in patients with axillosubclavian injuries including pseudoaneurysm, arteriovenous fistula, first-order branch vessel injury or avulsion, arterial intimal flap or focal arterial laceration (Figure 27-1).[33] With the advent of endovascular surgical suites, hybrid procedures can be utilized either for repair or even balloon occlusion in conjunction with primary repair. It is imperative that endovascular procedures not delay revascularization and ultimately conventional repair should be considered if there is inability to safely manipulate the wire to cross the affected lesion in a timely manner.

CONSIDERATION OF THE MANGLED UPPER EXTREMITY

The mangled upper extremity can be a complex problem resulting in profound lifestyle modifications. Significant traumatic injury can result in the mangled extremity secondary to tissue ischemia and direct skin, soft tissue, bone, and neurovascular destruction.[34] A variety of scoring systems have been utilized to aid in identification of patients that should undergo attempted limb salvage versus amputation including the Mangled Extremity Syndrome Index (MESI), the Mangled Extremity Severity

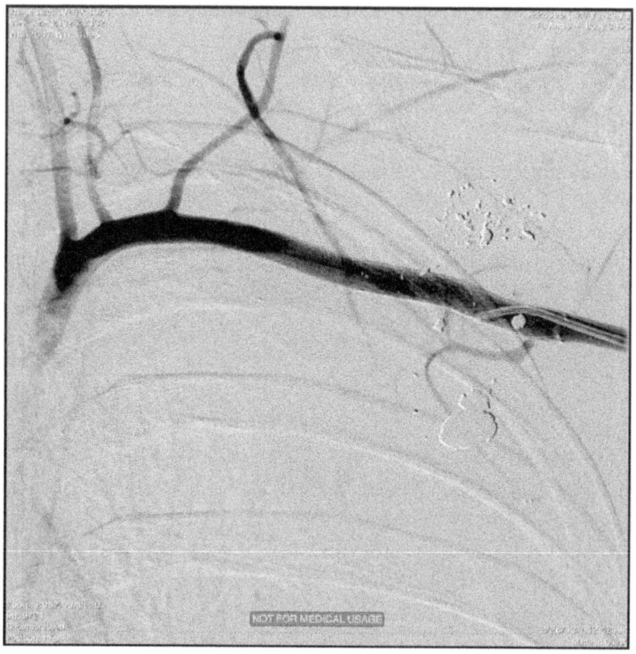

Figure 27-1. Successful deployment of a stent-graft (Viabahn, W.L. Gore & Associates, Flagstaff, AZ) from a transbrachial approach in a case of axillary artery transection from a gun shot wound.

Score (MESS), the Predictive Salvage Index (PSI), and the Limb Salvage Index (LSI).[35] Multiple studies have shown a MESS greater than or equal to 7 effectively predict amputation rates in the lower extremity.[36–37] However, given the significant morbidity associated with loss of an upper extremity every attempt should be made to salvage the limb with amputation as a last resort. The aforementioned scoring systems in additional to clinical stability should be used to assess attempts for limb salvage versus amputation.

CONCLUSION

Successful management of upper extremity vascular trauma requires a coordinated approach by multiple surgeons. Communication between surgical teams and prompt recognition are paramount to successful limb salvage and functional recovery. Most injuries are best approached via an open technique, although endovascular repair does have a utility in selected proximal cases.

REFERENCES

1. Rich NM, Mattox KL, Hirshbery A. In: Rich NM, editor. *Vascular Trauma*. Philadelphia, PA: Elsevier Saunders, 2004. pp. 223–40.
2. American College of Surgeons. *ATLS: Advanced Trauma Life Support for Doctors*. 8th ed. Chicago, IL: American College of Surgeons; 2008.
3. Hunt CA and Kingsley JR. Vascular injuries of the upper extremity. *South Med J*. 2000;93(5):466–8.
4. Zellweger R, Hess F, Nicol A, et al. An analysis of 124 surgically managed brachial artery injuries. *Am J Surg*. 2004;188(3):240–5.
5. Endean ED, Veldenz HC, Schwarcz TH, Hyde GL. Recognition of arterial injury in elbow dislocation. *J Vasc Surg*. 1992;16(3):402–6.
6. Graham JM, Feliciano DV, Mattox KI, Beall AC, DeBakey M. Management of subclavian vascular injuries. *J Trauma*. 1980;20:537–44.
7. McKinley AG, Carrim AT, Robbs JV. Management of proximal axillary and subclavian arterial injuries. *Br J Surg*. 2000;87:79–85.
8. Danetz JS, Cassano AD, Stoner MC, Ivatury RR, Levy MM. Feasibility of endovascular repair in penetrating axillosubclavian injuries: A retrospective review. *J Vasc Surg*. 2005;41:246–54.
9. DeBakey ME, Simeone FA. Battle injuries of arteries in World War II: An analysis of 2,471 cases. *Ann Surg*. 1946;123:534–79.
10. Graham JM, Mattox KL, Feliciano DV, DeBakey ME. Vascular injuries of the axilla. *Ann Surg*. 1982;195:232–8.
11. Flint LM, Snyder WH, Perry MO, Shires GT. Management of major vascular injuries in the base of the neck. *Arch Surg*. 1973;106:407–13.
12. Demetriades D, Chahwan S, Gomex H, et al. Penetrating injuries to the subclavian and axillary vessels. *J Am Coll Surg*. 1999;188:290–5.
13. Lin PH, Koffron AJ, Guske PJ, Lujan HJ, Heilizer TJ, Yario RF, et al. Penetrating injuries of the subclavian artery. *Am J Surg*. 2003;185:580–4.
14. Shackford S, Rich N. Peripheral vascular injury: *Trauma*. Feliciano DV, Moore EE, Mattox KL, (eds). Norwalk, Appleton and Lange, 3rd Ed, 1996, pp 819–51.
15. Percival TJ and Rasmussen TE. Reperfusion strategies in the management of extremity vascular injury with ischaemia. *Br J Surg*. 2012;99(S1):66–74.

16. McHenry TP, Holcomb JB, Aoki N, Lindsey RW. Fractures with major vascular injuries from gunshot wounds: implications of surgical sequence. *J Trauma.* 2002;53(4):717–21.
17. Bishara RA, Pasch AR, Lim LT, et al. Improved results in the treatment of civilian vascular injuries associated with fractures and dislocations. *J Vasc Surg.* 1986;3:707–11.
18. Karavias D, Korovessis P, Filos KS, et al. Major vascular lesions associated with orthopaedic injuries. *J Orthop Trauma.* 1992;6:180–5.
19. Zinman C, Norman D, Hamoud K, Reis ND. External fixation for severe open fractures of the humerus caused by missiles. *J Orthop Trauma.* 1997;11:536–9.
20. Luetic V, Sosa F, Tonkovic I, et al. Military vascular injuries in Croatia. *Cardiovasc Surg.* 1993;1:3–6.
21. Connolly J. Management of fractures associated with arterial injuries. *Am J Surg.* 1971;120–331.
22. Rich NM, Metz CW, Hutton JE, Baugh JH, Hughes CW. Internal versus external fixation of fractures with concomitant vascular injuries in Vietnam. *J Trauma.* 1971;11:463–73.
23. Mavrogenis AF, Panagopoulos GN, Kokkalis ZT, et al. Vascular injury in orthopedic trauma. *Orthopedics.* 2016; .http://dx.doi: 10.3928/01477447-20160610-06 [online advanced release].
24. Fox N, Rajani RR, Bokhari F, et al. Evaluation and management of penetrating lower extremity arterial trauma: An Eastern Association for the Surgery of Trauma practice management guideline. *J Trauma Acute Care Surg* 2012;73(5): S315–S320.
25. Vertrees A, Fox CJ, Quan RW, et al. The use of prosthetic grafts in complex military vascular trauma: a limb salvage strategy for patients with severely limited autologous conduit. *J Trauma.* 2009;66(4):980–3.
26. Dente CJ, Feliciano DV, Rozycki GS, et al. A Review of upper extremity fasciotomies in a level 1 trauma center. *Am Surg.* 2004;70(12):1088–93.
27. Feliciano DV, Cruse PA, Spjut-Patrinely V, Burch JM, Mattox KL. Fasciotomy after trauma to the extremities. *Am J Surg.* 1988;156(6):533–6.
28. Ritenour AE Dorlac WC Fang R, et al. Complications after fasciotomy revision and delayed compartment release in combat patients. *J Trauma.* 2007;64(2):S153–S162.
29. Tremblay LN, Feliciano DV, Rozycki GS. Secondary extremity compartment syndrome. *J Trauma.* 2002;53:833–7.
30. Nwakile OI, Sreenivasa AR, Christopher BT, Craig RS. A single volar incision fasciotomy will decompress all three forearm compartments: A cadaver study. *Injury.* 2012;43(11):1949–52.
31. Timberlake GA, O'Connell RC, Kerstein MD. Venous injury: To repair or ligate, the dilemma. *J Vasc Surg.* 1986;4(6):553–8.
32. Rich NM, Hughes CW, Baugh JH. Management of venous injuries. *Ann Surg.* 1970;171(5):724–30.
33. Danetz JS, Cassano AD, Stoner MC, Ivatury RR, Levy MM. Feasibility of endovascular repair in penetrating axillosubclavian injuries: a retrospective review. *J Vasc Surg.* 2005;41(2):246–54.
34. Bumbasirevic M, Stevanovic M, Lesic A, Atkinson HD. Current management of the mangled upper extremity. *Int Orthop.* 2012;36(11):2189–95.
35. Durham RM, Mistry BM, Mazuski JE, Shapiro M, Jacobs D. Outcome and utility of scoring systems in the management of the mangled extremity. *Am J Surg.* 1996;172:569–74.
36. Daines JK, Howey T, Hansen ST. The mangled extremity: Limb salvage versus amputation. *J Trauma.* 1990;62(6):563-563–76.
37. Kumar MK, Badole CM, Patond KR. Salvage versus amputation: Utility of mangled extremity severity score in severely injured lower limbs. *IJO.* 2007;41(3):183–7.

28

Outcome Comparison Between Open and Endovascular Repair of Axillosubclavian Arterial Injuries

Bruce L. Tjaden, Jr., MD and Naveed U. Saqib, MD

INTRODUCTION

> *As he piled wood on the fire he discovered an appreciation of his own body which he had never felt before. He watched his moving muscles and was interested in the cunning mechanism of his fingers. By the light of the fire he crooked his fingers slowly and repeatedly, now one at a time, now all together, spreading them wide or making quick gripping movements. He studied the nail-formation, and prodded the finger-tips, now sharply, and again softly, gauging the while the nerve-sensations produced. It fascinated him, and he grew suddenly fond of this subtle flesh of his that worked so beautifully and smoothly and delicately. Then he would cast a glance of fear at the wolf-circle drawn expectantly about him, and like a blow the realization would strike him that this wonderful body of his, this living flesh, was no more than so much meat, a quest of ravenous animals, to be torn and slashed by their hungry fangs, to be sustenance to them as the moose and the rabbit had often been sustenance to him[...] Never had he been so fond of this body of his as now when his tenure of it was so precarious.*[1]

The powerful passage above is taken from Jack London's classic serialized story *White Fang*. Though the prospect of being devoured by wolves is not common among our patients, the excerpt is still relevant. It captures the desperate realization of vulnerability of those who find themselves at risk of the limb loss or injury. Upper extremity vascular trauma and especially axillosubclavian arterial (ASA) injuries are particularly likely to lead to long-term morbidity and mortality. As vascular surgeons, we are uniquely poised to treat these injuries and to help our patients maintain their tenure of "the wonderful body of [theirs;] this living flesh." This chapter discusses both open and endovascular management of ASA injuries and compares the outcomes of these distinct, and sometimes complimentary, approaches.

BACKGROUND AND SIGNIFICANCE

It has been said that "[m]an has always had to face the problem of hemorrhage."[2] For thousands of years, the only surgical interventions performed were attempts at hemostasis. The development of modern vascular surgical principles and the lessons learned during the Korean and Vietnam Wars revolutionized the management of extremity vascular trauma. Still, extremity vascular injuries remain a significant source of morbidity and mortality in the modern era.

Five to nine percent of vascular trauma takes the form of ASA injury.[3,4] Unlike most civilian vascular trauma, they are usually due to penetrating injuries.[5,6] These proximal injuries are less common than more distal arterial damage, due to the relative protection offered by the bony thoracic cage protecting this location.[7] However, due to the risk of central hemorrhage and associated injuries to the brachial plexus, they carry a high morbidity and mortality rate.[4,8,9] Modern series report mortality rates greater that 20%.[3] Indeed, prehospital death rates can reach 80%,[6] and axillosubclavian vascular injuries requiring emergency department thoracotomy are almost always fatal.[4]

Traditional open surgical repair of axillosubclavian vascular injuries involves at least a periclavicular incision. Depending on the anatomy of the injury, more extensive exposures have been required, such as an anterior thoracotomy, midline sternotomy with or without cervical extension, sternoclavicular joint dissociation, and rarely clavicular resection. These extensive incisions may not only be associated with increased pain, opiate requirements, and length of stay, but also put neighboring structures at risk such as the vagus and phrenic nerves, thoracic duct, and brachial plexus.[10]

Due to these drawbacks of open repair, endovascular therapy has been increasingly embraced as an expeditious and minimally invasive management strategy for ASA injuries. Our institutional experience demonstrated an increase in endovascular interventions from 0.5% to 9% from 2002 to 2010.[3] This trend seems, by all accounts, to be continuing. Indeed, in a query of the National Trauma Data Bank spanning the years 2010–2012, utilization of endovascular repair of peripheral arterial injuries grew from 11.3% to 17.2%.[11]

Evidence suggests that this management technique is not only a rapid "damage control" strategy, but, in many respects, endovascular treatment is associated with superior outcomes when compared to open surgery. The following sections describe technical principles of open and endovascular repair of ASA injuries, and review the outcomes of the two strategies.

OPEN SURGICAL MANAGEMENT—TECHNIQUE

Traditionally, open surgical exposure for both proximal and distal control has been the mantra when approaching axillosubclavian vascular injuries. However, this is often easier said than done. The intrathoracic portion of the proximal subclavian artery, as well as the proximity of the proximal and mid portions to the brachial plexus and thoracic duct account for the difficult nature of its exposure and open vascular repair.

Many standard vascular surgery texts describe periclavicular incisions for mid or distal subclavian exposure on either side, and different approaches for proximal exposure depending on the side involved. Exposure of the right subclavian artery is usually described as a midline sternotomy for proximal control, with either a "hockey-stick extension" onto the right neck (overlying the sternal head of the sternocleidomastoid muscle) or an additional supraclavicular incision for distal control.[12] The proximal left subclavian artery is usually described as being approached via a left anterolateral thoracotomy through the fourth intercostal space. For example, a step-wise approach to a proximal left subclavian artery injury would be to begin with a left anterolateral thoracotomy for proximal control, followed by a supraclavicular incision distal control, with an upper midline sternotomy to connect these into a "trap-door" incision if further exposure or branch control is needed.[13] In a historic series, a periclavicular incision provided adequate exposure in 50% of ASA injuries, while the other 50% required an additional sternotomy or thoracotomy.[8]

Because the axillosubclavian segment is difficult to mobilize for end-to-end repair, injuries often require interposition grafting. When considering all extremity vascular traumatic injuries, there has been a suggestion that polytetrafluoroethylene (PTFE) underperforms when compared to autologous vein.[7] However, the high patency rates seen in synthetic conduits in the ASA location during elective cervical debranching and arterial thoracic outlet cases, it seems reasonable to consider its use if contamination is minimal in a trauma setting. Indeed, in a military series, PTFE was found to be equivalent to vein when used in the axillosubclavian segment, whereas more distally vein was a superior conduit.[14] A reasonable practice is to use autologous vein if it is available and the patient can tolerate the additional time needed for vein harvest, acknowledging that use of PTFE is entirely acceptable.[8]

ENDOVASCULAR MANAGEMENT—TECHNIQUE

A pint of sweat will save a gallon of blood.

—Austin O'Malley

Certain technical aspects of the endovascular repair of an ASA injury will be dictated by the anatomy of the lesion, the presence of other associated injuries, and the patient's body habitus. However, there are some universal principles that are helpful to consider in planning and executing these cases. We begin by describing one reasonable approach, and then will discuss possible variations from this strategy that may be needed.

Percutaneous puncture is used to establish access in either femoral artery with a 4 French (Fr) micropuncture sheath. This is then upsized to a 6 Fr sheath (rather than the usual diagnostic 5 Fr sheath, to permit the usage of widely available snares, if needed). A long 300-cm floppy tipped hydrophilic wire is advanced retrograde into the aortic arch, and an angled catheter such as a Glide or Bernstein is used to select the arch vessel of interest (the innominate or left subclavian depending on the side of the injury). A left-anterior oblique projection is ideal for this first-order cannulation. If an arch angiogram is required, a diagnostic catheter such a pigtail can be placed for an arch injection. Once the arch target is selected, selective angiography with a hand injection of dilute contrast can be used to establish the extent of the injury as well as the size of the proximal and distal arterial landing zones for stent-graft selection. Using the catheter and wire combination already employed, an attempt is made to cross the lesion in an antegrade fashion. If the wire can be advanced into the arm, the catheter should follow and allow for the wire to be replaced with a stiffer wire such as a Rosen to facilitate stent-graft placement.

The size of the proximal and distal stent-graft landing zones dictate the next sheath required—for most patients, a 90-cm stiff sheath such as a Terumo Destination will allow for brachiocephalic access from the groin. A sheath diameter of 7–9 Fr will usually suffice, depending on the device to be implanted. After stent-graft positioning and deployment, completion angiography is performed. If the result is satisfactory, hemostasis can be obtained with manual pressure or a closure device in the groin.

If the femoral wire coils within the associated hematoma and cannot be passed, a brachial cutdown should be performed and a 5 Fr sheath should be placed into the brachial artery. A 300-cm 0.018" wire and an angled catheter can be advanced through this to attempt to cross the lesion in a retrograde fashion, positioning this wire to be snared from the groin. The catheter should be used to protect the aortic arch as the wire is retrieved from the groin sheath. Through-and-through wire access may provide the support needed for stent-graft deployment, or the catheter which is now spanning the lesion can be used to exchange for a stiff wire. Device delivery can proceed from the groin, as described above, to avoid the need for large brachial sheath placement. The brachial arteriotomy is closed with interrupted 7-0 Prolene sutures.

The Gore VBX balloon-expandable stent-graft may be particularly useful in ASA injuries because of its ability to be postdilated and "flared." It is approved for the treatment of arteries ranging in size from 5 mm to 16 mm using only a 7 Fr or 8 Fr sheath, and can span lesions with proximal and distal diameter discrepancies of up to 8 mm.

Some authors have suggested that the passage of large sheaths, snares, and stent-grafts from the femoral approach may pose increased risk of stroke due to arch manipulation or bleeding via disruption of the hematoma at the injury site, and prefer a brachial access site for their primary working location, because bleeding may be controlled with an occlusion balloon placed centrally from the femoral access, leaving its guidewire to be snared via the arm.[15] These points are certainly valid. However, the risks of brachial artery dissection or thrombosis due to the placement of large sheaths and devices may outweigh the benefits of its routine use. If the patient is felt to be at particularly high risk for complications from antegrade device passage (i.e., at high risk for atheroembolism due to a shaggy aorta or thoracic aortic aneurysm, or at high risk for major bleeding due to a history of massive hemorrhage with hemodynamic instability or a large surface wound), it may be worthwhile to minimize these risks by performing an initial brachial cutdown and attempting a retrograde-first approach, with wires, catheters, snares, and devices passed via this direction.

COMPARATIVE OUTCOMES: OPEN VERSUS ENDOVASCULAR REPAIR

As there are no randomized controlled trials to compare the outcomes of open and endovascular interventions for ASA injuries, we must turn instead to published case series on the subject and attempt to derive a "big-picture" perspective from them.

Open Surgical Outcomes

Hyre et al. published a series of 35 open repairs for axillosubclavian vascular traumas encompassing 30 arterial injuries. There was a 6% rate of surgical site infections after open vascular repair. One patient died after successful arterial repair due to sequelae from hemorrhage, for an overall arterial-injury related mortality of 3%. In patients that survived, there were no early or late graft thromboses.[16] Demetriades et al. also contributed a sizeable historical series of open repairs for axillosubclavian vascular trauma. In their cases, lone arterial injuries were associated with a 20.5% mortality rate, and combined arterial/venous injuries were associated with a 45% mortality rate.[8] Another large series by Lin et al. consisted of 54 patients undergoing open repair for ASA injuries. They noted an early graft thrombosis rate of 9%, and each of these patients underwent reoperation. Importantly, they noted a very sobering mortality rate of 39%. A third of these mortalities were actually intraoperative deaths associated with exsanguination after arterial repair.[9] The single largest series of open repairs for ASA trauma comes from McKinley et al., consisting of 260 patients. They noted a 10% rate of bypass graft thrombosis, with 17% of these occlusions requiring repeat operation. They reported a 12% mortality rate, half of which were intraoperative.[17]

Starting in the early 2000s, surgeons began publishing small series comparing their institutional experiences with open and endovascular interventions for ASA trauma. The first of these was produced by Xenos et al. Their patients treated with open surgery did very well overall with 0% surgical site infections, 0% graft failure rates, 0% limb loss, and 0% mortality. Notably, this was a selected subset of patients who were stable enough to undergo preoperative diagnostic angiography (to determine their candidacy for endovascular or open repair). This triage strategy ruled out patients with "extensive injuries" and may account for the markedly lower mortality rate than seen in other open series.[18] Shalhub et al. described 16 open repairs for ASA injuries. One patient (6%) developed a graft infection, early graft thrombosis, and ultimately lost their upper extremity.[19] Our own published experience with open revascularization for ASA injuries includes 135 patients from our institution and a collaborating center. There were no complications in these patients noted during follow-up.[3]

The long-term fate of open ASA repairs is not well characterized. Postoperative follow-up is notoriously poor in trauma patients, resulting in only limited reliable data on patency rates. Each of the publications discussed above was characterized by a large portion of patients being lost to follow-up. However, there were no reported late thromboses in any of the series discussed above.

Endovascular Surgical Outcomes

The 2003 series by Xenos et al. mentioned above was the first to describe a series of endovascular repairs for ASA injuries. Each repair was performed using a Wallgraft endoprosthesis (composed of braided steel and Dacron). They found no access site or graft infections and no early failures. One patient (14%) had a late stent-graft failure, which did not result in limb-threatening ischemia, but required open bypass for claudication. Even in this small series (seven endovascular and 16 open repairs), they noted statistically significantly shorter procedures and less blood loss in cases managed endovascularly. While two of these patients (29%) died during follow-up, neither death was related to the device or related to hemorrhage associated with their vascular injury (one death was due to complications of HIV, and the other was a suicide).[18]

Piffaretti et al. published a series of endovascular interventions for a variety of peripheral arterial injuries, four of which were in the axillosubclavian segment. The repairs involved one Wallgraft device for pseudoaneurysm and three Luminexx (nitinol) stents placed for dissections. They noted no infections, early failures, late failures, or conversions to open surgery. There were no mortalities. Notably, unlike virtually every other study of ASA trauma, they had a 100% follow-up rate with a mean duration of 16 months.[20] du Toit et al. reported their outcomes of a large series of 57 endovascular repairs of subclavian arterial injuries. No patients managed endovascularly required transfusions. They found a 5% rate of stent-graft occlusions within the first 30 days, all of which were managed with endovascular rescue. Beyond 30 days, a total of 20% of patients experienced significant in-stent stenosis requiring retreatment, and an additional 12% experienced stent occlusions which were managed without reintervention. No open conversions were performed, no immediately threatening episodes of limb ischemia occurred, and no limbs were lost. There were no deaths during postoperative surveillance. They reported an impressive mean follow-up duration of 49 months (though only 45% of patients were ever seen in follow-up after their procedure). Their publication is the first to note that the rates of stent-graft occlusions seemed directly related to the material makeup of the implanted device—50% of the Wallgraft devices failed, whereas 0% of the Hemobahn (nitinol) devices failed.[21]

Carrick et al. described a small series of six attempted endovascular repairs in which half were characterized as endovascular failures. However, the details of these failures warrant discussion. One case was considered a "failure" because the stent-graft was landed in a suboptimal seal zone in order to spare the dominant vertebral artery. This lead to a Type Ia endoleak into a pseudoaneurysm, and a decision was made to follow this patient clinically. The patient remained symptomatic for more than three years of follow-up at the time of their publication. Another case was deemed a failure when a wire placed via the femoral artery could not cross the lesion, but no attempt to cross the lesion in a retrograde fashion from the arm was made. One case was considered an endovascular failure because the patient died poststent-graft implantation, yet autopsy revealed pulmonary embolism as the likely source of death. Discounting the death due to pulmonary embolism, their failure rate would be 2/6 (33%). Neither of these failures led to limb loss or additional reported complications.[22] A 2011 publication by Shalhub et al. described their endovascular management of 12 patients. They found a statistically significant decrease in operative time in their endovascular interventions compared to their open surgeries, along with less blood loss, and less intravenous fluid requirements. They noted no infections, thromboses, or limb loss in their endovascular patients, and the endovascular cohort had no deaths associated with their vascular injuries.[19] Leong et al. reported a small case series of three endovascular interventions with no reported complications over a two year mean follow-up.[23] Another small endovascular case series was produced by Chopra et al., encompassing 10 patients. Median follow-up was 117 days, with 70% of patients lost to follow-up. No mortalities occurred in their cohort, and no limbs were lost. However, one patient (30%) developed device occlusions during follow-up, and one (10%) required open bypass for claudication.[11]

An excellent review of the literature on the endovascular management of ASA injuries between 1996 and 2012 by Dubose et al. summarizes the results of 32 publications. One hundred sixty patients were treated in total. Initial technical success rates averaged 96.9%. There were no infections or episodes of limb threatening ischemia noted during follow-up. Only two patients (1.2%) required a repeat endovascular intervention, and only one patient (0.6%) required a subsequent open surgery. There were no mortalities related to endovascular treatment reported in any publication.[24]

Our institution contributed to the largest modern study comparing endovascular therapy to open surgery for ASA injuries. Two hundred and thirty-four patients from the Memorial Hermann Hospital at the Texas Medical Center in Houston and the University of Arizona Medical Center were treated and screened for inclusion, ultimately resulting in 153 suitable study patients with 72 patients treated endovascularly and propensity-matched for statistical analysis. The study period spanned 2003–2013. All endovascular repairs were performed via percutaneous femoral and/or open brachial access. Repairs were carried out with 6–10 Fr sheaths and an assortment of Viabahn (nitinol), Wallstent (steel), and/or iCAST (steel) devices, with standard 10%–20% oversizing and a standardized surveillance protocol at 1, 3, 6, and 12 months postoperatively. We found that patients treated endovascularly received a fewer packed red blood cell and plasma transfusions. These patients also had statistically significantly fewer surgical site infections (0.0% vs. 25.5%, $P < 0.021$, odds ratio (OR) 0.3, 95% confidence interval (CI) 0.1–0.9). A trend toward fewer episodes of sepsis and fewer ventilator days was also noted among endovascular patients, though this did not reach statistical significance. Follow-up data were available for 88.2% of endovascular patients, with a range of 1–30 months, median eight months. Two patients (2.8%) experienced stent-graft failures, both of which were treated with open surgery. There was a statistically significant decrease in mortality for patients treated endovascularly compared with their open surgery counterparts (5.6% vs. 27.8%, $P < 0.04$, OR 0.7, 95% CI 0.6–0.9). We concluded that endovascular repair for ASA injuries was associated with decreased complication rates and decreased mortality over mid-term follow-up.

DISCUSSION

Due to the relatively low frequency of ASA injuries, the evidence available to compare the outcomes of open and endovascular repair is limited. Furthermore, the emergent nature of many of these cases and the requirement for the treatment of other concomitant injuries means that standardization of treatment strategies is difficult. A randomized controlled trial has never been carried out. However, some obvious trends can be generalized from the literature reviewed above.

1. Open repair of ASA injuries is certainly more invasive, and carries with it the substantial risk of morbidity associated with large incisions and soft tissue dissection, such as infection. While the rate of surgical site or graft infection appears low (<5%) after open surgery, it is not zero. By comparison, no studies reported infections associated with endovascular repair.
2. Open repair is associated with excellent short-term and long-term success, with most studies reporting no episodes of graft thrombosis or required reinterventions. This compares favorably to the reported failure rates of approximately 15%–40% for endovascular interventions. However, the evolution of endovascular devices forces us to carefully consider these failures. Several, but not all, of the publications discussed above provide details regarding the specific devices implanted in each case and their outcomes. When considering all cases in which

the necessary information is available to categorize their successes or failures, only 3/54 nitinol devices ever failed (5.6%) compared to 12/33 non-nitinol devices (36.4%).

3. Even if endovascular interventions are more likely to fail than an open bypass, these failures are often amenable to an additional minimally invasive revascularization such as thrombectomy, angioplasty and repeat stenting, and rarely require open surgery.
4. In none of the aforementioned publications was a stent-graft failure associated with acute limb ischemia, limb loss, or death. In effect, no bridge was burned by attempting an endovascular repair as the initial management in patients with suitable anatomy.
5. In studies that examined intraoperative and postoperative resource utilization, endovascular interventions were found to be associated with less blood loss, shorter procedures, and shorter hospitalizations.
6. Finally, and most importantly, it seems that endovascular intervention is associated with a decreased mortality rate compared to open surgery, with most series reporting 0% mortality in endovascular cohorts compared to the historic 10%–30% reported for open cohorts.

One immediately obvious problem with interpreting the morbidity and mortality results of the nonrandomized literature discussed above is that selection bias certainly plays a major role in skewing the results. Patients who are unstable after traumatic injury (and especially after poly-trauma) are usually taken to a dedicated trauma operating room for exploratory laparotomy, thoracotomy, aortic cross-clamping, and/or open cardiac massage when indicated. Most trauma operating rooms are not fully equipped for sophisticated angiographic imaging and endovascular interventions, and therefore are better equipped to handle open vascular repair, making it more likely these patients will be treated in this manner. In addition, these critically injured patients who are already in extremis may be subjected to more blood loss, hypothermia, and anesthesia time during attempts at damage control, and may be predestined to experience a complicated postoperative course after open vascular repair.

As endovascular capabilities become more widespread, it will more often be possible for vascular surgeons to perform endovascular repair of an ASA injury in an operating room that also allows for adequate resuscitation by anesthesia, operative intervention by other teams such as orthopedics and trauma, and rapid transport from the emergency department and to a waiting trauma intensive care unit. For example, at our institution, we recently managed a hypotensive poly-trauma patient successfully with endovascular intervention, but this required close coordination with multiple operative teams. First, the orthopedic service splinted unstable fractures in the emergency room, then the trauma team performed a mini-laparotomy to rule out intra-abdominal hemorrhage, and then the neurosurgery service performed a decompressive burr-hole in the endovascular suite immediately prior to our ASA stent-grafting. This allowed for successful control of hemorrhage and rescue of an acutely ischemic limb in a patient who would have been extremely difficult to repair via open techniques given his body habitus and other injuries (Figures 28-1–28-3).

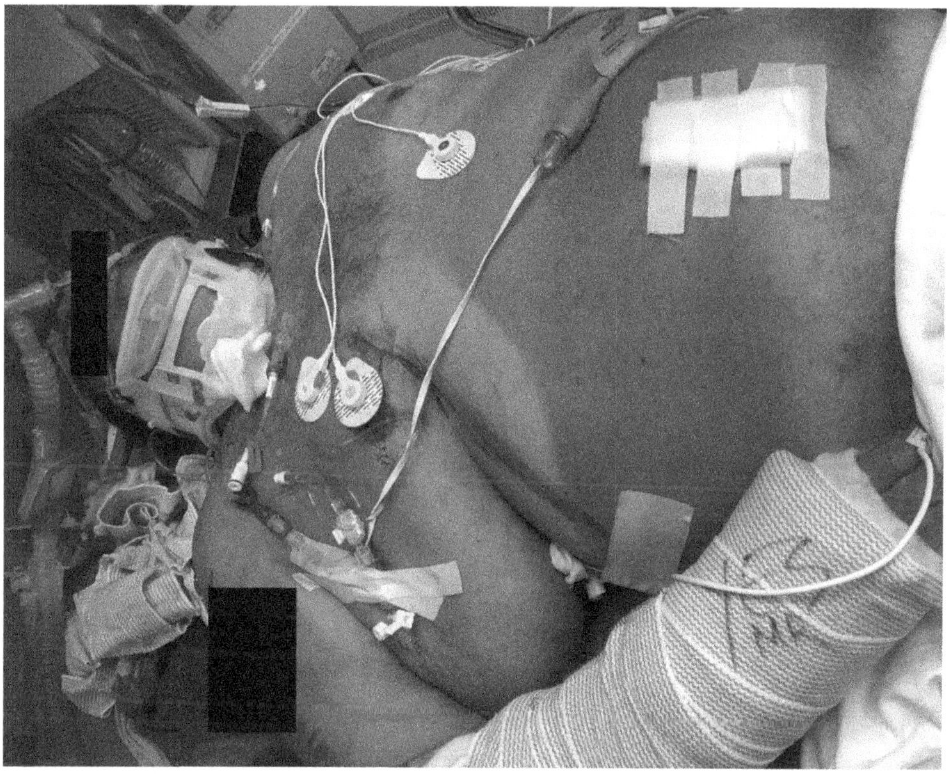

Figure 28-1. A morbidly obese male involved in a high-speed motorcycle crash sustained a right scapulothoracic dissociation as well as right radial and ulnar fractures. No brachial, radial, or ulnar pulses were detectable by palpation or Doppler interrogation on the right side.

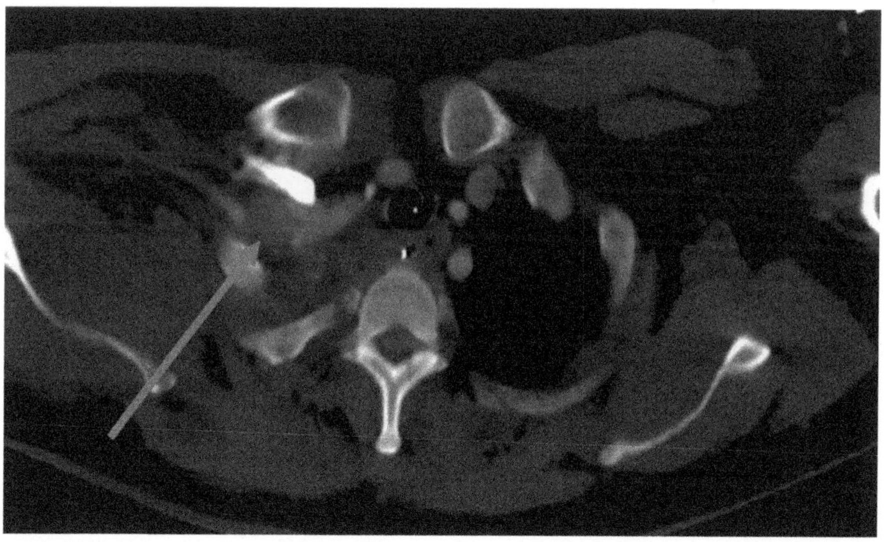

Figure 28-2. Computed tomography (CT) showed a right subclavian arterial injury.

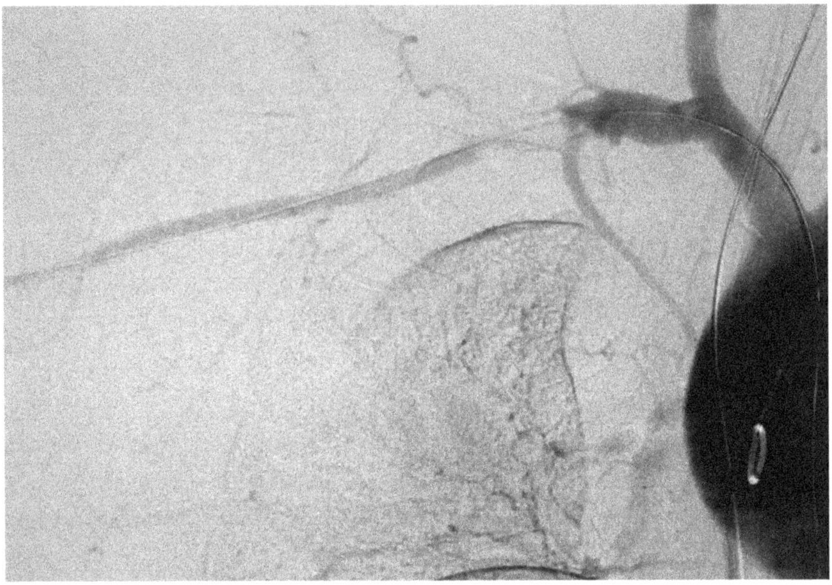

Figure 28-3. Diagnostic angiography via the right femoral artery confirmed the presence of a right subclavian artery transection, which was crossed via a retrograde approach.

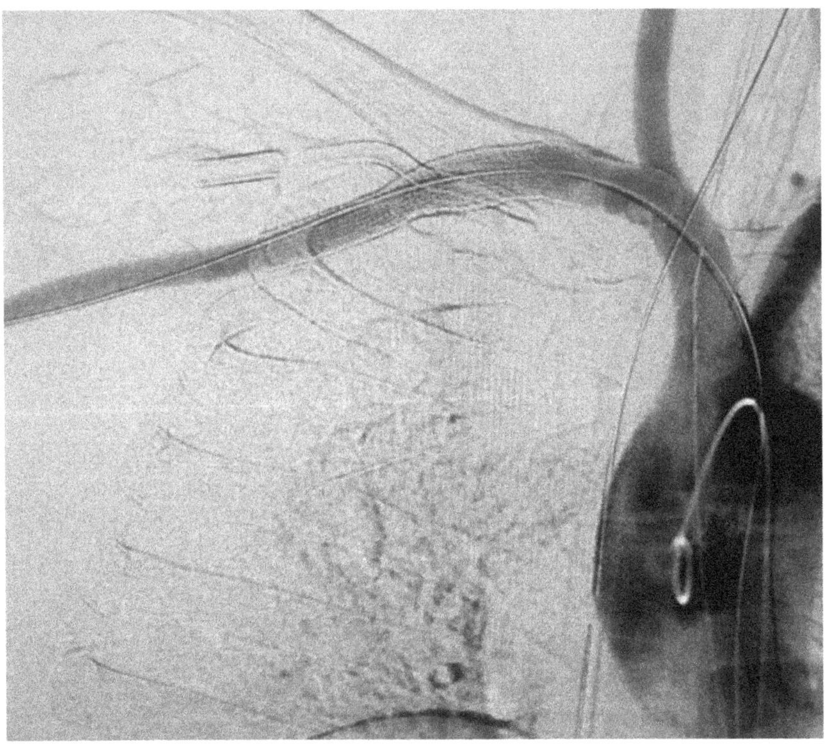

Figure 28-4. Three Viabahn stent-grafts (9 mm × 5 cm; 11 mm × 5 cm; 13 mm × 5 cm) were placed via a 12-French sheath and an open brachial artery exposure, in order to span the injury and account for the size discrepancy between the distal and proximal landing zones. The patient had a palpable pulse at the completion of the case.

CONCLUSION

ASA injuries remain a challenging problem facing by vascular surgeons. Endovascular interventions for these injuries are becoming increasingly common. Drawing conclusions about the outcomes of endovascular versus open repair is difficult, due to inherent selection bias in treatment choice and the lack of randomized studies. However, it can be reasonably concluded that the endovascular repair of ASA injuries can be performed more rapidly than open repair, with less blood loss, fewer infections, a low failure rate, and without preventing additional attempts at a later open repair, if needed. With the increasing application of resuscitative endovascular balloon occlusion of aorta (REBOA), more and more hemodynamically unstable patients may be stabilized without an open surgery, and may be excellent candidates for a minimally invasive endovascular repair of their peripheral arterial injuries.[10] We believe that for patients who are suitable anatomic candidates, endovascular surgery should be considered the first line of treatment for ASA injuries.

REFERENCES

1. London J. *White Fang*. New York, NY; 1906.
2. Friedman S. *A History of Vascular Surgery*. Vol 7. 2nd ed.; Wiley Blackwell Publishing (Futura), USA; 2005. doi:10.1002/9780470750773.
3. Branco BC, Boutrous ML, DuBose JJ, et al. Outcome comparison between open and endovascular management of axillosubclavian arterial injuries. *J Vasc Surg*. 2016;63(3):702–709. doi:10.1016/j.jvs.2015.08.117.
4. Danetz JS, Cassano AD, Stoner MC, Ivatury RR, Levy MM. Feasibility of endovascular repair in penetrating axillosubclavian injuries: a retrospective review. *J Vasc Surg*. 2005;41(2):246–254. doi:10.1016/j.jvs.2004.11.026.
5. Martin M, Long W. Vascular trauma—epidemiology and natural history. In: Cronenwett JL JK, ed. *Rutherford's Vascular Surgery*. 8th ed.; 2014:2422–2437. https://www-clinicalkey-com.ezproxyhost.library.tmc.edu/#!/content/book/3-s2.0-B9781455753048001552.
6. Starnes B, Arthurs Z. Vascular trauma: head and neck. In: Cronenwett K, Johnston K, eds. *Rutherford's Vascular Surgery*. 8th ed.; 2015:2438–2450.e2.
7. Kauvar D, Kraiss L. Vascular trauma—extremity. In: Cronenwett K, Johnston K, eds. *Rutherford's Vascular Surgery*. 8th ed.; 2015:2485–2500. https://www-clinicalkey-com.ezproxyhost.library.tmc.edu/#!/content/book/3-s2.0-B978145575304800159X.
8. Demetriades D, Chahwan S, Gomez H, et al. Penetrating injuries to the subclavian and axillary vessels. *J Am Coll Surg*. 1999;188(3):290–295.
9. Lin PH, Koffron AJ, Guske PJ, et al. Penetrating injuries of the subclavian artery. *Am J Surg*. 2003;185(6):580–584. doi:10.1016/S0002-9610(03)00070-9.
10. Branco BC, DuBose JJ. Endovascular solutions for the management of penetrating trauma: an update on REBOA and axillo-subclavian injuries. *Eur J Trauma Emerg Surg*. 2016;42(6):687–694. doi:10.1007/s00068-016-0739-5.
11. Chopra A, Modrall JG, Knowles M, Phelan HA, Valentine RJ, Chung J. Uncertain patency of covered stents placed for traumatic axillosubclavian artery injury. *J Am Coll Surg*. 2016;223(1):174–183. doi:10.1016/j.jamcollsurg.2016.02.007.
12. Shalhub S, Azizzadeh A. Vascular trauma: thoracic. In: Cronenwett J, KW J, eds. *Rutherford's Vascular Surgery*. 8th ed.; 2015:2451–2465.e3.
13. Wind G, Valentine R. *Anatomic Exposures in Vascular Surgery*. 3rd ed.; 2013.
14. Watson JDB, Houston IV R, Morrison JJ, Gifford SM, Rasmussen TE. A retrospective cohort comparison of expanded polytetrafluorethylene to autologous vein for

vascular reconstruction in modern combat casualty care. *Ann Vasc Surg*. 2017;29(4):822–829. doi:10.1016/j.avsg.2014.12.026.
15. Shalhub S, Starnes BW, Tran NT. Endovascular treatment of axillosubclavian arterial transection in patients with blunt traumatic injury. *J Vasc Surg*. 2011;53(4):1141–1144. doi: 10.1016/j.jvs.2010.10.129.
16. Hyre CE, Cikrit DF, Lalka SG, Sawchuk AP, Dalsing MC, Schuler JJ. Aggressive management of vascular injuries of the thoracic outlet. *J Vasc Surg*. 1998;27(5):880–885. http://www.embase.com/search/results?subaction=viewrecord&from=export&id=L28394432%0A http://sfx.library.uu.nl/utrecht?sid=EMBASE&issn=07415214&id=doi:&atitle=Aggressive+management+of+vascular+injuries+of+the+thoracic+outlet&stitle=J.+Vasc.+Surg.&title=Jou.
17. Mckinley AG, Carrim ATOA, Robbs J V. Management of proximal axillary and subclavian artery injuries. *Br J Surg*. 2000;87(1):79–85.
18. Xenos ES, Freeman M, Stevens S, Cassada D, Pacanowski J, Goldman M. Covered stents for injuries of subclavian and axillary arteries. *J Vasc Surg*. 2003;38(3):451–454. doi:10.1016/S0741-5214(03)00553-6.
19. Shalhub S, Starnes BW, Hatsukami TS, Karmy-Jones R, Tran NT. Repair of blunt thoracic outlet arterial injuries: an evolution from open to endovascular approach. *J Trauma Acute Care Surg*. 2011;71(5). http://journals.lww.com/jtrauma/Fulltext/2011/11000/Repair_of_Blunt_Thoracic_Outlet_Arterial_Injuries_.66.aspx.
20. Piffaretti G, Tozzi M, Lomazzi C, et al. Endovascular treatment for traumatic injuries of the peripheral arteries following blunt trauma. *Injury*. 2007;38(9):1091–1097. doi:10.1016/j.injury.2007.02.044.
21. du Toit DF, Lambrechts AV, Stark H, Warren BL. Long-term results of stent graft treatment of subclavian artery injuries: management of choice for stable patients? *J Vasc Surg*. 2008;47(4):739–743. doi:10.1016/j.jvs.2007.11.009.
22. Carrick MM, Morrison CA, Pham HQ, et al. Modern management of traumatic subclavian artery injuries: a single institution's experience in the evolution of endovascular repair. *Am J Surg*. 2010;199(1):28–34. doi:10.1016/j.amjsurg.2008.11.031.
23. Leong BDK, Naresh G, Hanif H, Lee SK, Zainal AA, Sara CM. Endovascular management of axillosubclavian artery injuries: report of three cases. *Surg Today*. 2013;43(8):918–922. doi:10.1007/s00595-012-0330-6.
24. DuBose JJ, Rajani R, Gilani R, et al. Endovascular management of axillo-subclavian arterial injury: a review of published experience. *Injury*. 2012;43(11):1785–1792. doi:10.1016/j.injury.2012.08.028.

Index

Note: Page numbers followed by f and t refer to figures and tables respectively

A

Abdominal aortic aneurysms, 12
Abduction and external rotation (AER), 220, 221, 224
ABS. *See* American Board of Surgery
Access preservation
  AV fistulas in kidney transplant, 168
  following renal transplantation, 167t
  spontaneous fistula closure, 168–169
Accredited Council of Graduate Medical Education (ACGME), 260
ACGME. *See* Accredited Council of Graduate Medical Education
ACS. *See* American College of Surgeons
Activated clotting time (ACT), 191, 202
Acute finger ischemia (AFI), 181
  adjunctive treatments, 196–197
  algorithm for patients, 192f
  anatomic classification, 182, 183f
  anatomic imaging, 186–189
  approach and technical considerations, 194–195
  catheter angiography, 187, 188f, 189–192
  catheter-directed thrombolysis for, 192–193, 193t
  clinical presentation, 183
  contrast arteriography, 189
  cross-sectional contrast imaging, 187
  diagnosis and treatment, 181
  diagnostic testing, 189
  differential diagnosis, 184t
  duplex ultrasound, 187
  echocardiography, 189
  electrocardiogram, 189
  epidemiology, 182
  etiology, 190
  history and physical examination, 183–185
  ischemic finger symptoms, 181
  laboratory testing, 185, 186t
  outcomes, 197, 198f
  patient care and monitoring, 195–196, 196f
  physiologic testing, 185–186
Advanced Surgical Skills for Exposure in Trauma (ASSET) course, 262–263
AER. *See* Abduction and external rotation
AFI. *See* Acute finger ischemia
Allen test, 19, 184–185, 202, 213
Allogenic graft, 83
Allograft dialysis access development, 79–80
Alteplase, 194, 196
AMA. *See* American Medical Association
American Board of Surgery (ABS), 1, 260, 261t
American College of Radiology, 89
American College of Surgeons (ACS), 245, 262
American College of Surgeons Advanced Trauma Life Support, 267
American Medical Association (AMA), 89
American Society of Diagnostic and Interventional Nephrology, 102, 176
Amputations, 214
  digital, 214
  limb salvage *vs.*, 271, 272
AnastoClips, 48, 51, 52
Anastomotic angle, 36, 39–41. *See also* Autogenous arteriovenous fistulae
Anesthesia, 21, 232, 282
Aneurysmal dilatation, 160, 164
Angiography, 92, 213. *See also* Catheter angiography
Angioplasty, 61, 90, 92, 99
Antecubital fossa, 136, 156, 255
Anterior scalene muscle, 231–233
Antithrombin III, 69

Arch angiogram, 277
Arch angiography, 191
Arch aortography, 191
Artegraft®, 78, 79
Arterial endothelial cells, 37–38
Arterial line complications, 209–210
Arterial system, 132
Arterial thoracic outlet syndrome, 229, 250
Arterial thrombosis, 204–205, 213
Arteriotomy, 132, 215
Arteriovenous access (AV access), 98–99, 101, 102, 160, 169
  age and life expectancy, 18
  algorithm for planning, 25–26
  anastomosis for, 52
  anesthesia, 21
  brachial artery aneurysms with, 163
  brachiocephalic fistula, 22
  central vein stenosis, 20, 24
  chest wall/truncal, 25
  cosmetic deformities associated with, 159f
  diabetes mellitus, 17
  duplex ultrasound, 19
  end stage renal disease, 16–17
  factors, 20–21
  general algorithm for, 15, 16t
  guidelines for managing, 170
  Hemodialysis Reliable Outflow graft, 24
  hypotension, 18
  inflow artery aneurysmal dilatation, 164
  lower extremity, 24–25
  management, 160
  non-diabetic patients, 17
  obesity, 18
  patency rates, 17
  planning, 15
  prosthetic upper extremity, 23
  radiocephalic fistula, 21–22
  transposed brachial-brachial fistula, 23
  transposed brachiobasilic fistula, 22–23
  venography, 19–20
  venous exam and, 19
Arteriovenous access-associated hand ischemia, 135
Arteriovenous anastomoses, 45, 52
  categories, 45
  constriction, 47
  empiric and human data, 48
  end-to-side, 45, 46f
  intimal hyperplasia, 47
  nonpenetrating clips, 48
  penetrating clips, 48
  penetrating continuous *vs.* nonpenetrating interrupted, 49–51, 50f, 51f
  penetrating continuous *vs.* penetrating interrupted, 48–49
  penetrating interrupted *vs.* nonpenetrating interrupted, 49
  theoretical and animal data, 47–48
Arteriovenous fistula (AVF), 136, 160, 163, 164, 204. *See also* Autogenous arteriovenous fistulae
  closure, 170
  femoral, 118
  for hemodialysis access, 151
  patency rates, 50f, 51f
  upper extremity, 77, 123
  utilization, 55, 65, 107
Arteriovenous grafts (AVG), 55, 62, 65, 77, 79, 80, 83, 107, 109, 118
  advantages, 56, 66
  bacteriology, 130
  bovine carotid artery, 58
  bovine mesenteric vein, 58–59
  configuration and location, 59–61
  cryopreserved femoral vein, 58
  early access grafts, 57–58
  with focal hemorrhage, 131
  for hemodialysis, 132
  indications for placement, 56
  infection, 129–130, 131f
  partial graft excision, 132
  patency rates, 50f, 51f
  perigraft response, 67
  polytetrafluoroethylene grafts, 57, 130, 130f
  prosthetic cuff infection, 132
  prosthetic material use, 66
  secondary interventions, 61
  subtotal graft excision, 132
  total graft excision, 131–132
ASA injuries. *See* Axillosubclavian arterial injuries
ASSET course. *See* Advanced Surgical Skills for Exposure in Trauma course
Atherectomy, 91, 189
Atheroembolism, 203, 205
Atherosclerosis, 20, 37
Autogeneous upper limb fistulae, 35
Autogenous arteriovenous fistulae, 35
  anastomotic angle, 36, 39, 40
  end-to-end, 36
  end-to-side, 36, 37f, 39
  failure, 35, 38
  hemodynamics
    with computational modeling, 35–37
    and vessel wall remodeling, 37–38
  implications for hemodialysis patients, 38–39
    follow-up, 39
    patients and design, 39
    surgical procedures, 39
  outcomes and definitions, 36, 39–40
  results, 40–41

Autogenous bypass graft, 255
AV access. *See* Arteriovenous access
AVF. *See* Arteriovenous fistula
AVG. *See* Arteriovenous grafts
Axillary artery percutaneous access, 202, 202f
Axilloaxillary loop graft, 25
Axillosubclavian arterial (ASA) injuries, 271, 275
  comparative outcomes, 279–281
  endovascular repair, 276, 277–278, 282
  morbidity and mortality, 276
  open revascularization, 279
  open surgical management, 276–277, 281–282
  patency rates, 277
  polytetrafluoroethylene, 277
  vascular trauma, 276

B

Balloon angioplasty, 41, 107, 109
Banding, 139–140
Basilic vein fistula, 30
Basilic vein transposition, 29
  elevation technique, 32–33
  one-stage *vs.* two-stage technique, 29–32, 31t
  primary and secondary procedure, 31
BCA. *See* Bovine carotid artery
BCF. *See* Brachiocephalic fistula
Bergan, John, 2, 2f, 8f
Bernstein catheter, 277
Bioengineered vascular grafts (BEVGs), 77
  allograft dialysis access conduit development, 79–80
  application, 82, 83
  durability, 81, 82, 84
  emergence and clinical use of, 80–83
  heterograft dialysis access conduit development, 78–79
  historical context, 78–79
  human implantation of, 82
  limitations, challenges, and future directions, 83–84
  manufacturing process, 81
  selection criteria, 80
  technical modification, 82
  3D printing, 84
  utilization, 79–80
BioPolyMeric®, 78–79
Bioprosthetic graft devices, 84
Bioreactor, 81
Blood pressure cuff, 130
BMV. *See* Bovine mesenteric vein
Bovine carotid artery (BCA), 58
Bovine mesenteric vein (BMV), 58–59
Brachial arteriotomy, 132, 278
Brachial artery access, 201–202
  AngioSeal for, 202
  aortic cases, 211
  arterial thrombosis, 204–205
  arteriovenous fistula, 204
  atheroembolism, 205
  closure devices, 202–203
  complication rate for, 203
  for endovascular therapies, 211–212
  to femoral access, 203
  hematoma formation, 204
  for iliac interventions, 211
  independent factor, 203t
  pseudoaneurysm, 204, 211
  risk with, 204t
Brachial artery aneurysms, 163
Brachial artery diameters, 163t, 164
Brachial artery dilatation, 160–164, 161f, 162f, 163t
  brachial artery aneurysms, 163
  dilated brachial artery, 161f
  distal embolic occlusions, 161f
  fusiform brachial artery aneurysm, 162f
Brachial artery dissection, 278
Brachial artery exposures, 261–262
Brachial artery thrombosis, 211
Brachial-brachial fistulas, 18, 20
Brachial cephalic fistula, 29
Brachial plexus, 232, 233, 252
Brachiobasilic AVFs, 59–60
Brachiocephalic fistula (BCF), 18, 20, 22
Brachiocephalic vein, 113, 114
Buttonhole technique, 32, 152, 153, 153f

C

Candida albicans infection, 133
Cardiac devices, implantation of, 98
Cardiac implantable electronic devices (CIED), 97, 102
  central venous stenosis, 97–99, 101
  chronic kidney disease patient progression, 102
  end-stage renal disease patients, 102–103
  insertion sites
    cephalic vein, 99
    epicardial leads, 101
    femoral vein, 99–100
    internal jugular veins, 100
    subclavian vein catheters, 99
    subcutaneous devices, 101
  surgical management, 102–103
  vascular access patency, 98
Carmeda BioActive Surface (CBAS), 70
Catheter, 277–278
Catheter angiography, 187, 188f, 189–192, 194
Catheter arteriogram, 221
Catheter-associated upper extremity deep vein thrombosis (CA-UEDVT), 173, 178
  acute, 177, 177t

bleeding risk, 177
incidence and clinical significance, 174
prophylaxis against, 176
risk factors, 175t
symptomatic, 176
treatment, 176–177
Catheter-directed arteriography, 268
Catheter-directed thrombolysis (CDT), 222, 255
acute finger ischemia, 192–193, 193t
for acute UEDVT, 177
Catheters, 121–122
CA-UEDVT. *See* Catheter-associated upper extremity deep vein thrombosis
CBA. *See* Conventional balloon angioplasty
CBAS. *See* Carmeda BioActive Surface
CBAS-ePTFE grafts, 70
CCJ. *See* Costoclavicular junction
Center for Medicare and Medicaid Services (CMS), 89, 93
Central-line-associated blood stream infection (CLABSI), 173
Central vein stenosis (CVS), 20, 97, 101, 113
after CIED lead placement, 98–99
treatments, 24
Central venous catheters (CVC), 117, 123, 173
Central venous obstruction (CVO), 117–118, 122
Cephalic arch, 108–109
Cephalic/basilic vein, 113
Cervical ribs, 249, 254
brachial plexus compression, 252
C7 transverse process, 249
embryologic development, 249
excision, 255
incidence, 253
subclavian artery, 250, 251f, 252
types, 250
Chronic hemodialysis, 107
Chronic ischemia, 215
Chronic kidney disease (CKD), 16, 17, 55, 97
CIED. *See* Cardiac implantable electronic devices
CKD. *See* Chronic kidney disease
CLABSI. *See* Central-line-associated blood stream infection
Clopidogrel, 68, 212
Closure devices, 202
CMS. *See* Center for Medicare and Medicaid Services
Committee on Trauma (COT) leadership, 262
Compartment syndrome, 269, 270
Contralateral insertion, 99
Contrast arteriography, 189
Conventional balloon angioplasty (CBA), 111
Coronary arterial models, 109
Cosmetic concerns, 159, 159f
Costoclavicular junction (CCJ), 24
COT leadership. *See* Committee on Trauma leadership
Cox model, 41
CPT. *See* Current Procedural Terminology
CPT code 35476, 90
CPT code 36147, 90, 94
CPT code 36148, 90
CPT code 36870, 90
CPT code 36901, 92, 94
CPT code 36902, 92
CPT code 36903, 92
CPT code 36904, 92
CPT code 36905, 92
CPT code 36906, 92
CPT code +36907, 92
CPT code +36908, 92
CPT code +36909, 92
CPT code 37238, 90
CPT code 37241, 91
CPT code 37799, 91
CPT code 75791, 90
CPT codes 35475, 90
Cryopreserved femoral vein, 58, 79
CryoVein®, 79
C7 transverse process, 249
Current Procedural Terminology (CPT), 89
CVC. *See* Central venous catheters
CVO. *See* Central venous obstruction
CVS. *See* Central vein stenosis
Cytograft®, 82

D

DAC. *See* Dialysis Access Consortium
Daley, Richard M., 2, 3f
Dardik Biograft®, 79
DASH. *See* Disability of the Arm, Shoulder, and Hand
Dean vortices, 36
Deaver retractor, 230
Decellularization, 81
Delphi approach, 262
De Takats, Geza, 2, 3f
Diabetes mellitus, 17
Diabetic *vs.* nondiabetic patients, 17
Dialysis access coding, 89–90
implications of new codes, 94
new coding family, 91–93
previous coding convention, 90–91
work relative value units, 91
Dialysis Access Consortium (DAC), 60
Diastolic hypotension, 18
Digital amputations, 214
Digital subtraction angiography (DSA), 19–20
Digital ulcers, 183
Dilated brachial artery, 161f
Diligent pulse assessment, 269
Disability of the Arm, Shoulder, and Hand (DASH), 241
Distal limb hypoperfusion, 125
Distal revascularization/ interval ligation (DRIL), 125, 136, 142–143, 146

Distal stent-graft, 278
Disturbed flow, 38
Doppler ultrasound, 102
"DOQI Guidelines," 160
DRIL. *See* Distal revascularization/interval ligation
Drug-coated balloons (DCBs)
  AVF and AVG stenosis, 111–113
  balloon angioplasty, 109
  clinic experience, 114
  definitions and statistical methods, 112t
  hemodialysis access, 107
  Lutonix balloon, 110–111
  overview, 110–111
  PACT Admiral balloon, 110–111
  stenosis, 108–109
  target lesion revascularization, 112
DSA. *See* Digital subtraction angiography
Duplex ultrasound (DUS), 19–20, 39, 170, 187

E
Early access grafts, 57–58
Echocardiography, 166, 189
ECM. *See* Extracellular matrix
Effectiveness-per-protocol (EPP), 110
Electrocardiogram, 189
Elevation techniques, 32–33
Embolectomy, 255
Embolic phenomena, 215
Embolization, 91
End-hole catheter, 194
Endothelial nitric oxide synthase (eNOS), 38
Endovascular reconstructive procedures, 255
Endovascular repair, ASA injuries, 276–281
Endovascular therapies
  brachial artery access for, 211–212
  radial artery access for, 208, 210–211
  repeat brachial access, 212
  upper extremity arterial access for, 207–208
End-stage renal disease (ESRD), 16–17, 55, 56, 58, 65, 77, 82, 97, 107, 117, 118
End-to-side anastomoses, 45, 46f, 47
eNOS. *See* Endothelial nitric oxide synthase
Epicardial leads, 101
EPP. *See* Effectiveness-per-protocol
ePTFE. *See* Expanded Polytetrafluoroethylene
ESRD. *See* End-stage renal disease
Expanded polytetrafluoroethylene (ePTFE), 57, 62, 65, 77, 78, 118, 122, 125
  heparin-bonded, 69–70
  neointimal hyperplasia, 68
External jugular veins, 100
Extracellular matrix (ECM), 81, 84
Extremity vascular injuries, 276

F
Family of codes, 89, 91, 93
Fasciotomy, 260, 262, 263, 270
fAVG. *See* Forearm AVG
Fellowship program, 259
Femoral access, 118–119, 123, 126, 201, 209
Femoral arteriovenous graft (fAVG), 118–119
Femoral artery, 190, 203, 208, 215, 277
Femoral catheters, 123
Femoral vein approach, 99–100
FGF. *See* Fibroblast Growth Factor
Fibroblast Growth Factor (FGF), 69
First rib resection, 24, 232, 233–234
First rib resection and scalenectomy (FRRS), 243, 244
Fistula anastomosis, 35
Fistula First Initiative, 55, 56
Fistulogram, 90, 91, 94
Flow to the fistula, 137–138
Flow to the hand, 138
Fluoroscopy, 90, 191, 201
Focal gangrene, 183, 184
Focal hemorrhage, 131
Forearm AVG (fAVG), 56, 59–61
FRRS. *See* First rib resection and scalenectomy
Fusiform brachial artery aneurysm, 162f

G
GFR. *See* Glomerular filtration rate
Glide catheter, 277
Glomerular filtration rate (GFR), 165, 185
Gore VBX balloon-expandable stent-graft, 278
Gram-negative bacilli, 133

H
Haimovici, Henry, 1
HAV. *See* Humacyte acellular vessel
HD access. *See* Hemodialysis access
Hematomas, 204, 215
Hemodialysis access (HD access), 65, 77, 79, 107, 117, 118, 129, 151
  and arterial reconstruction, 83
  arteriovenous access. *See* Arteriovenous access
  BEVGs utilized for, 84
  conventional balloon angioplasty for, 113
  history of steal, 17
  and non-HD patients, 102–103
  "off-the-shelf" conduit for, 82
  patency, 112
  stenotic lesions, 111
Hemodialysis catheter, 121
Hemodialysis Reliable Outflow (HeRO) grafts, 24, 117
  advantages and disadvantages, 122
  avoiding bridging catheters, 121–122
  central venous obstruction, 117–118, 120, 122
  components, 119f, 125
  configurations, 123–124
  end-stage renal disease patients, 121
  femoral AVG, 118–119
  hemodialysis access algorithm, 118–120
  inflow and arterial considerations, 121

maintenance, 124–125
outcomes, 120t
salvage of existing access, 122–124
steal syndrome, 121
systolic blood pressure, 121
thrombectomy, 124–125
venous outflow component, 125–126
Hemodynamic monitoring
purposes of, 208
radial artery cannulation, 213
radial artery line placement, 208–210, 212
upper extremity arterial access for, 207
Hemopneumothorax, 268
Hemorrhage, 130, 259, 269, 279
Hemostasis, 152, 278
Heparin, 69, 202, 214
Heparin-bonded ePTFE graft, 69–70
clinical outcomes, 70–71, 71t
experimental studies, 69–70
Heparin bonding, 70
HeRO grafts. *See* Hemodialysis Reliable Outflow grafts
Heterograft dialysis access development, 78–79
High flow access, steal, 148
High-pressure balloon angioplasty (HPBA), 112
HLA sensitization. *See* Human leukocyte antigen sensitization
Hoover, Jack, 6–7, 6f
HPBA. *See* High-pressure balloon angioplasty
Humacyte acellular vessel (HAV), 83, 84
Human leukocyte antigen (HLA) sensitization, 83
Hypercoagulability, 245
Hypotension, 18
Hypothenar hammer hand syndrome, 221

I
Implantable cardioverter-defibrillators (ICDs), 97
Inferior vena cava (IVC), 118, 123, 124
Internal jugular veins, 100
International Society for Cardiovascular Surgery (ISCVS), 1
Intimal hyperplasia, 220
Invasive therapies, for ischemia, 214
Ischemic monomelic neuropathy, 17
ISCVS. *See* International Society for Cardiovascular Surgery
IVC. *See* Inferior vena cava

J
Juxta-anastomotic stenosis, 35, 39, 40–41, 108

K
KDOQI. *See* Kidney Disease Outcomes Quality Initiative
Kerrison bone rongeur, 233
Kidney Disease Outcomes Quality Initiative (KDOQI), 16, 19, 21, 22, 65, 66, 107
Kidney transplants, 160
AV fistulas in, 168
for fistula closure, 166
Krüppel-like factor-2 (KLF2), 38

L
Laminar flow, 38
Large anastomoses, 45
Lass, Donald, 6–7, 7f
Lateral intermuscular approach, 255
Left anterior oblique, 277
Left axillobrachial artery, 161f
Left ventricular ejection fraction (LVEF), 121, 167
Left ventricular end-diastolic diameter (LVEDD), 165, 166, 169
Left ventricular end-systolic diameters (LVESD), 169
Left ventricular hypertrophy (LVH), 164–166
Left ventricular mass index (LVMi), 165–169
Lesions, types, 114
Lifeline® graft, 82, 83
Ligation
access, 166, 167
advocating, 165–167, 165t
Limb ischemia, 254
Limb loss, 252
Limb salvage *vs.* amputation, 271, 272
Long-segment plication (LPS), 140–142, 146
Lower extremity bypass grafts, 83
LPS. *See* Long-segment plication
Luminexx (nitinol), 280
Lutonix balloon, 110, 111, 113
LVEDD. *See* Left ventricular end-diastolic diameter
LVEF. *See* Left ventricular ejection fraction
LVH. *See* Left ventricular hypertrophy
LVMi. *See* Left ventricular mass index

M
Mangled Extremity Severity Score (MESS), 271–272
Mangled Extremity Syndrome Index (MESI), 271
Massive hemorrhage, 278
McCleery's syndrome, 245
Medicare Physician Fee Schedule (MPFS) Proposed Rule, 90
Mentorship program, 12
MESI. *See* Mangled Extremity Syndrome Index
MESS. *See* Mangled Extremity Severity Score
Metabolic syndrome, 133
Middle scalene muscle, 233

Minimally invasive limited ligation endoluminal-assisted revision (MILLER) procedure, 136, 139, 140, 140f, 145
Modern Trends in Vascular Surgery, 4
Multihole microcatheters, 215
Mural thrombosis, 68
Myofibroblasts, 109

N
National Institutes of Health (NIH), 12
National Kidney Foundation Kidney Disease Outcomes Quality Initiative Guidelines, 55, 60, 151, 160
National Surgical Quality Improvement Program (NSQIP), 245
Neoendothelial healing, 68
Neointimal hyperplasia (NIH), 107–109
Neurogenic quadrilateral space syndrome
  antiinflammatory agents, 222
  axillary nerve, 224
  case report, 223–224
  electromyography, 222, 224
  fibrous bands, 220
  magnetic resonance imaging, 222, 224
  physical therapy, 222
Neurogenic thoracic outlet syndrome, 229
  compression of brachial plexus, 234
  operations performed for, 230
  transaxillary approach for, 230
Neurolysis, 224
NIH. *See* National Institutes of Health
Non-operative management, 259, 270
Non-progressive stenosis, 36
Non-viable soft tissue, 269
Normal flow access, steal, 148
Northwestern Vascular Fellowship (1981–82), 11
Northwestern Vascular Symposium, 1, 4
  books produced in, 4t–5t
  format, 2
  Hoover, Jack, 6–7
  Lass, Donald, 6–7
  success, 8
  vascular surgeons by, 3t
  W. L. Gore & Associates, 6–7
NSQIP. *See* National Surgical Quality Improvement Program

O
Obesity, 18
Occlusion, 208
One-stage *vs.* two-stage technique, 29–32, 31t
Open surgical management, ASA injuries, 276–277, 279, 281–282
Orthopedic fractures, 269

P
Pacemakers (PMs), 97
Paclitaxel, 110
PACT Admiral Balloon, 110, 111
Paget–Schroetter syndrome, 237, 245
PAI. *See* Proximalization of arterial inflow
Patch angioplasty, 223
PCHA. *See* Posterior circumflex humeral artery
Pearce, William H., 11, 11f, 12, 13f
  clinical, 13
  education, 12
  humanitarian, 13–14
  research, 12
Percutaneous access, 201, 203
Percutaneous balloon angioplasty, 101, 102
Percutaneous puncture, 277
Percutaneous transluminal angioplasty (PTA), 107, 118
Peri-anastomotic vein, 108
Periclavicular incisions, 277
Peripheral arterial revascularization, 202
Peripheral artery disease (PAD), 123
Peripherally inserted central catheters (PICC), 173, 175f, 176, 178
Permissive hypotension, 267
Phrenic nerve, 232
PICC. *See* Peripherally inserted central catheters
Pigtail catheter, 277
Plain old balloon angioplasty (POBA) patency rates, 111
Poiseuille's law, 136, 137
Polytetrafluoroethylene (PTFE) grafts, 57, 65, 66, 77–79, 114, 121–122, 269, 277
  failure rate of, 67
  neo-endothelium in, 67
  outcomes, 57
  patency rate, 62
Posterior circumflex humeral artery (PCHA), 219, 221f, 223–224
  endovascular exclusion of aneurysmal, 222
  proximal and distal ligation, 222
  thrombosis, 220
Postoperative anticoagulation, 222
Postoperative infection, 133
Precision banding, 140
ProCol®, 79
Progressive stenosis, 36
PROPHET-II randomized controlled trial, 214
Prophylactic fasciotomy, 270
Prosthetic grafts, 29, 68, 107, 269
Prosthetic upper extremity AV access, 23
Proximal arch vessel disease, 191
Proximalization of arterial inflow (PAI), 125, 135, 144, 145f, 146
Proximal left subclavian artery, 277

Proximal stent-graft, 278
Proximal subclavian artery, 276
Pseudoaneurysms, 164, 203, 204, 211–213, 215, 280
PTA. *See* Percutaneous transluminal angioplasty
PTFE grafts. *See* Polytetrafluoroethylene grafts
Pulsatile laminar flow, 38

Q
QS. *See* Quadrilateral space
QSS. *See* Quadrilateral space syndrome
Quadrilateral space (QS), 219
Quadrilateral space syndrome (QSS), 219, 224. *See also* neurogenic quadrilateral space syndrome; vascular quadrilateral space syndrome
  catheter directed thrombolysis, 222
  demographic breakdown, 225t–226t
  posterior circumflex humeral artery. *See* Posterior circumflex humeral artery
  preponderance, 220
  suspicion, 224
  work-up and treatment algorithm, 225t

R
Radial artery access, 202, 207
  complications in, 208
  endovascular therapy, 208, 210–211
  hemodynamic monitoring, 207
Radial artery cannulation, 213
Radial artery line placement, 208–210, 212
Radial artery occlusion, 208, 209
Radiocephalic fistulas (RCF), 18, 19, 21–22, 29, 36, 39, 41
Randomized controlled trials, 19
RAND/UCLA Appropriateness Method, 56
Ratio of flow, steal, 146t
Raynaud syndrome, 254
RCF. *See* Radiocephalic fistulas
REBOA. *See* Resuscitative endovascular balloon occlusion of aorta
Recombinant variants of t-PA (rt-PA), 194
Relative value units (RVUs), 94
Renal Physicians Association, 89
Renal replacement therapy (RRT), 77, 84, 125
Renal transplantation, 159, 160, 168
  access preservation following, 167t
  AV fistula closure, 160
  left ventricular hypertrophy after, 165
  ligation following, 165t
  spontaneous fistula closure, 169
  systematic AV access closure, 170
Resident Review Committee (RRC), 1
Resuscitative endovascular balloon occlusion of aorta (REBOA), 285
Retrograde flow, 135, 139, 142, 144
Revascularization using distal inflow (RUDI), 135, 143–144, 146
Rib resection, 233
Richardson retractor, 233
Right subclavian artery, 277
  angiography, 284f
  computed tomography, 283f
RIVAL trial, 207
Royal College of Surgeons of England, 259
RRC. *See* Resident Review Committee
RRT. *See* Renal replacement therapy
rt-PA. *See* Recombinant variants of t-PA
RUDI. *See* Revascularization using distal inflow
"Rule of 6s" guidelines, 151, 155
RVUs. *See* Relative value units
RVU Update Committee (RUC), 89, 93

S
Salvage of AV Fistulae (SAVE) trial, 153, 154
sBP. *See* Systolic blood pressure
Scalene fat pad, 232
Shear stress, 36–39
Sheet-based tissue engineering, 81
Short form 12 (SF-12), 241
Sibson's fascia, 231
Small anastomoses, 45
Smooth muscle cell (SMC), 69, 109
Society for Interventional Radiology, 89
Society for Vascular Surgery (SVS), 1, 89, 93
Society of Vascular Surgery Vascular Quality Initiative (SVS-VQI) data base, 203
Solcograft-P®, 78
Sorbitol/polysorbate, 111
Spontaneous fistula closure, 168–169
Staphylococcus aureus, 130, 133
Staphylococcus epidermidis, 130
Steal, 135
  flow to the fistula, 137–138
  flow to the hand, 138, 139
  patients with high-flow access, 139
    banding, 139–140
    long-segment plication, 140–142, 146
  patients with normal-flow access, 138–139, 142
    distal revascularization/interval ligation, 142–143, 146
    proximalization of arterial inflow, 144, 145f, 146
    revascularization using distal inflow, 143–144, 146
  treatment
    action and outcome, 147t
    high flow access, 148
    normal flow access, 148
    ratio of flow, 146t
Steal syndrome, 121, 125
Stenosis
  balloon angioplasty, 109
  pathophysiology, 108
  types, 108–109

Stent grafts, 109
Stent placement, 90, 98, 101
Sterile ruler, 39
Subclavian artery, 231, 250–252, 251f, 254–256
Subclavian vein, 99, 175f, 243
Subcutaneous implantable cardioverter-defibrillators, 101
Superficialized cephalic fistulas, 154
Superior vena cava (SVC), 120
Supraclavicular approach
 for neurogenic TOS, 234
 to thoracic outlet decompression, 232–233
Surgical Skills Committee (2005), 262
Surgical training, 259
SVC. *See* Superior vena cava
SVS. *See* Society for Vascular Surgery
SVS-VQI data base. *See* Society of Vascular Surgery Vascular Quality Initiative data base
Synergraft®, 79–80
Systematic approach, 267
Systolic blood pressure (sBP), 121

T
Target lesion revascularization (TLR), 112
TBBF. *See* Transposed brachiobasilic fistula
TDC. *See* Tunneled hemodialysis catheter
Teflon, 57
Terumo Destination, 278
Thoracic outlet syndrome (TOS), 221, 229, 249, 254
 arterial, 229, 253, 254, 256
 development, 250
 forms, 229
 neurogenic, 229, 230, 254–256
 subclavian artery, 250, 251
 supraclavicular approach, 232–234
 surgical treatment, 229–230
 symptoms and signs, 252
 transaxillary approach, 230–231, 234
 types, 253
 venous, 229
Thrombectomy, 223
Thromboembolism, 222
Thrombolysis, 215
Thrombolytic therapy, 194, 214
Thromboprophylaxis, 176
Thrombosis, 222, 278
Tissue plasminogen activator (t-PA), 194
TLR. *See* Target lesion revascularization
TOS. *See* Thoracic outlet syndrome
Transposed brachial-brachial fistula, 23
Transposed brachiobasilic fistula (TBBF), 22–23, 154
Transverse skin incision, 230
"Trap-door" incision, 277
Trauma, 223
Traveling Fellowship, 7
Tunneled hemodialysis catheter (TDC), 118
Two-stage technique, one-stage *vs.*, 29–32, 31t

U
uAVG. *See* Upper arm AVGs
U-clips, 48
Ultrasonography, 157
United States Food and Drug Administration (FDA), 118
United States Renal Data System (USRDS), 18, 154
Upper arm AVGs (uAVG), 56, 59–61
Upper extremity arterial access, 207
 arterial anatomy of hand, 208, 209f
 arterial line complications, 209–210
 brachial artery access, 211–212
 for endovascular therapies, 207–208
 occlusion, 208
 radial artery access, 210–211
 risk factors for complications, 212–213
 strategies for prevention, 213–214
Upper extremity arterial civilian injury, 267
 approach and considerations, 270t
 endovascular repair, 271
 hard and soft signs, 268
 mangled, 271–272
 open revascularization, 269–270
 revascularization, 268
 subclavian and, 268
 venous injuries, 270
Upper extremity central venous obstruction, 118, 121, 122
USRDS. *See* United States Renal Data System
U.S. Renal Data System Annual Data Report, 35

V
Vascular access patency, 98
Vascular access stenosis, 109
Vascular endothelial cell growth factor (VEGF) expression, 68
Vascular forms of TOS, 230
Vascular quadrilateral space syndrome
 case report, 222–223
 clinical signs, 220–221
 computerized tomographic arteriogram, 221
 direct contrast arteriogram, 221
 hypothenar hammer hand syndrome, 221
 intimal hyperplasia, 220
 magnetic resonance angiogram, 221
 mechanical stress, 220
 stretch trauma, 220
Vascular surgery, 259–261
Vascular trauma, 259, 261, 276
Vascular tube, 80
VCS, 48
VEGF. *See* Vascular endothelial cell growth factor expression
Venogram postvenoplasty, 240f, 241f

Venogram prevenoplasty, 240f
Venography, 19–20
Venous injuries, management of, 270
Venous thoracic outlet syndrome (vTOS), 24, 229, 237, 246
  arm swelling, 239
  controversies, 243–245
  definition, 237
  first rib resection and scalenectomy, 243–245
  multiple treatment algorithms, 242t
  outcome for, 237–238
  patency outcomes, 243–245
  presentation, 238–239
  protocol, 239f
  removed rib, 242f
  stricture location, 238f
  surgical approaches for, 239, 243
  treatment algorithms, 239–241, 246
  venogram postvenoplasty, 240f, 241f
  venogram prevenoplasty, 240f
Venous Window Needle Guide (VWING), 32, 151–152, 152f, 156f
  alternative role for, 155
  fistula cannulation, 152, 153f
  implantation, 153–155
  Kaplan–Meier survival curves, 155f
  patients with, 154
  primary patency rate, 154
  Salvage of AV Fistulae trial, 153, 154
  techniques, 155–157
Vessel wall remodeling, 36, 37–38
Viabahn (nitinol), 281
vTOS. *See* Venous thoracic outlet syndrome
VWING. *See* Venous Window Needle Guide
V wing procedure, 32, 33

W

Wallgraft device, 280
Wallgraft endoprosthesis, 279
Wallstent (steel), 281
Wearable cardioverter defibrillators, 102
W. L. Gore & Associates, 6–7
Work relative value units (wRVUs), 91
Wylie, E. J., 1, 7

Y

Yao, James S.T., 11, 11f